PRAISE FOR OUR HEARTBREAKING CHOICES

This book is a collection of writings by parents, about babies who were loved and wanted. This book is also about the parents themselves, who faced a most agonizing decision before their baby's birth. For these families, the "right" choice was to terminate the pregnancy. Their written narratives demonstrate the honest, soul-searching deliberation required for making such a solemn decision. They looked into their hearts, examined the evidence before them, and based their decision on their assessment of realities—their emotional, physical, medical, financial, familial, cultural, social, spiritual, educational, and logistical realities. And all of these parents came to the conclusion that the better path for their babies was to end their pregnancies and say goodbye to the precious life they'd conceived.

After meeting the challenge of deciding and carrying through, these parents still face the challenge of living with their decision. While every story is unique, parents share an emotional common ground of grief, coping, adjustment, and healing. If you too terminated a pregnancy, you can see yourself reflected in various aspects of these parents' experiences and perspectives, and find comfort in the realization that you are not alone. If you question their decision, you may come to understand that these parents bravely and unselfishly entered the suffering of grief in order that their babies be spared another kind of suffering. If you work with parents who face the decision to terminate a pregnancy, reading this book can sensitize you to the emotional aspects of this kind of perinatal death. Listening to these parents' stories can inform the way you deliver care and inspire you to approach these families holistically and as a collaborator in their care. If you are a policy maker, these narratives can provide you with the awareness and education you need to advocate for better care and support for parents who face heartbreaking choices. You will be inspired by the courage and strength these parents demonstrate.

To comfort, inform, inspire, and improve care – this book's heart is in just the right place, and is a powerful legacy for these babies. What an honor to meet their parents.

—**Deborah L. Davis, Ph.D.**
Author, *Empty Cradle, Broken Heart* **and** *Loving and Letting Go*

A woman's story is her truth, and the truth about the heartbreaking choices described in this book is that once you've heard the stories, you will never think the same way about abortion again. *Our Heartbreaking Choices* is more than a book; it is a solace to those faced with similar situations, a lesson in empathy for those inclined to judge women's childbearing choices, and a message of healing and peace for all.

—Gloria Feldt, author, activist, former president Planned Parenthood Federation of America

Women who have made the agonizing decision to terminate a pregnancy for fetal or medical indications often feel bereft, isolated and unsupported. *Our Heartbreaking Choices* provides much needed solace and comfort to women and their families as they navigate these truly treacherous waters.

For those lucky enough not to have faced these difficult issues, this book will be an eye-opener and a heart-opener. Forty-six women courageously tell us stories of great hardship, courage and ultimately, love. As an abortion provider, I am so gratified that this book has been written. I highly recommend it to all who want to have a more complete understanding of abortion, in all its complexity.

—Dr. Shelley Sella, MD
Women's Health Care Services

Appendix A of *Our Heartbreaking Choices* is a very thorough overview of prenatal testing and screening options over the years with detailed information of the process from discovery of abnormalities in the pregnancy through the options, costs, and laws. And then the stories…46 courageous families pour out their stories from very obviously-broken hearts. The stories are hard to read because they demand an emotional response that we (health care providers) are often trying to control in our interactions with patients, but they fulfill a need for families entering into and attempting to heal from this gut-wrenching process.

—Sally Shields, RN, CGC

Our Heartbreaking Choices

Our Heartbreaking Choices

✦

Forty-Six Women Share Their Stories of
Interrupting a Much-Wanted Pregnancy

Christie Brooks

iUniverse, Inc.
New York   Bloomington

Our Heartbreaking Choices
Forty-Six Women Share Their Stories of
Interrupting a Much-Wanted Pregnancy

iUniverse books may be ordered through booksellers or by contacting:

iUniverse
1663 Liberty Drive
Bloomington, IN 47403
www.iuniverse.com
1-800-Authors (1-800-288-4677)

Because of the dynamic nature of the Internet, any Web addresses or links contained in this book may have changed since publication and may no longer be valid. The views expressed in this work are solely those of the author and do not necessarily reflect the views of the publisher, and the publisher hereby disclaims any responsibility for them.

ISBN: 978-0-595-53047-2 (pbk)
ISBN: 978-0-595-63100-1 (ebk)

Printed in the United States of America

Cover image © S. Newman, 2008.
www.ourheartbreakingchoices.com

This book is dedicated to all of the women and men who have had to make the heartbreaking choice to end a much-wanted pregnancy due to a fetal anomaly or due to a complication with the mother's health.

And to our sweet angels who graced our lives too briefly, but whose presence left an everlasting impact on our lives and the lives of those around us. May their spirits soar…until we meet again.

ACKNOWLEDGMENTS

The evolution of this book, from a thread on a message board to an actual published book, was rather long and daunting. I had witnessed many similar book concepts come and go over a period of four years. So when the idea was reintroduced on a message board in early 2007, I was cautiously optimistic that this time, hopefully, we could finally pull it all together.

I have many people to thank for helping to bring this project to fruition. First and foremost, to Ayliea—thank you for your leadership, guidance, expertise, encouragement, and support from start to finish. Your assistance was critical and there is no way this book would have happened without you. To Catherine, Nicole, Ayliea, Julie, Jen, Sara, Marissa, and the rest of the ladies who helped to edit the stories—thank you for your diligence, your hard work and your thoroughness. To Marsha—thank you for your hard work in creating the support resources Appendix, and for being my sounding board and trusted guide over the past few years. To S. Newman—thank you for your beautiful and poignant cover art. You poured your heart and soul into its creation, and for that I am so very grateful.

A heartfelt thank you to all of the ladies who so courageously shared their very personal and private stories for use in the book; this book could not have been created without the cooperative effort of each and every person involved. Thank you for assisting me in assembling the additional parts of the book, and for encouraging me to stick with it even when obstacles were thrown my way.

A very special thank you to Deborah L. Davis, Gloria Feldt, Dr. Shelley Sella, Sally Sheilds, and Dr. Nancy Stanwood for taking the time out of their demanding schedules to review the manuscript and provide feedback. Your wisdom and guidance were invaluable.

To the *A Heartbreaking Choice* and *BabyCenter.com* message boards— thank you for providing us with a safe haven to meet, to grieve, to support, to encourage, and to inspire one another.

To my parents—thank you for raising me to have the courage and the confidence to stick to my guns, to put my nose to the grindstone, and to follow my heart.

To my husband and living daughters— thank you for your patience, understanding, and support, not just during the creation of the book, but over the past five years as I muddled my way through my grief, found a new focus for my life, and devoted myself to helping a group of virtual "strangers" over the Internet. None of this would have been possible without your support and encouragement.

Contents

PREFACE

Abortion is a topic on which most people have very passionate, though sometimes private, views. They either support the right of a woman to choose to end a pregnancy or they do not. There usually is not much middle ground. People's views on abortion can be driven by religion, by political affiliation, by society and the media, or by personal experiences. The Guttmacher Institute estimates that nearly 22 percent of all pregnancies (excluding miscarriages) will result in an abortion (Jones, Zolna, Henshaw and Finer 2008). Furthermore, more than one-third of all American women will have had an abortion by the time they reach the age of 45 (Guttmacher 2006). The vast majority (about 90 percent) of all abortions are for reasons not related to the physical health of the baby or of the mother. We do not judge those who choose to abort for non-medical reasons. We stand together with all women who make the decision to end a pregnancy, regardless of their reasons. This book, however, was created as a place for women like us who comprise the other 10 percent to share our stories.

The women who have contributed to this book are the *other* face of abortion. We are your next-door neighbor, your child's teacher, your attorney, your family physician, and your personal trainer. We are stay-at-home moms, artists, librarians, scientists, computer programmers, waitresses, and policy analysts. But most importantly, we are moms. We are moms who loved our precious babies enough to let them go far sooner than we ever wanted to. We took on the possibility of a lifetime of emotional pain so that our little ones would not have to feel one moment of physical pain.

The contributors come from varied upbringings, varied religious backgrounds, and varied family circumstances. Some of us are single women in committed relationships; some of us are married. Some of us have only the angel children we conceived; some have living children. We span all age, geographical, racial, educational, and socioeconomic status demographics. We are not evil or uneducated; we are not callous or insensitive. We are just people—people who when faced with a tough decision bravely shouldered the responsibility for that decision rather than do nothing (which is in itself a decision.)

We came together to write this book for several different reasons. The first reason was to help other women (and men) who have faced a similar loss to feel less alone, less isolated, and less stigmatized. No parent should ever have to grieve for a child silently, without support, without empathy from others, or without the assistance and kindness of others who have already walked that same path. Our hope is that by courageously sharing our stories here, thousands of others who find themselves facing a similar loss will not feel *quite* so alone. We hope to break the conspiracy of silence and shame that surrounds the decision to terminate a pregnancy for medical reasons. And we hope to give a voice to all those parents who are too fearful or too apprehensive to speak openly about their own losses.

The second reason we decided to write this book was in response to the almost complete absence of media coverage and societal support for losses like ours. There is no way to know with certainty the frequency of abortions which occur in the United States each year due to a poor prenatal diagnosis or serious maternal health complication. There are problems with reporting these types of losses at the local and federal level, and even if we were to use statistics based on gestational age at the time of the abortion there is no way to know for sure how many of those were actually for medical reasons. Based upon the most recently published studies, one can estimate that terminations for medical reasons account for somewhere between 5–11 percent of all abortions (based on gestational age at the time of the termination, five percent being 16 weeks gestation or more and 11 percent being more than 13 weeks gestation) (Strauss 2007). Given that there were an estimated 1.2 million abortions performed in the United States in 2005 (Jones, Zolna, Henshaw and Finer 2008), that could mean there are between 60,000 to 130,000 terminations for medical reasons each year in the United States alone. Even though so many families are seemingly affected each year by a termination due to a poor prenatal diagnosis, there have been very few magazine or newspaper articles and even fewer televised news segments for those who "electively" abort due to fetal anomalies. Although there have been celebrities and other high-profile individuals who have spoken out about their own abortions for non-medical reasons, there has not been a high-profile person in the United States who has admitted to ending a pregnancy for medical reasons. This disregard for our losses extends to the lack of community-based support available. There are no nationwide organizations or associations which support those who have ended a pregnancy due to a fetal anomaly. There are no hospice-types of support programs, no international alliances, and there are no hospital-based symposiums or workshops. Even so, we do have the ability to connect with and support one another via online resources. We have web sites such as *A Heartbreaking Choice* and some Internet-based support message boards, such as on *BabyCenter.com, P.A.S.S.,* and *BabyFit. com,* which are specifically for those who terminate for medical reasons (see Appendix B). In the stories that follow, you will read time and again how these online resources were instrumental to the emotional healing of so many of the contributors. Despite our own efforts to actively seek out support, and given that our numbers are so large, the amount of media and community-based attention given to situations such as ours is suspiciously low. Quite frankly, the silence is deafening.

The third reason we decided to write this book was to try to show those people who view abortion as a black-and-white, right-or-wrong issue that there are shades of gray. There are circumstances in which an abortion can be the most appropriate and most moral option. We are not so delusional as to think that our little book could change anyone's fundamental views on abortion. But we do hope that our book can shed some light on those who choose abortion as the least worst option. Many of us had assumed that we would never end a pregnancy, either due to our religious beliefs or because of our stable life circumstances. But one truly never knows what one will do unless faced with a situation where a choice must be made, and must be made relatively quickly. Some people are pro-choice in theory—we are pro-choice in practice.

Unfortunately, many politicians who do not support a woman's right to choose have been unable to see in these shades of gray that we so deeply understand, and have consequently supported the *Partial-Birth Abortion Ban Act of 2003,* upheld by the United States Supreme Court in 2007. While there are still two other procedures available to women undergoing pregnancy terminations past the first trimester (labor and delivery and dilation and extraction; see Appendix A for more details), the use of a third option, intact dilation and extraction (D&X) has been greatly restricted for political, not medical, reasons. Its use has been limited to cases where a mother's *life* is in danger, despite the fact that many lower courts have concluded that, in certain cases, a D&X *is* the safest option to preserve a woman's *health* (Center for Reproductive Rights 2003). Since not every case is the same medically, when facing a surgical abortion ultimately only our doctors know once in the operating room which procedure is safest in maintaining *our* health and *our* lives. By leaving out an exception for the *health* of the mother, outlawing D&X procedures essentially downgrades the importance of the life of the woman undergoing the abortion. We would like anyone reading this book to understand that everyone deserves access to the safest health care possible—and that only our doctors know what is safest for us.

The fourth reason we decided to write this book was to honor the babies we lost. We hope this book can be a testament to the legacies that their brief existences left behind. Although their time here on Earth was far too short, they have, through us, made significant contributions to this world. They have motivated us to continually give of ourselves and reach out to others in need. They have inspired us to be kinder, more compassionate, and less judgmental. And they have reminded us and those closest to us how truly blessed our lives are. We realize that by referring to our lost little ones as "babies" or "angels" instead of as "fetuses" we are challenging the platform of some in the pro-choice movement who wish to downplay the "humanness" of the unborn. But to us they always were, and will always be, our precious babies.

The final reason we decided to write this book was to inspire and give hope to those who are in the depths of their despair and cannot foresee finding their way out. We want to convey to those experiencing a similar loss that you CAN get through this tragic time, you CAN be happy again, and you CAN live and laugh again. Though some would like to believe that we live our lives after our abortions filled with guilt and regret—the truth is that, for most of us, we do not. We do not regret our choices, because they were made out of love.

Some people view abortions in instances of rape, incest, or fetal anomaly as more "acceptable" abortions. From our experiences we have learned that all abortions, when made with careful consideration and soul-searching, are acceptable abortions. We do not draw a line between "us" and "them"—between those who terminate due to unwanted pregnancies, financial concerns or family constraints, and those who choose to terminate due to fetal anomalies or complications with the mother's health.

We did *not* come together to write this book in an effort to convince or persuade people to end problem pregnancies. We hope that all men and women facing a problem pregnancy will seek out information from a wide variety of sources in order to make a truly *informed* decision. We encourage people to seek out second and third medical opinions, to connect with parents who are raising children with the same disorder or defect, and to invite their clergy into their decision-making process.

This book has been a cooperative effort of women who connected with each other on the *A Heartbreaking Choice* and *BabyCenter* Internet message boards. We each found our way to the message boards after suffering our own loss, and joined in the virtual chain of support with those who had walked the same path before us. We have been there for each other through the darkest of days immediately after a loss, during the anxiety-filled months of trying to conceive again, and, for some, throughout the bittersweet experience of a subsequent pregnancy.

Convincing people to share their most intimate and heartbreaking stories for the book was a difficult challenge at times. But it was a challenge that turned into a cathartic and liberating experience for many, and one that hopefully will bring comfort to those who read our stories.

Some names and other identifying facts have been changed in order to protect the privacy of the contributors. In an effort to preserve the unique voices of the contributors, most of the stories are largely unedited.

In closing, we would like to extend our heartfelt thanks to all of the healthcare professionals who have had to deliver the devastating news of a poor prenatal diagnosis with honesty, compassion, empathy, and grace; to all of the healthcare professionals who have held our hands, stroked our brows, embraced our anguished souls, and cried alongside us as we said goodbye to our much-loved babies; and to our family and friends who enveloped us in support, love, and kindness when we needed it the most.

1

Abby's Story "Dear Isaac…"

Wednesday, August 22, 2007

Dear Isaac,

I am sitting in the room that was to be your bedroom; it is just one week after you were born 18 weeks too soon. By now, it would have been getting filled with baby furniture and supplies. Your grandmother and I would have painted a Winnie the Pooh mural on the wall over your changing table. Our plan was to wait until my summer school teaching was complete, have our ultrasound to learn your gender, and begin preparing for your arrival in less than four months. That's not what happened, though.

Two weeks ago, I hopped into the shower at about 6:30 AM, mindful of the two pints of water I was explicitly instructed to drink at 7:15 AM. I was grooming myself for a very special day, a day we had been told to look forward to at each of our prenatal visits: "That's the most exciting visit," our OB or physician's assistant would say. "That's when you finally get to see the baby!" We could hardly wait.

I could hear your dad rustling under the sheets, waiting for his alarm clock to signal it was time to roll out of bed and walk the dog before his customary three-minute shower.

We were out the door that morning by exactly 7:45 AM. We were so eager to finally see you. As we waited in the reception area, I could hardly stay seated. I asked for an early admission form that I could fill out in the weeks remaining before I went into labor with you; everything was to work smoothly. I was paging through yet another baby publication at the hospital, noting which coupons could be cashed in and new web sites could be explored. I didn't know then that I would go home that day and throw away the magazine and all the others that had accumulated in neat stacks on every surface of our home.

As the ultrasound technician escorted us to the exam room, she commented that I seemed nervous and assured me that everything would be fine. I didn't know why I was so anxious. Maybe I was too excited to finally see you? Maybe I knew something was wrong?

I got on the table, and the technician started the exam. Something was very strange. She showed us your brain, your heart, your upper arms and thigh. She measured your strong heartbeat. I spotted your spine—you looked like a tiny fish on your side. But something wasn't right. Instead of talking about you, the technician kept making small talk. That was supposed to be our magical ultrasound appointment. Why didn't she focus on you, as I wanted her to?

There was one screen view that she kept coming back to. I didn't know what it was, but I'll never forget how it looked. There were several dark masses in a cluster, each slightly different in size. She kept studying it, looking at it closely. Finally, she said she didn't want to alarm us or put needless fear in our minds but that something didn't look right to her. She excused herself from the room to get a doctor because she wasn't sure what she was seeing. The doctor came in and looked for only a few seconds at the pictures the technician had taken. The doctor used a term I couldn't quite understand, something about kidney disease. I thought that might mean you'd need a kidney transplant. I immediately envisioned multiple trips to the state university hospital, making sure you received the best care.

By 9:15 AM, when we should have been celebrating your gender and upcoming birth, we sat and listened as the OB again repeated that confusing term: bilateral multicystic dysplastic kidney disease. She added that the condition was 100 percent fatal and explained that "these babies" often don't survive in the womb because the lack of amniotic fluid leads them to crimp their umbilical cord. I thought of you dying inside me, cut off from the essential life support I had worked so hard to provide over these many weeks. I know the doctor said some other things, but I didn't want to listen. I wanted to run away or go back to earlier that day and do things over. None of this could be happening. The doctor explained that we were being referred to another facility for a higher definition ultrasound to confirm the diagnosis. "Until then," she said, "I'm afraid there's nothing more we can do for you."

We told my parents that evening. We drove the hour and a half to their house. First we told them about the ultrasound and about seeing you. We showed them the pictures of you and pointed out your head, nose, arm, and tiny hand. Then I told them what I had not yet processed in my own mind or heart—that you would probably not live. We explained that we were going to confirm the ultrasound findings and explained everything as best we could. It was so difficult to tell everyone because everyone thought I was having twins. The Nurse Educator had mentioned it within the first few weeks of my pregnancy because my hCG levels were so high. The Nurse Practitioner had mentioned it at 18 weeks because I had felt you move so early. And I was gaining a lot of weight (at the high-end of average), which could indicate twins. And there are two sets of twins on the paternal side of your dad's family tree and two sets on the maternal side of my family tree. So I thought we might have twins—how exciting! But instead the ultrasound showed that the reason I felt you move so early was because, without amniotic fluid, my uterus was so close to you all the time that I constantly felt you move. (How I miss your tiny kicks!) And each time we told another family member about your condition, they were sure we were sitting them down to announce we were having twins. Instead, we would be bringing no baby home at all.

That night I could not sleep. I woke up at 3:00 AM and searched the Internet for hope. If there was one working kidney, I learned, they could have done surgeries that might have allowed you to grow and develop. But you had no kidney function. I learned the chances of this fetal anomaly were one in 20,000. One in 20,000! I saw other ultrasound images and pictures from autopsies that looked like the screen everyone had stared at the day before. The tell-tale "cluster of grapes" presentation, it was called. I read over and over that when the disease affects both kidneys, it is 100 percent fatal. All I could do was hope that the high-definition ultrasound would find a working kidney.

As we drove to our appointment the next morning, your dad talked about the faintest glimmer of hope we clung to that you would be okay. I have no idea what I said. I know I cried a lot. It was a two-hour drive through beautiful farmland. All I could think of was how beautiful you were to me before I even saw you. Since about 11 weeks I felt you moving. Now I worried constantly whenever you moved. I thought you might be cramped without amniotic fluid or that you might be in pain. I must have asked your dad 20 times that day whether he thought you were in pain. He said you weren't. I kept trying to be calm so you would be calm. I kept thinking about the Monday morning a few weeks earlier when I was startled by our next-door neighbor starting his motorcycle at 5:00 AM. I jumped in bed. As I laid there for a few seconds trying to drift back to sleep, I felt you leap from the adrenaline. You moved around inside me all day long. Oh, how I dread the day when I can no longer remember those precious movements! But now I was suddenly afraid that with each movement you would crimp your umbilical cord and suffer. What a change! The day before, we had left our house expecting to return home with a narrower field of names in mind and nursery plans taking shape. This day was filled with dread and overwhelming sorrow. The months I had spent filled with joy at your every movement were now eclipsed with the (probably irrational) fear that these same movements would end your life.

When we finally arrived at the hospital, we were taken to see a genetic counselor who explained a range of possibilities our ultrasound might reveal. She took a pregnancy history, and I puzzled over how, after being so careful not to inhale exhaust of passing cars or smoke from passersby (I myself have never smoked), after months of not having a drop of caffeine or alcohol, after months of avoiding all medications and herbs, and after shunning nitrates and nitrites in processed meats, anything could have happened to you, my precious son?

After lunch, we watched the same images as the day before cross the ultrasound monitor. The technician narrated each perfect part of your body as she scanned. Then she conducted an arduous search with the ultrasound wand for any amniotic fluid or the missing second kidney. I held my head close to your dad's and tried to be brave, tried not to cry, and tried not to think about what the tell-tale "cluster of grapes" that was still there would mean. A perinatologist who had been reading our ultrasound scan in the next room came in and confirmed the diagnosis made the day before.

We moved back to the genetic counselor's office where we talked about "options." None of these seemed like "options" to me because I hated all of them. (1) We could carry you to term, providing you would live that long; your only moments outside my body would be full of struggle as you tried to breathe with lungs that could never form for the lack of amniotic fluid and as your body filled with its own poisons. (2) We could go to a special clinic across town for a dilation and extraction (D&E), which at 21 weeks gestation was too difficult for me to think about. (3) We could have a potassium chloride injection, be induced into labor, and deliver you stillborn (L&D).

Please understand, my sweet son, that none of these was what we wanted. We wanted to be able to give you a rich, full life. We wanted to bring you home. We wanted to watch with wonder as you grew. We loved you so very much. So much. But how could we let you be born only to suffer? How could we watch you not be able to breathe? How could we see the pain as (without kidneys) your own body's poisons filled you? Well, we couldn't. How selfishly I wish for those moments of holding you in my arms, feeling your warmth, your movements outside my body. But I could not bear to think of you suffering.

Our doctors and genetic counselor explained that, because we were already at 21 weeks, we would have only a few days to think about what we wanted to do. The laws in our state allowed termination only before 23 weeks. We didn't need a few days, though. We already knew. When we were left alone in the next room waiting for another doctor, we knew the only option that was right for us. I hated it! HATED it! I still hate it now. But it was the only thing we knew to do for you, little one.

I tried to pay attention through the rest of the day. A doctor came to explain what little science is understood about the disease. I reeled with pain as our social worker made suggestions for how we might make "a special good-bye" with you. I couldn't look at your dad. I could hear him and feel him gently weeping. He's so strong, he never cries. But that was a day for tears.

We also had to sit and listen as a form, required by the state legislature, was read to us by the attending OB and our social worker. It was supposed to make us acknowledge that we understood our decision. By signing the form we acknowledged that we had heard your heartbeat and knew we were agreeing to end your life. I wanted to note on the form that these all were things we knew too well.

The next days were spent telling family and our closest friends our very sad news. But there was still joy for you, too, Isaac. One night in particular—that Friday—we went to a party for two of our colleagues celebrating promotions. Everyone chattered about the two infants, Helen and Harry, who attended with their tired but jubilant parents. One mom, Chrissy, said that in a few years you would seem to be the same age as they would be. Everyone made fun of my pregnant clumsiness and encouraged me to have a second helping of everything served, since I was "eating for two." They eagerly asked us about names. Your father told them some names we had considered, though by that time we knew you would be named Isaac. For one more magical night, we were the happy pregnant people. I'll always remember that night. As I looked at baby Helen sleeping peacefully across the room, I thought of you at peace.

I want to tell you about your name, Isaac, which was among our favorites from the beginning. But we chose it because of the story of Isaac in the Bible. Isaac's father and mother waited until his mother Sarah was 99 years old before their son was born…a miracle! We waited for what felt to me like that long for you, sweet child. Then one day when Isaac was a boy, God tested Abraham's faith by commanding him to sacrifice his son Isaac as a burnt offering. Abraham did not understand why he would be asked to make such a sacrifice, but he obeyed. He had faith, even in the grimmest of situations. For that, Isaac, the Lord appeared in a burning bush and told Abraham to stop, not to sacrifice his son Isaac. For you, Isaac, it was very different. There was no burning bush. There was no miracle. We did not understand the sacrifice we had to make, but we made it with faith that it was the only right choice for us.

We are getting our pictures of you back today, Isaac—the only pictures we'll ever have of you. Before I see those pictures, I want you to know how amazingly beautiful you were, my sweet little one. How I wish I could hold you again now. I knew from the moment you were born I wanted to hold you immediately. I wanted to remember you soft and warm, as you had been inside of me, though that time was too, too short. I remember how sweet you felt at the instant you were born as your skin brushed against mine.

The nurse brought you back to us, wrapped in a blanket with pastel-colored animals and shapes. Your dad sat right next to me in a chair by my bed. I looked down at you, not sure what to expect. They had told us how small you'd be. We thought you might not look like a baby at all, but like an alien (as your dad said). But Isaac, you didn't! You looked just like the tiny baby that you were. Just like our baby. How I loved you!

As we held you, I touched your soft forehead in awe that something so beautiful could have come from us. Dark buds showed where soon your hair would grow. Your eyes were closed peacefully with a slight wrinkle in your brow, just like your dad's. I kissed that soft, sweet brow so many times! Then I began to notice how many ways you looked exactly like your dad. I can't even express the tenderness and joy of seeing another tiny person who looks just exactly like the person you most love.

Laurie, a hospital chaplain, came during the time you were with us. You were her first baptism. She said you had such a strong name. She scooped water into a tiny seashell and dripped some onto your precious forehead as she said a blessing. Your dad wrote your name on the dry-erase board in our room: "Son: Isaac." We were so proud of you, my precious first-born son. You were so brave and beautiful. How I miss you now. How empty my heart feels.

We held you for two hours—though it seemed like less than five minutes—knowing it was the first and last time, the only time. I didn't cry while you were in the room with us. You were pure joy to me, and I drank you in. Your father told you as many important things as he could think of that a little man like you should know—how to drive a stick shift, to remember Achilles was the greatest hero, that you should always be gentle and kind to others; so many things that I can't remember them all. The last time he held you, he sang his favorite song to you, while I whispered the words, too. I couldn't look in his eyes, only at you. I watched as one tear soaked into his Detroit Tigers t-shirt while he held you and said good-bye, tenderly singing, "Oh, oh, come take my hand, riding out tonight to case the promised land."

When they took you from the room, they told us that we could see you again before we left the hospital in the morning. But we knew we had said our good-byes.

The next week, we drove to pick up your ashes at a funeral home near the hospital. When they brought out the tiny urn, I could not believe it! It was in a red velvet pouch that fit in the lady's hand. She set your remains so carefully onto the table. I wanted to scream! No! No! No! But what could we do? We paid for your cremation and took you out to the car. During the two-hour ride home I held you deep in my lap, where you had been while you lived inside me.

When I look at your tiny urn on our mantle—so tiny it looks like a toy—I think of how unfair it all is. By the time your tiny ultrasound image was real to us, even by the time your kicks and squirms could be felt, your body had already turned against itself. Still, though I know what we chose was the best for us, it hurts like hell. I miss you so much.

It is so difficult to accept the logic of it, to know that the world is not perfect. To know that, even though you were perfect in almost every way, there was one tiny part that did not work quite right. You could never breathe; you could never drain toxins from your body. How could that be? I remembered the morning that I took a home pregnancy test—we had only had time to "try" once that month, and I didn't think there was any way you were coming. But there was the sharp pink line. I cried. When I told your dad, as soon as he woke up, he gave me a high-five and a hug. We waited and planned until the time was just right for you. But that was not to be.

Oh, Isaac, how I wanted you to be my Christmas elf! You'd have been a reminder of the baby Jesus to everyone who saw you at that time of year. But instead you were born during the driest July of my 33 years on earth, and with our sorrow for you the whole earth spilled forth rain. Today is the first day in over eight weeks that we have had rain. It pours like my tears for you.

Love,

Your Mamma

Saturday, September 22, 2007

Dear Isaac,

It has been a few weeks since I have written to you. Please don't think that it's because I've forgotten you. On the contrary, you are what I think of at every waking moment and dream of still at night. I miss you so.

I will admit that I have tried to force away the tears these weeks. There have been concerns about work to distract me. Sometimes, I just push everything else away, though, and all I feel is you.

Today should have been your first baby shower, Isaac. Your "Aunt" Pam and I had already talked about it so much. I had registered for so many gifts for you. I had researched different baby products for months. I'd finished just two days before we learned you'd never live outside of me. I never looked at the registries again. Do you think anyone else found the notation in their calendar about the shower and thought of you and me? Do you think they care?

And, as if some cruel joke of the cosmos, today I also got my first period since you were born. It hurts in a way I have never hurt before. I'm just so sad. And I'm so scared now. I thought I'd have at least three more weeks before having to think about whether to start trying to get pregnant again, like last November when I miscarried. It's just too soon. I'm so scared of forgetting you, Isaac. I'm afraid others will forget you, too. I'm also so fearful of another pregnancy, of more complications. I'm even more afraid everyone will think everything is okay now. But it never will be. You were stolen from me, Isaac.

I have to tell you why I am so afraid. I have to tell you what I have been so afraid to remember. It was so impossibly difficult to lose you, Isaac. But I want to remember it all, good and bad, joyful and terrifying.

We arrived at the university hospital at 10:45 AM, 15 minutes before our appointment. We were taken to an ultrasound exam room where I tried not to notice several very long needles laid out on the counter beneath the supply cabinets and a tray with syringes. Barb, our ultrasound technician, did a scan as your dad held my hand. I asked her whether, by some miracle, there was any amniotic fluid or if she could perhaps find one kidney. She looked down at me sadly and said, "I'm afraid not."

By 11:20 AM, two ultrasound technicians and two doctors crowded into the room. We were participating in the Wisconsin Stillbirth Project, so the doctors had to take a cord blood sample (since there was no amniotic fluid) before injecting the potassium chloride that would stop your heart. The social worker and genetic counselor had told us that it would take about 20 minutes. The doctors needed to get everything in position so that the two ultrasound monitors they were using would be in place for the percutaneous umbilical blood sampling (PUBS) test. Because the exam room we were in was quite small, though, I had to get up off the table so they could move it into a better position. Then they inserted the needle. They found the PUBS sample was difficult to collect because you were lying so low in my abdomen, the cord was wrapped around you, you covered the site where the umbilical cord attached to the placenta, and because you could not move from that position since there was no amniotic fluid. The needles were in my abdomen for about two hours while they tried to collect the sample. I tried very hard to relax and lie still, but the needles had caused contractions. I had never felt contractions before and they scared me. I just laid there unable to move and tried not to cry. I felt like a fish on a chopping block; I wanted to die there. Suddenly, they were finished as quickly as they started. Barb, our ultrasound technician leaned over and whispered to me that they were done. I asked if *everything* was done. She said it was. You were gone. I sat up and just sobbed and sobbed. None of this could be happening.

At about 2:20 PM, your dad and I were taken to a second room where another perinatologist began inserting laminaria into my cervix. It wasn't painful, just uncomfortable. When they had placed as many laminaria as they could, we were told we could leave until that evening when I would be checked into the hospital for delivery. We went to a Peruvian restaurant around the corner from the hospital with my husband's best friend who had driven up from Illinois to be with us. Then we went and sat in a park overlooking the lake until it was time to check in. I tried so hard not to think about the fact that you had already passed away inside of me.

I checked in to the hospital, and we were escorted to a room at the end of the hall on the high-risk pregnancies floor. There was a tiny butterfly on the door jamb of our room that I knew must have been a signal to the staff that you had died. The nurse who checked us in had a packet of paperwork for us to look through. That evening, the doctors removed the laminaria and began to insert Cytotec (misoprostol) suppositories. A hospital chaplain came by to talk with us, but I didn't really see the point in talking with him. You were already gone. I slept restlessly from 10:00 PM until 2:00 AM when they inserted more Cytotec, and again at 6:00 AM. We ate breakfast and watched movies we had brought with us. At some point in the late morning, I called the nurse when my mucous plug fell out in the toilet when I used the bathroom (I didn't know what it was).

By 1:00 PM, my contractions were about 20 minutes apart, so I decided to take a short nap. Afterward, I asked your dad to help me walk around our floor at the hospital. As we passed each room, I couldn't help but notice no one else had a butterfly on their door jamb. By 4:30 PM, I was very uncomfortable and frightened. I had never given birth before and our childbirth classes had not been scheduled to begin for another two months, so I did not know what to expect. The nurse gave me a half-dose of a narcotic for the pain (if I had wanted an epidural, I would have to be moved to another floor of the hospital for monitoring). Your dad and I walked around our floor again, which I had read somewhere might make things progress more quickly. I tried to ignore the parents holding babies in the hallways and outside the nursery. I tried not to notice whenever someone would look at my undergrown bump and smile.

By 6:30 PM, I was again in a lot of pain. The nurse, Whin, suggested that your dad massage my back to give me some relief. It felt good to have him touch me, but I felt like I needed something to focus on. I began writing down how far apart my contractions were. I didn't have any idea how close together they should be before I should expect something to happen. At 7:15 PM or so, I called the nurse because I felt very uncomfortable again. She asked whether I wanted more painkillers. I kept saying, "I don't know… I don't know…." When she touched my arm to comfort me, I basically screamed at her not to touch me.

When asked whether I needed to use the bathroom I said, "I might." Whin and your dad helped me out of bed. But instead of needing to use the bathroom, the pressure I felt was actually you coming. I yelled for the nurse. She told me it was okay. They had placed a "hat" in the toilet because apparently it's very common to deliver in the bathroom. The nurse reached down between my legs and told me to push, which I was surprised I knew how to do. Two doctors, the nurse and I were all in the tiny bathroom now. They cut the cord, and the doctor helped me back into bed while Whin cleaned you a bit. The doctor quickly examined me, and Whin announced we'd had a baby boy. The ultrasound images had not been clear enough to detect your gender because of the lack of amniotic fluid, but I had known since I found out I was pregnant that you were a boy. Within a few minutes, I delivered the placenta. It was over.

I've already told you how we held you and how you were baptized. We took pictures of you ourselves, and Whin took a few pictures of you, too. A professional photographer came and took photos of our family for free. When those pictures arrived a few days after you were born, though, I was so shocked to see how you looked. You didn't look like that to me. I've never looked at them again.

So much of it seems like it never happened. Yesterday I was cleaning and came across the pot that had held the Stargazer lily your dad had brought home for me on Mother's Day. By now, the pot is completely dry. I pulled apart the soil mound, hoping that I would find the fleshy bulb still inside. But it had dried up. Nothing was left. I was so very sad to find nothing there. It made me think of you, Isaac. I thought I would have you forever, but the fleshy part of you is gone. All I have now is your memory.

Love,
Your Mamma

Monday, October 22, 2007

Dear Isaac,

I just wanted to write you a short note this month. I wanted to tell you that your dad and I have agreed to start trying to have another baby. Don't be angry, little one, okay? You will always be my first-born son. And we will never forget you. I know you are always here.

It might seem a little bit crazy, but I imagine you are the morning star, Isaac. Every morning, I look up at you when I am on my walk at 5:30 AM. When I walk up the stairs, I glimpse you shining down through the window. It gives me strength to know you are here with me. It reminds me you will always be with me, that you will always be my son.

Please know that I am thinking of you and that I will always hold you close to my heart. Please keep shining down on me.

Love,

Your Mamma

Thursday, November 22, 2007

Dear Isaac,

Today is Thanksgiving. I am trying hard to find things to be thankful for. I guess I am thankful that we knew what was wrong with you, that we didn't go to the hospital expecting to bring you home but return without you. But it's hard to be thankful for anything.

This morning I walked down to the river for the first time in ages, since over a year ago when we first started to try to get pregnant. Striding along the bank and looking at the watery expanse took me back to that time, Isaac, when you were just a dream. Never was a baby more wanted than you were, my precious child! I was over 350 pages into my dissertation when we decided to start trying to get pregnant. I was to defend my dissertation by December, and your dad had always said we would try to get pregnant when both our dissertations were finished. I don't think either of us knew then how long it would take us to finish, but we finally were finished. Autumn leaves were falling. What beauty! I was so hopeful for the future.

But that month I had a very early miscarriage. Before I even knew I was pregnant, I began spotting and had cramping, which I had never experienced before. I thought it might have been an ectopic pregnancy, so I called the doctor. I went in that same morning. When the nurse came in with the blood test results, she said, "Well, you are pregnant." I burst into tears. I was pregnant, but I knew something was wrong. By that time, I was bleeding.

My doctor put me on bed rest and continued to monitor the hormone levels in my blood for a few days, but the levels were steadily falling. I was so incredibly sad.

That spring, we started trying again. In February I got my period. I didn't think there was any way I could be pregnant in March because I had very bad allergies and we had been visiting colleagues over Spring Break, so we had only had intercourse once. But that was apparently all it took!

I woke up early on the morning I was expecting my period and took a home pregnancy test. It was positive! I was so excited that I took a picture of the stick. It was a Monday, so I called as soon as the doctor's office opened to schedule my first prenatal exam. I was surprised that they wanted to see me in several weeks' time rather than right away since I had had the miscarriage in November.

Within two days, I was devastated to discover that I was spotting. I called a nurse who had seen me when I went for my follow-up appointment after my miscarriage. She asked the doctor on call to write orders for a blood test. I began having my hCG levels checked every other day, and although the spotting continued for over 10 days, my hCG levels continued to climb. By the time I went in for my nurse educator's meeting, she suggested that I might be having twins since my hCG levels were so high. Because of the ongoing spotting, I had a transvaginal ultrasound as soon as a heartbeat might be detectable. I was very nervous during the scan, but it turned out I had nothing to worry about. There it was! Your loud, strong heartbeat was clearly detectable. And there it was each month when we went back for our appointments. Your dad used to imitate the quick beat of your tiny heart as we'd walk to the car after each appointment. What joy that was! I wonder whether I'll ever feel real joy again.

There was never any clue that anything would be wrong with you, Isaac. We opted not to have a chorionic villus sampling (CVS) test or a quad-screen test because if anything had been wrong with you we felt strongly that we would have done our best to care for you and raise you. If we had done one of those tests, they might have found the lack of amniotic fluid and detected the problems sooner. But I'm so glad they didn't because it meant you were with us a little longer. It meant that finally one day while we were laying on the living room floor together your dad got to feel you kick inside me. It was two days before we terminated. You started kicking. So often your dad would put his hand on my abdomen to feel you kick and you would stop. Did he comfort you? I think he pressed too hard. So I held his hand just far enough away so he could feel the tiny rhythm of your movements. Sometimes I still feel those movements as if you are inside me. I've read that others feel these "phantom" movements. They make me miss you so!

I guess that is one thing to be thankful for this year. I'm thankful for the time that we did have with you, however short. I'm thankful that the dream of you finally pushed me to finish my dissertation. I'm thankful that you are my son.

Love,

Your Mamma

Saturday, December 22, 2007

Dear Isaac,

This is the week you were to be born. But today, the darkest day of the year, I sit with empty, aching arms that never were to hold you while you were alive. The holidays seem so impossible to deal with. No one knows what to say, really. What can they say? Only a handful of people have even acknowledged that this is the week we were to bring you home.

I wish there were some profound peace or sense of closure that would have come with this week. But there isn't. It is just what it is. A startling sense of reality. The semester has ended. All of the papers are graded. The shopping is done. There is nothing to do now but face the rest of my life without you.

I bought you a Christmas ornament. Is that crazy? It is Winnie the Pooh on a rocking horse. I hung it over the mantle next to your urn. It reads "Baby's First Christmas." But you never will have a Christmas, Isaac.

I wish it were easier in one way, and I'm glad it isn't easier in another way. Sometimes, I wish the earth would open and swallow me up to end the horrible aching grief. At other times, I am thankful that this is the way things have worked that we might remember you.

You might have noticed that I haven't mentioned a brother or sister on the way yet. That's because there isn't one yet. Maybe you already know that where you are? Right now we are trying to get pregnant again. Do you think we will be pregnant this month? It's only the second month of trying. If you know that we will be, or when we might be, I wish you could tell me. Will you be happy to have a brother or sister?

If I do get pregnant again, I think it will be a girl next time. I have felt that way since August when you left us. Maybe I'm just hoping not to give the world anything to compare you to. You might already know, wherever you are, that my goddaughter Chavalah died when she was just nine weeks old. She would be three years old now. Her mom and dad had another little girl, Eliana, a week before what should have been Chavalah's first birthday. Everyone talked about how they were "replacing" her. I don't think they were. They just needed to fill the awful void, the overwhelming emptiness. They wanted a child, not a replacement. I never want anyone to think that we are replacing you.

I forgot to tell you that in October, after we had decided to start trying again, I did something about my fear that people would think we had forgotten you. I started a page for you on the *March of Dimes* web site. The program is called "Banding Together." It shows a little hospital bracelet with your name on it that reads, "Born 18 weeks too soon." I invited our family and a lot of our friends to make contributions. Many of them did. So many, in fact, that we have raised almost $1,000.00 for the March of Dimes. I hope to invite a few people to contribute each year so that we can continue to raise funds in your honor. It seems like so little, but it is a start.

I think I have been dealing with things about as well as anyone could expect, though. Your dad and I went to grief counseling for a while, but I don't think it helps very much. I have meant to go to a support group, but have missed it each month so far. I think I'm afraid of hearing others' sad stories and of others judging us for not carrying you to term. I have found support online. It is useful to hear others' struggles and to have others, who have a good idea of what I'm feeling, offer something in response. But I think it will take time. Not time to forget, for I never will forget. It will take time to accept what has happened and to find peace. It still feels impossible right now, but I hope one day I will find it.

Love,
Your Mamma

2

Adrianne's Story "I Am a Good Mom"

When I was 23 years old, my husband and I found out I was pregnant. I had been off any sort of birth control for almost two years, and I was beginning to worry that I might never get pregnant. After I took a home pregnancy test and saw a positive result, I called pretty much everyone in my address book. We were so excited!

We had a sonogram to determine how far along I was, which put me right around seven weeks. We saw the heartbeat, and as far as anyone could tell, things were progressing well.

At 18 weeks we went to the hospital for the "big" ultrasound. We were going to find out the sex of our baby, and the whole way there we argued over different names. The technician that did the ultrasound was great. She was so nice, and while she was doing the sonogram, she asked us a bunch of questions about ourselves. Since it was our first pregnancy, I didn't really know what to expect, so I certainly didn't think there was anything weird about the questions.

She got really quiet after a couple minutes, but I was still clueless. I remember my husband commenting, "Wow, the baby has a big head like me!" She asked if we had tested for spina bifida. That's when I started to worry. After a couple more minutes of looking, she said she wanted to call in the doctor, saying she suspected the baby may have Turner syndrome.

The perinatologist came in and looked at the pictures, and agreed with the technician. That's when it hit me. He showed us where the kidneys were supposed to be, and explained that he couldn't see them or a bladder. The body was covered with something called fetal hydrops, which he explained was basically fluid-filled sacs. He explained that the heart/lung cavity was so full of fluid that the heart and lungs would be prevented from developing, and our little baby would die. "Incompatible with life," was the phrase he used. It still haunts me.

We were stunned, to say the least. Neither of us knew what to say, or what questions to ask. All I could think of was how much I wanted the doctor to be wrong. Maybe if it wasn't Turner syndrome, as he thought, our baby wouldn't die.

I had an appointment with my obstetrician the next day, and all our hopes were dashed. Basically, he told us that he thought it was Turner syndrome, but no matter what the diagnosis, with such severe physical problems our baby wouldn't live. He urged me to go for an amniocentesis, but made it clear that it was only for a definite diagnosis, not in order to give us any hope. That was when we first discussed termination. I had the choice of a dilation and evacuation (D&E), or labor and delivery (L&D). I decided I couldn't make myself go through labor, knowing my baby would die. My husband and I talked about it at length, and although I felt it was selfish on my part, I simply knew I couldn't put myself through that.

I started doing research on Turner syndrome, which was when it hit me that I hadn't even asked whether our baby was a boy or girl. Because of the genetics of the condition, I learned our baby was a girl. I learned what all of the things on the ultrasound that had been pointed out to me meant—the hydrops, the uncertainty if a bladder was present, and the inability of the heart and lungs to grow. It meant that my baby was in pain. If she wasn't already in pain now, she would be soon. All I could think to compare it to was pneumonia—on the inside. I couldn't comprehend it. I still can't, actually.

My obstetrician said he could perform the D&E procedure in a hospital if I wished, but assured me that the doctor at the clinic was the best he knew. I decided to go to the clinic.

On the first day, October 28th, 2005, I met with a counselor. My doctor had already called her, so she was aware of our situation, and she was very understanding. She knew how wanted our baby was, and it was very obvious to my husband and me, even in our grief-filled state, how badly she felt for us. She explained the procedure to us, and we decided to start it that day.

The laminaria were inserted, and I got all my instructions on what to do. I was numb. I just went through the motions. It didn't really hit me until that night what was really happening: my cervix was being forced to dilate, so it would be easier to get my baby out. I felt so guilty.

The next morning we got up early and made the hour drive back to the clinic. My husband's best friend came with us, to support my husband while I was in having the procedure done. There were protestors outside the clinic, and we could hear them screaming all the way inside the clinic. I found out later that my husband went out and yelled at them while I was inside, and I think that if it weren't for his friend, he probably would have ended up in jail that day.

The actual procedure went a lot more quickly than I expected. I remember a lot of pain, then getting a shot of something that took the pain away. I remember asking the doctor if she could tell my baby was a girl, since at that point we didn't have a definitive diagnosis of Turner syndrome. She couldn't tell.

Afterward, I was wheeled into a room with four other women. After a few minutes, a nurse came in and made us eat a few crackers. As soon as she was sure we could keep them down, we were given prescriptions for birth control pills, along with a free one-month supply of birth control pills. We were sent off to the bathroom to get changed, and then we were ushered out. I forgot my prescription by the nurse's desk. A nurse chased after me with it, saying "Don't forget these. We don't want to have to go through this again!" It took all of my self-control not to hit her. I wasn't there for the same reason as most of the other ladies. I wanted my baby; my baby was planned! It didn't occur to me until later that the other ladies there were probably feeling just as sad and guilty as I was about what we had just gone through.

My husband met me in the waiting room with a big hug. We found out a week later that the definitive diagnosis was Turner syndrome.

I know in my heart that we made the right decision. We chose to stop the suffering of our child. We didn't look at it as having to make a decision—it was made for us when we heard the horrible news.

I now have a healthy nine month old son, and as I write this, am 23 weeks pregnant with a little girl. They will both know about their big sister, and know that they will always have a guardian angel watching out for them. I still have days when I feel guilty, but I know it's because that's how I was conditioned to feel, and that my husband and I put our child's feelings before our own.

That's how I know I'm a good mom.

3

Amanda's Story "An Angel is Born"

All along, we knew we'd have a family. Before we got married, we had agreed we wanted two or three kids. For as long as I can remember, I wanted a boy and two girls, in that order. We wanted to wait a few years after getting married to start a family so we could have some time just the two of us—to go to dinners and travel and really just enjoy each other.

After about two and a half years of marriage we started thinking about having a family a lot more, and we began to feel more ready to have a baby. We wanted to take some big trips before the babies came, and decided we'd try to squeeze a few in and then start a family in the summer of 2008. I think we both started feeling a bit anxious, and so we decided to start trying the fall before. Everyone knew of our plans to try the next summer, so we decided not to tell them about the change in plans. We wanted to be able to surprise everyone when we announced that we were pregnant. We started trying in November 2007 and became pregnant in December 2007. We found out the day after Christmas and were both so excited and a little nervous too. But more than anything, we were just really excited. Our little family was growing to three!

I had a lot of spotting around the time we found out I was pregnant, so that worried us some, but the books and the doctors told us that it could be normal and wasn't necessarily a bad sign. We knew that there was an increased risk of miscarriage early in pregnancy, so we thought that if I did miscarry, we would be sad but accept that something just wasn't right. And we would be glad to know that at least we'd be able to have children. By six weeks, I started having strong feelings that the baby would be a boy. I was getting more and more excited. All I could think about was little baby clothes, and my tummy getting big. I wanted to shop for maternity clothes, even though I knew I wouldn't need them for a long time yet. I was just so excited and so looking forward to the little baby on the way.

When I was finally eight weeks along, I went to see my doctor and have my first ultrasound. Again, we knew there was a possibility that we would find our baby didn't make it, so we were trying to be prepared in case they said something was wrong. When the technician said she saw the heart beating, we were so excited! She turned the screen so we could see, and I cried when I saw my baby. I couldn't believe there was a little baby in my tummy that we were seeing for the first time! We felt like we had made it through the first hurdle and we were excited to share our news. At that point, only our parents knew, and I was starting to let it "slip" to more people because of my excitement. We called both our parents and gave them the green light to tell the rest of the family. We both also told all our friends and everyone at work.

At 11 weeks I had a tiny bit of spotting, and just felt a little weird. I called my doctor and she wanted me to come in for an ultrasound just to make sure everything was okay. We went in and they immediately said the baby was fine. The technician asked if we wanted to do the nuchal fold test, which was typically done at 12 weeks. We asked for an explanation of the test, and the technician explained that it's a screening for certain chromosomal disorders. She explained that they measure the nuchal fold, which is the thickness of the skin at the back of the baby's neck, and then draw a little bit of blood from me to look at my hormone levels. We said sure, sounds great! It would be nice to have some reassurance that the baby was healthy and it sounded like a simple enough test with no risk to the baby. The technician began trying to do the measurement on the screen, but said our baby wasn't big enough to perform the test accurately. She said they'd re-do the test when I came back the next week for my 12-week appointment. We later learned that that was a lie, and that she had been able to get a measurement, but it was abnormal, and she and my doctor thought we should wait until the next week to see if it got bigger or smaller.

The next week, at our 12-week appointment, the technician did the measurement again, and when we finished the ultrasound we were moved into another room to be seen by my doctor. My doctor seemed to take awhile to come in, and when she came in she asked how I was feeling and if I was having any more spotting. I hadn't been. The 11th week was the last time I had any spotting, and even then it was almost none. She told us that unfortunately things didn't look good on the ultrasound. What could she possibly be talking about? I remember thinking, it must be something small that they can fix, everything is going to be okay. She went on to say that the nuchal fold was very large at 4.4 mm (they considered the high range of normal to be 2.5 to 3 mm). She explained that about 50 percent of the time when they saw nuchal folds over the normal measurement, it indicated that the baby had a chromosomal disorder, which usually was trisomy 13, trisomy 18 (both incompatible with life), trisomy 21 (Down syndrome), or Turner syndrome. The other 50 percent of the time, it was a heart defect or a variety of other rare disorders that were not chromosomal. Or it could possibly be nothing. She said that she expected me to miscarry, and I should be prepared for that happening.

We couldn't believe it. I felt completely blindsided and didn't understand what was going on. How could our baby not be perfect and healthy? I was still holding the ultrasound pictures they had given us, and the baby looked perfect! I think I was extremely naïve and never really fully understood that everything might not be perfect with my pregnancy. My doctor said that in the event we didn't miscarry we could do an amniocentesis to get a definitive diagnosis to find out what if anything was wrong. She asked if we would consider doing anything to interfere with the pregnancy in the event we discovered something was definitely wrong. I knew she was referring to terminating, and I told her absolutely I would not do anything, no matter what the tests showed. I couldn't imagine ever doing anything to end my pregnancy. I thought that if I was meant to not have the baby, then God would take it from me naturally, because He knew what was best for us and for the baby, and I shouldn't interfere. My doctor referred me to a perinatal specialist, who dealt with high risk pregnancies and saw these situations more often than she did.

On the way back to the car, I cried a lot. I was still absorbing everything we'd been told, and I don't think it was completely sinking in yet, but already we were devastated. I just couldn't believe that was happening. That was a Thursday, and we got an appointment to see the specialist scheduled for the following Monday. Over the weekend, my husband and I cried a lot, and spent most of our time researching the Internet for what the increased nuchal fold could mean. We were searching for stories of people who had been told the same things we had and turned out to have perfectly healthy babies. We did find some stories like that, but we read a lot of stories that didn't turn out so well too. We were just so upset and so worried about our baby. We debated whether or not we would do an amniocentesis, and through our research learned of the chorionic villus sampling (CVS) test. I was worried about the risk of miscarriage, but we decided that we needed all the information we could get, and we were pretty sure we would do invasive testing, whether it was CVS or amniocentesis.

On Monday, we went to see the specialist, where they again measured the nuchal fold. We had said prayers all weekend that it would have resolved itself, or at least gotten smaller, but instead it had gotten bigger. It was now measuring 5.3 mm. I asked during the ultrasound if the nasal bone was present, as I knew the absence of one was an indicator for Down syndrome. The technician said yes, it was present. We saw the doctor next, and she went over the pictures with us. She talked about the nuchal fold, and discussed with us whether she thought it would be considered a cystic hygroma, which was considered more severe. She said she couldn't be sure. She also said she was concerned about the ultrasound pictures of the baby's brain, and wasn't sure if the brain looked normal or not. She thought there might be fluid in the brain, but later said she thought it looked normal, although she couldn't be sure. She again explained what the increased nuchal fold could mean for the baby, and explained that she recommended an amniocentesis. We decided that we would do the amniocentesis, so that we could prepare for the baby and get the best possible care knowing exactly what was going on. She asked us if the amniocentesis showed a bad result if we would consider terminating, and again I said absolutely not. When we left, we scheduled an appointment to do the amniocentesis two and a half weeks later. I would have to wait until I was at least 15 and a half weeks along.

We spent the rest of the week frantically researching and praying. We met with our pastor and talked a lot to our parents. We were looking for help. At that point, we were basically in a holding pattern until we could do the amniocentesis and find out what was going on. At the beginning of the next week, my 14th week, we got the results back from the blood work done at the 12-week appointment. My hormone levels and the nuchal fold measurement had been combined together to give us odds for some of the most common chromosomal abnormalities. The test results showed that the chance of our baby having trisomy 13 or 18 was one in 826, which was not considered to be an increased risk. But the chance of our baby having Down syndrome was one in less than five, which is the highest chance the test would show. So with that, we basically knew we were only looking at Down syndrome. My hormone levels were consistent with what is typically seen in a Down syndrome pregnancy. I also learned that with my hormone levels the way that they were, the baby was at an increased risk for being delivered premature, having a low birth weight and having intrauterine growth restriction. We were terrified.

We started talking a little more about termination, but I didn't know if I could bring myself to do that. I was, for the first time, willing to consider it though. I still didn't really think it was the right thing to do, but I was scared and scared for my baby and for our future children. At 15 and a half weeks, on a Thursday, we went in for the amniocentesis. They did a level II ultrasound before the amniocentesis to try to look at the baby's anatomy.

Overall, they said the anatomy looked great! There were no markers seen for Down syndrome and everything seemed to be forming as it should for that stage of development. We also found out that the baby was a BOY! From very early on I had been convinced that it was a boy, and I cried when the technician said it was. My husband looked very happy too, but we still knew there could be something terribly wrong with him. He was moving around a lot in that ultrasound, and he looked so cute and sweet. The doctor came in and talked to us a little more about the anatomy, and then performed the amniocentesis. It really wasn't bad at all.

Afterward, we went home and I rested the remainder of the weekend to try to reduce the potential risk of miscarriage. We made it through the weekend and were dying to hear the results of the test. We had the FISH test done with the amniocentesis, and were expecting the results at the beginning of the week. On Tuesday morning, March 18th, the doctor called to tell us the FISH confirmed that our baby boy had Down syndrome. We knew there was a good chance that would be the finding, but it was still so crushing to hear the diagnosis. We couldn't believe it was happening to us, the odds were so against anything like that happening. We prayed together and cried for our baby. My husband had to get to work, and left. I just lay in bed for a while crying and called my mom to tell her. I felt like I had to get out of the house, so I went to work, not knowing what else to do. I knew if I stayed at home I'd go crazy and cry all day. So I went to work that day, and I think I was pretty bitter. Even though I went to work every day that week, I didn't get any work done. I spent each of the days researching online for all the information I could find, and was reading a lot of Internet message boards. For the first time, I allowed myself to read posts on the termination for medical reasons message boards. I had never allowed myself to look there before because I was so hoping that was not something we would have to consider. I also read messages on the Down syndrome boards, which I had also never allowed myself to do. I now knew I had to become informed, and wanted to see both sides.

That afternoon my husband and I went to see a genetic counselor, and she was no help at all. After the appointment we went home, and weren't really sure what to do. We talked to our parents and cried a lot. In the mail that day, we got one of the junk catalogs that we somehow had gotten on the mailing list for. On the front cover of the catalog was a ring, which had inscribed on the inside a prayer that I had always loved. It was a prayer that was on a plate that hung on a wall in my grandma's house, and I remember reading it when I was little and really liking it. It was the serenity prayer, "God grant me the serenity to accept the things I cannot change, the courage to change the things I can, and the wisdom to know the difference." I thought it was interesting that I saw that prayer, and I wondered what it meant. I wondered if God was sending me a message that I needed to be courageous, as this was something that I could do something about. What was really weird was the very next day, in my searching every web site under the sun for answers, I saw the same prayer again. I really felt like God must be trying to guide me by showing me that prayer two days in a row, and again I wondered what it meant that I saw it again. I kept looking at the "courage to change the things I can" line.

My husband and I started seriously thinking of terminating, and I think during that week we both were feeling that that was what we would end up doing. We were scared for what our baby would go through, and what health problems he might have. We were also scared that if his health problems were really severe, that we may never get around to having more children, and I so wanted to have more kids. We were worried too that if we did have more kids, that their childhoods might be limited if we were restricted in what we could do because of our oldest child. We were also scared for ourselves and our marriage, and I thought about the possibility that our baby might never be able to live on his own, and might be living with us for the rest of our lives. And in thinking about that, we worried about who would take care of him in his adulthood after we were gone. I think we both had a lot of reservations about terminating, but were scared of having a special needs baby.

I read about the two different options I would have for terminating, and we knew right away that I couldn't go through the labor and delivery (L&D) procedure. If we were going to do this, I knew it would be by dilation and evacuation (D&E). I just didn't think I could bear to go through 20 hours of labor to deliver my baby that would never make it. I also didn't think I could handle seeing my baby. I thought about having future children, and I didn't want my memories of labor to be ones of sadness in delivering a baby asleep when I was delivering my living babies.

I called my doctor and talked to her about the options, mostly about the D&E option. She said that if we chose to do that, she would perform the procedure herself in the surgery clinic next to her office. She made me feel better about the procedure for a lot of reasons. First of all, I think my doctor is amazing. She is very warm and compassionate, and she really makes me feel better about things. Plus, I liked that she didn't do these procedures all the time, only in cases like mine. I appreciated that. I also liked that I wouldn't have to go to a clinic. My husband and I discussed it, and we knew that if we did decide to do this, that would be the way we'd do it. But we still had a lot of reservations about making that decision. I thought over and over, how are we ever going to figure out what to do? How are we ever going to know what's the right thing and what's best for our baby? We were very worried about the baby's health, and knew there was so much we wouldn't know until after the baby was born. We prayed and prayed for an answer, or guidance on what to do. We so desperately wanted to know what God would want us to do, and what the right thing to do was. We knew that even if we thought terminating was best, if we didn't feel that God was leading us there we wouldn't terminate. We knew that whatever we decided to do would be where we felt led by God. So we kept praying and praying for an answer, but so far, didn't feel like we were getting one. We also had decided that we absolutely could not make a decision out of fear—either way. We were both very concerned that the reasons we were thinking of choosing to terminate were very selfish reasons. I knew that it was not something I could do for selfish reasons, and I didn't know how to rectify the two.

If we were not going to terminate we would have to make a clear, conscious decision of that, and reclaim our pregnancy. I continued to read messages on the Internet board for mothers expecting their babies the same month I was, because there was such a big part of me that still wanted to pretend I was having a normal pregnancy. It was sort of refreshing to read posts of women concerned about whether or not it would be appropriate for them to wear bikinis to the beach all summer. I so wished that I too thought that was a big issue. Over the weekend, I remember we cried a lot, but I did notice that all of it was bringing us a lot closer together and closer to God. On Sunday, Easter, we went to church, and afterwards went to brunch. At brunch, we were seated at a table right next to another family. One of their children clearly had Down syndrome. He looked about 15 or so, and they had two other children with them, who also looked to be teenagers. I couldn't help but watch them, and to me, they looked like just a regular family having brunch together on Easter. I started thinking that didn't look so bad at all. The rest of that day I thought that maybe we could do it. Maybe we could have the baby and everything would be okay. I started thinking maybe having the baby really was the right thing to do. I started talking about having the baby more and more, and my husband started thinking more and more maybe it was the right thing to do too.

That Tuesday, we got back the full amniocentesis results. My doctor called me at work and said that, as expected, the results showed that our baby did indeed have Down syndrome. I was prepared for that, and accepted that. But then she said something that I was not prepared for. She said the results showed a translocation, which shocked me. We had been told briefly that in rare cases of Down syndrome, the third 21 chromosome is stuck to one of the other chromosomes, and that it could be something passed from a parent. My doctor wanted us to talk to our genetic counselor again, and have our chromosomes tested to see if we were a carrier. It was pretty late in the day, and I got upset about the new information and left work.

We continued to consider having the baby, and thinking that we could handle having a special needs child. I figured we'd just know up front what one of our challenges in life would be, and we'd get through whatever problems came before us. I talked to my husband more about having the baby, and he was also willing to consider it. I even started looking at nursery items online a little. I started thinking about all the cute little clothes and getting excited again. I started thinking about holding my baby and dressing him and what he would look like. But every time I pictured him, he looked like a normal healthy baby. I suppose that's partly because I didn't know how to picture him any other way. But something was still really holding us back. I was still scared of that decision too.

I posted messages on the Down syndrome message boards, explaining our situation and that we were thinking of having the baby and that we were scared. The women were so supportive, and I was really surprised at how many of them responded so quickly to my post. I think I got about 15 responses in two days, and all but one or two said they had found out after their babies were born that they had Down syndrome. That surprised me a little. And pretty much all of them advised me to stop reading so much online about Down syndrome and to take it a little at a time. That was hard for me to consider doing, because basically what they were saying is you don't know what you're going to be faced with, so don't worry about it. But how could I not worry? How could I not read about all the health problems my baby might face? We talked about that some, and I realized that the people whose babies are diagnosed after birth do not benefit at all from worrying about what their baby's health will be like in 10 or 20 years. They can't think that far down the road. They can't think about college and marriage and independence. They have to think about getting them to nurse, and whether they need surgery for a heart defect, and how many surgeries they're going to need this year. After that they can focus on how to get them to sit in their highchair and eat their food without throwing it on the floor. I was worried about all those things, but I knew there was still a choice we had to make that hadn't been made yet, and to make that choice, we had to consider the long term things we would face down the road. Otherwise we were just burying our heads in the sand to pretend that those things might not be there. So I knew in that way things were different for us than for most of those other women. I knew that I had to think about my baby's future.

By the next weekend, I was starting to feel the baby kick, which was something I had been so excited for. Now it was very bittersweet. It had been almost two weeks since we had received the diagnosis, and I started again feeling like I didn't know what to do. I didn't know what was right and what would be best for our baby. My husband and I had been pretty sure we would terminate the first week and then we really wanted to have the baby the next week, and I felt like I'd come full circle again and just wasn't sure what to do. We had determined that raising a special needs baby was something we *could* do, but that didn't necessarily mean I thought it was the *right* thing to do. I started feeling more and more like it wasn't fair for our baby, and I just wanted our baby to be healthy and live a normal life. I wanted that SO badly, and I knew it was the one thing I couldn't have. I just felt lost again. And I knew that we were getting close to the point where we would have to come to a decision. I wasn't sure how we'd get to one. My mom flew in on Sunday for support. My husband and I knew that we needed to make a decision soon, and I was getting worried that if we chose to terminate that it would end up falling very close to my birthday, which was in a week and a half. We were talking more about terminating, and I was again starting to feel like that was what we'd end up doing.

I took the following week off from work to stay home and think and be with my mom. On Monday, I went to the lab to have my blood drawn for the chromosomal test to see if I was a carrier for translocation Down syndrome. That afternoon, my mom and I sat outside and talked for a long time. I kept thinking about the fact that the day our baby would be born, unless he had a heart defect that had to be treated immediately, he would be the same as all the other babies—needing to be fed and changed and held. But as he continued to get older, the gap between him and others his age would continue to grow. I was really worried about that, and worried about him wanting to be able to keep up with the other kids his age and not being able to more and more. I just felt so bad for our baby—this was so unfair to him. I didn't understand, and I'm sure I never will, why this had to happen to him. My husband had also told me that his thoughts were that if you find yourself going down one path and you continually run into obstacles and resistance, you can keep plowing down that path, or you can take that as a sign that maybe you're not on the right path, that you're meant to turn around or look for an alternate path. Maybe that was what was happening to us. We also considered that all along we had thought we wouldn't get pregnant until the summer, and maybe we weren't meant to try for a baby when we did. Maybe it wasn't meant to happen until the summer after all. I continued to pray for some epiphany and a clear message of what we were meant to do. And I actually did have an epiphany of sorts, just not like what I'd been praying for. Instead, it really hit me HARD how much I truly loved our baby, and that I would do absolutely anything I could for him that I felt like was the best thing for *him*. I couldn't believe how much love I had for him, and still do have for my child. And even though it made me a little sad,

I loved feeling my baby's kicks and movements. It made me feel closer to him. And at times he kicked pretty hard!

Tuesday night when my husband got home, we went into our room to talk. It had been two weeks exactly since the FISH results had confirmed that our baby had Down syndrome. We decided to come to a decision that night before we went to bed. It really didn't take us long, because deep down we both already had decided for ourselves what we thought was best. It was just hard to admit it and have a decision made to terminate. Plus I hated to think that we'd only have days left before I would no longer be pregnant and the baby wouldn't be with me anymore. But we made our decision that we'd say goodbye to our baby and let him go to Heaven to be in a better place, where he'd be whole and healthy. In some sense it was a relief to have a decision made and not feel like we were standing still anymore. We had come to a decision and would move forward, no matter how difficult. I felt like we were moving from a place of constant stress and worry into a place of resolution and sadness. We decided to sleep on our decision and make sure we were still comfortable with it the next day.

The next day we both told our parents of our decision, and I called my doctor to see about scheduling the procedure. Because I had never had a baby before, she thought they would need to insert laminaria sticks into my cervix, beginning two days before the actual procedure, to get it dilated enough to perform the procedure. Because of that, she said they couldn't get me in until the following week. I made the appointments for the laminaria insertion on Monday and Tuesday (my birthday), and for the procedure on Wednesday. So now everything was set. That made me a little sad, but I still really thought we were doing what was best. I kept hugging my tummy and talking to my little boy some. I knew that he'd only be with me one more week, and I knew I'd miss him very much. Even though I knew my baby couldn't understand me, I thought he could probably hear us, and I wanted to make sure he heard his mommy and daddy tell him how much we loved him. My husband and I said prayers and talked to our baby and told him how sorry we were and how much we loved him. I was actually glad that I had a whole week left with him, because I think it helped me to be able to spend that time with him. On Sunday night, we talked to our baby again and said more prayers that we were making the right decision and that our baby would go to Heaven and everything would go smoothly. Monday was the point of no return, but we still felt comfortable that it was the best thing.

On Monday, my mom went with me to the appointment. The nurse took me back into the office and went over with me what would happen. I started crying, and the nurse was very warm and comforting, which helped. I kept thinking that after that, I couldn't turn back, but I knew I had to keep moving forward. The doctor came in, and I was given a cervical block to help with the pain. My doctor inserted several laminaria sticks into my cervix to get it to start dilating. It really wasn't painful having them inserted. When she had gotten in all that she could, she filled me up with gauze as she said I might have some bleeding. I felt a little lightheaded, but there wasn't too much pain. I was supposed to have gone back to work that day, but obviously with the decision we'd made, I'd be out all week. Everyone knew I'd had a doctor's appointment that morning and would be in late. When I got home, I got on instant messenger and told a few people at work that I'd lost the baby and wouldn't be in and to start spreading the word since everyone at work knew I was pregnant. I was really worried about going back to work and someone saying something to me about the baby, not knowing I wasn't pregnant anymore.

Everyone was really supportive, and they sent flowers. My husband also shared with everyone he worked with that we'd lost the baby, and he came home mid-afternoon. It felt a bit strange because we were telling everyone we'd lost the baby, but we hadn't yet. We were telling almost everyone a lie. I felt pretty good physically. I took some light pain medications, but it was much more bearable than I thought it would be.

The next day, Tuesday, was my 29th birthday. My husband stayed home from work that day and went with my mom and me to my second appointment for the laminaria insertion. It was much more painful than having the laminaria inserted the first time. Once my doctor was finished, the pain did get better. I spent most of the rest of day on the couch. That night, the three of us went to dinner to celebrate my birthday, although it was a very somber night.

It was really important to me to take time to spend with the baby that night, since that was the last night he'd be with us. When we got home, my husband and I spent some time together talking to our baby and telling him how much we loved him. I didn't feel him moving much that day, or the few days prior, but that may have been partly because of the pain medication I was on. It was a really sad night, and I had a hard time going to sleep, knowing I had just hours left with my little boy. All I could think about was how much I loved him and how much I was going to miss him and how sorry I was for all of it. I just wished so badly he could be healthy and I would get to hold him in my arms.

The next morning, my husband's mom flew in, and my husband, my mom and I picked her up at the airport. We went straight from there to the surgery center where I would have my procedure done. I wasn't really sure what to expect when I got there and I didn't know if anyone would be able to go back with me. When we checked in, a nurse took all four of us back into a small office to fill out paperwork and go over what would happen. She had me change into a hospital gown, and drew some blood. The nurse was very comforting and warm. We spent a lot of time in the office just waiting. The anesthesiologist came in and introduced himself to us and told us I was in good hands and not to worry. My doctor came in shortly after and talked to us briefly. She also gave us the news that my results were back from my chromosomal testing and I was not a carrier for translocation Down syndrome. That was a great relief to hear before I went in for the procedure. We still had to wait on my husband's results, but we knew that if either of us were a carrier, it was much more likely to be me. My doctor said that we were almost ready to get started and left the room. The four of us remained in the little office, and I asked my husband to say a prayer for us before I went into the operating room. We were all crying as he asked God to look over me and the baby, and to take the baby into Heaven. It was extremely emotional. The nurse came back and led us down a hallway towards the operating room. We got to the double doors leading to the OR, and I hugged my husband, my mom and my mother-in-law before they went back to the waiting room.

I walked through the double doors and into the operating room. It looked like something on television. I'd never been in an operating room before, and it was very frightening. And I was scared for what I was about to go through, and for my baby. There were several nurses in the operating room, all in surgical gowns with their faces covered. They had me lay down on the bed and covered me with blankets. They hooked me up to all the machines and my IV. I closed my eyes and started to pray for my baby. I prayed that I was doing the right thing and that God would accept our baby into Heaven and that he wouldn't suffer. I had been concerned about what our baby would feel during the procedure and if he would be in pain. My doctor had reassured me that she would cut his umbilical cord first, and he would go quickly. I prayed that he would not feel pain. The anesthesiologist told me he was putting something into my IV, and it would burn a little at first. I thought it was probably the drug that would put me to sleep, but I wasn't sure. I felt a warming sensation in my arm and then a little burning feeling wash over my face.

The next thing I remember is being wheeled into another room. I faded in and out some, but I was in recovery. I think the procedure only took about 30–45 minutes. I woke up again and could see a clock, and was trying to figure out how much time had passed. I felt my tummy and knew I wasn't pregnant anymore. I hoped and prayed my baby was safe in Heaven. My doctor sat by me and told me everything had gone smoothly. She said I had bled more than usual, but she didn't think it was anything to be too concerned about. A nurse noticed I was awake and asked if I was in pain. I was, and she gave me something that made it much better very quickly. She asked if I wanted to see my family and I said yes. They all came back and had tears in their eyes and asked how I felt. After about 20 minutes the nurse helped me get dressed and get to the car. We got home and all had lunch outside. We sat outside for a long time not saying much. I was surprised at how well I seemed to be doing physically, because I wasn't groggy and tired like I expected to be. I kept thinking about our little boy and how he was gone. The next day, my husband went back to work, and my mother-in-law flew home. The day after that my mom flew home.

Over the weekend, it was just my husband and me again. I think we did pretty well emotionally during that time, all things considered. I think it helped us tremendously that we had three full weeks to make our decision after we got the diagnosis before we terminated. I think that helped us to work through our feelings about terminating and feel confident that it was the right thing for us to do for our baby. We got my husband's results back from his chromosomal test and learned that he was also not a carrier, so we were told that our chances of having another baby with Down syndrome were very small. That was somewhat comforting, but I still couldn't understand how it could have happened for this baby. Over the weekend, my milk also came in, which I knew was a possibility. It was physically painful, but luckily that only lasted a few days.

Over the next few weeks, we had up moments and down moments. It has been difficult, but it is getting better. We are very anxious to be able to try for another baby soon, and my doctor has said that we need to wait at least two cycles. I am a little worried about having another baby who also would have problems, but I know that the chances of that happening are very small. I somehow feel like our next baby will be healthy. We think about our baby often, and are still really sad that he's not still growing and developing inside of me. But I keep reminding myself that he's in Heaven, in a place where Down syndrome doesn't exist. I hope he is running and playing and smiling with the sun shining on him. I hope we have done the right thing for him and that he is happy. We both love him so much, and hope he knows that and is proud of us. We will always remember him and think of him, and look to the future for our family. It's only been three weeks since we terminated, even though it feels like it's been a lifetime. I have noticed that each week seems to get a little easier. But we will get through. I can say, this has brought my husband and me closer, and I know one day soon we will welcome a healthy baby into our lives, which I look forward to.

4

Amy's Story "A Heartbreaking Choice and Twin Reduction: Kayla's Story"

Realizing my dream of becoming a mother came later in life for me, as I became pregnant for the first time at age 41. I wasn't even supposed to get pregnant on that first cycle, as some tests had indicated that I had blocked fallopian tubes. Not only did I conceive, but I conceived twins!

Of course my husband and I were thrilled. We were pregnant on our first try and with twins—how lucky could we be?!

My pregnancy was pretty easy. I had no morning sickness and felt great—albeit tired early on. I did have some spotting during the first two months, and that was scary. But each time ultrasounds showed that my little ones were fine; they were nestled in with strong heartbeats. I looked forward to "showing" and especially looked forward to feeling my babies move!

All of our family and friends were ecstatic for us, and along with us, were eager to find out the gender of our children.

Knowing the statistical odds for genetic issues were higher for advanced age moms, we did opt to have an amniocentesis. But even before the results came in, there was an indication that something was wrong with our little girl via the ultrasound. The lateral ventricles of her brain were enlarged, a condition known as ventriculomegaly. We were told this condition would, in the least, result in mild learning disabilities. We held on to that, and read everything we could on it, hoping that there was no other reason for concern.

But there was reason for concern…and the dreaded phone call came from my obstetrician. You know, the one where the doctor (not the nurse) calls you directly and as soon as you hear his voice, your heart drops into the pit of your stomach? That call. The news wasn't good—our little girl was a trisomy 21, or Down syndrome, baby.

I think here is where selective memory, or perhaps post-traumatic stress syndrome, can be a blessing. I do remember crying so much that I didn't know if I'd ever stop. I remember crying together with my husband and crying with friends and family. I remember the emotional pain and shock, coupled with fear. I remember we had to make a decision—the right decision for all of us.

We did a lot of research, and talked with a number of professionals before making our decision. Firsthand accounts of some of the incredibly difficult health issues that these children face were paramount in our decision. The public only really sees those who are coined as "happy" children. But those who are subjected to countless surgeries and ailments are not exposed. While our decision was truly ours, having a pediatric nurse as a very close relative was incredibly helpful as he was able to share these firsthand accounts of the difficulties many babies and children with Down syndrome face. Incredibly difficult to hear, but equally just as helpful.

Once we made the decision to reduce, I really wanted it over and done with so I could move forward. While we had already consulted with the specialists, we still had to wait a few days for the actual procedure, and that wait was excruciating. Little did I know that moving forward would really take quite some time.

Choosing to terminate for medical reasons is very difficult *regardless* of the circumstances. The big difference with a selective reduction is that there is no true closure until the healthy baby is delivered at full term. While there is grieving, it is also very hard to continue looking forward to the birth of the healthy baby, knowing you've lost one. Continuing to carry both babies causes an entirely different set of issues and questions. Will reducing cause me to lose both? Will my remaining baby continue to thrive? Will I still be able to carry to term?

The reduction itself was no different than an amniocentesis physically. Emotionally it was a different story. I wanted to be anywhere but there—and cried the entire way to the hospital. Once it was over, I just wanted to disconnect for a while and try to heal.

Moving forward was difficult though—the guilt was overwhelming at times. I questioned myself often, even knowing that the decision was the right one for Kayla, her twin brother, and us. I know that Kayla has a "do over" and that she will always be a part of our family.

I do think of Kayla often, and look forward to the time when we can take her sweet little urn and release her remains in the ocean near where her daddy and mommy were married.

Postscript: It's been two and a half years now since we faced the pain of having to reduce. Time does heal though. Today, Kayla's twin brother is a thriving two-year-old full of energy. He has his own sense of humor and there's nothing better than hearing him laugh! He brings us great joy every day—along with many hugs and kisses. We'd love to add to our family and give him a sibling, but have not had any luck with that yet. We're still hopeful, but if not, we are thrilled to have such a happy, healthy, fun-loving little boy in our lives!

5

Ayliea's Story "My Miracle Baby"

When I was 30 years old, I went off the birth control pill. My husband and I had recently finished building our home, and we were ready to have children. I had a sister who had been in and out of drug rehab and had two children of her own; Emily was three years old and Brandon was four and a half years old at that time. I was awarded partial custody of her children and since I did not get pregnant right away, I figured that God meant for me to be available to help take care of her kids.

Fast-forward 10 years: My nephew Brandon came to live with us permanently at age 14. Although I still had not been able to conceive I wasn't very upset about it. My husband and I had come to terms with the fact that maybe we could not have children of our own. We felt that taking care of my nephew was what we were supposed to do.

I never even knew I had endometriosis until right before Brandon came to live with us permanently. I had a laparoscopy done in January 2004, and Brandon moved in one week later. Shortly thereafter I began going through endometriosis treatment.

Everything was fine until March 2004, when I ended up spending 12 hours in the hospital with a burst ovarian cyst. The ER doctor was about as sensitive as a post. He actually told me, "It's only a small cyst—it shouldn't hurt that bad."

I went to my gynecologist the very next day to ask her about treatment for another small cyst they found on the same ovary that had not yet burst. She suggested that I go on Lupron treatment; it would help to clear up the cyst and also completely get rid of the remaining endometriosis. During my earlier surgery she had found tissue attached to my bowels that she could not remove for fear of rupturing my intestines. I had initially hesitated going on Lupron because of the negative side effects of it—it puts you in a menopausal state and can cause hot flashes and mood swings. I eventually agreed to the Lupron treatment. I completed six months of treatment and my regular monthly cycle returned two months after my last shot was administered. I had regular periods for the next two months, and in the third month I missed my period. I assumed it was the effects of the Lupron messing up my cycles. To be safe and because I had been on antibiotics for a sinus infection, I called my general practitioner and asked him if I should be taking antibiotics if there was a possibility I might be pregnant. He told me to stop taking the antibiotics immediately, and to take a home pregnancy test. I did both.

My initial reaction to the positive pregnancy test was disbelief. After 10 years of no birth control, no initial symptoms of endometriosis, and no pregnancies, I was shocked. I showed my husband the pregnancy test results, and he said, "Take another one just to be sure." He couldn't believe it either. I took the second pregnancy test the next morning, and it was also positive! I called the doctor to go in and have a blood test done and to get some advice. I did not have morning sickness, and had only a little breast tenderness. After learning from the doctor that everything should be all right with my pregnancy, I scheduled my first prenatal check-up with the OB/GYN recommended by my general practitioner.

My husband went with me to the first appointment because the doctor was going to do an ultrasound. I was just nine weeks along at the time, but because of my age they wanted to make sure everything looked all right. The baby was so tiny and at that stage only looked like a little tadpole, but we were so excited and happy that after all those years we were going to be parents. We told all our family, and of course they were thrilled. My mother-in-law Lillie, for whom our daughter would be named, was so joyful; she had wanted us to have children for so long and thought we'd make great parents.

The first doctor's appointment went well. The only cause for concern was that I had just turned 40 years old and there was an elevated risk of the baby having Down syndrome. Our OB/GYN suggested we might want to have a prenatal test, and since I was already at nine weeks, I could schedule a chorionic villus sampling (CVS) with a perinatologist. There was only one doctor in our area who performed the CVS.

We scheduled the CVS, never thinking there was anything to worry about. We arrived for our appointment and went through the genetic counseling. Since neither of our families had a history of chromosomal abnormalities, we weren't too worried. The ultrasound went well and we saw our beautiful, perfectly healthy looking baby in 3-D! Unfortunately, my placenta was turned so the doctor could not do the CVS. He said it was like trying to bend a wire around a corner, and he couldn't get a sample of the placenta without risk to the baby, so we could not continue. I was a little relieved, because I'd read that there was a slightly higher risk of miscarriage with CVS than there was with amniocentesis, and I had some concern about it.

We scheduled an amniocentesis for March 11, 2005, since on March 16th we would be leaving for a trip to Central America, where we were in the process of building a vacation home. As things turned out, our insurance would not pay for that doctor to do the amniocentesis since he was not on our "preferred providers" list. They had only approved him for the CVS because he was the one doctor in the area who did CVS's. So we cancelled all the appointments with him, and I tried to schedule an amniocentesis with my regular OB/GYN. Unfortunately, he was not available, so his office got me scheduled with another OB/GYN who could do the amniocentesis on March 15th, the day before we left for vacation.

My husband couldn't go with me to the amniocentesis appointment since we were leaving the very next evening, so I asked my mother to go with me. She was very excited and sat through another genetic counseling session with me. We both thought there shouldn't be any problems.

We went in for the ultrasound, and there again was my perfect looking baby. The technician kept taking "slices" of ultrasound images, but she didn't say anything about them. She did say she thought the baby was a girl, even though I was sure it would be a boy. After about a half-hour of scanning, she excused herself and told us the doctor would be right in to do the amniocentesis. Strangely, a different technician came in and took over the ultrasound while the doctor did the amniocentesis. The amniocentesis went alright, but it took the doctor two tries to get through the placental wall into the amniotic fluid. Both my mother and I were a little concerned as he did the procedure because we could see on the screen the needle coming close to my baby's little hands; the baby had been moving around a lot and we were afraid the doctor might hit her with the needle.

He finished the amniocentesis and told me to take bed rest for 24 hours. He said that, since I would be flying to Central America within that 24 hour period, I should not walk around the airports, but my husband should transport me in a wheelchair. The doctor told me that we should have the results of the test by the time we got back from our trip.

Everything seemed fine while we were in Central America. We got back on March 24th and took the 25th off from work with plans to relax and do some baby shopping after we got the amniocentesis results. On the morning of the 25th, I called the doctor's office to get the results. The nurse told me that the initial results were fine but that they did not have all the results back yet. She said that they were waiting on confirmation of the baby's sex. I wasn't at all sure that the technician who told me it was a girl was correct, since the entire pregnancy I could have sworn the baby was going to be a boy. We even had a boy's name picked out, and then decided that if it was a girl we would name her after her grandmother "Lillie."

After a very long wait, the doctor finally called back with the results. He said the baby was a girl and that she had Down syndrome. I was shocked. How could the nurse tell me that everything was fine and they were just waiting for the results on the baby's sex to come back? Why would she say that everything was okay, and then have the doctor tell me my daughter had trisomy 21? I asked the doctor if it could be accurate—if it could be bad lab results, or maybe someone else's results had been mixed up with my own. It just couldn't be my little girl!

I was so upset that I handed the phone to my husband and broke down. It couldn't be right—the baby we had waited 10 years to conceive and wanted so much had Down syndrome. As if that wasn't bad enough, when my husband got off the phone he explained to me that not only was it trisomy 21, but that the ultrasound showed signs of developmental problems in her digestive tract and her heart showed signs of congenital heart failure.

The doctor told my husband that if I was able to carry the baby to term the possibility of her survival was slim; she would need immediate heart surgery and reconstructive surgery on her digestive system. I cried and cried. I called my sister, who was in town, to give her and the rest of my family the news. We called our general practitioner and our OB/GYN (we had an appointment scheduled with the OB/GYN a few days later), and discussed our options. We also called our insurance company to see if they would cover a termination, and to find out where we could have the procedure done in case that was the route we decided to go. We decided to wait until the appointment to make the final decision, but we checked on making arrangements in case we needed to.

After speaking with our regular OB/GYN at the appointment and consulting with the doctor who originally was going to perform our CVS (who was the doctor who would be performing the termination) we went ahead and scheduled the termination. We were told by all three doctors that the prognosis was not good, and that even if Lillie did make it to term (which was unlikely in their opinions) she would need immediate heart and digestive surgery, not to mention that she would be mentally disabled.

On March 29, 2005 I went in for the laminaria insertion to begin the process of opening my cervix. The procedure itself was not very painful for me—it was like having a pap smear. But that night when the contractions started, it was agonizing. The doctor gave me a pain killer, but it couldn't take away the emotional pain of my impending loss. I cried very hard as I lay there with the most severe cramps I have ever had in my life.

The next day I went in to the hospital to have the dilation and evacuation (D&E) and was treated kindly, but wasn't given a lot of information. I initially told the doctor that I wanted my daughter's remains, thinking that the hospital would have them cremated for me. We learned that the hospital would just release her remains to us—not cremate them. My husband did not think either of us was up to taking care of her remains ourselves, so we had the hospital bury her with the other lost babies.

After struggling with our loss of Lillie, we decided to try again. My pregnancy with her made me believe that I could bear children after all. We tried for three months on our own, from May to August of 2005. In August I sought out my reproductive endocrinologist (RE) to ask if there were any tests that could be done to help us conceive. I was tested for follicle stimulating hormone (FSH), thyroid, and luteinizing hormone (LH) levels and I had a hysterosalpingogram (HSG) test, which all came back normal. The doctor then put me on Clomid to induce ovulation. I was on Clomid for three months, to no avail. I then went on a mixture of Clomid/Bravelle for three months and did an intrauterine insemination (IUI). Still no luck, and I was 41 years old. After talking again to my RE in December 2005, he put me back on the Lupron treatment for three months. After coming off the second Lupron treatment, we tried to conceive for another three months. In July 2006 I became very depressed and sought counseling.

I then turned to the Nevada Center for Reproductive Medicine. After my initial consultation in August 2006, my husband and I went ahead with the testing for my FSH again. Since I was 41, they needed to check to see if my eggs were good. Since my FSH came back at 8.0 and was within low enough levels to use my own eggs, we went ahead with the cycle. We were lucky to retrieve 22 eggs; 17 were mature and 11 were fertilized using intracytoplasmic sperm injection (ICSI). Out of the 11 fertilized eggs, eight made it to day three for preimplantation genetic diagnosis (PGD). We had already decided we would do the PGD, since my chances of having another trisomy 21 baby at age 41 were quite high. Out of the eight that made it to PGD, seven of the eight were chromosomally abnormal! We discovered that although my ovaries stimulated well, my eggs were old. We then looked into donor eggs. After some trepidation and a lot of discussion, we went ahead with a donor egg cycle.

Our donor produced 60 eggs, but only approximately half of them were mature. After fertilization (we did natural fertilization that time since we used a donor) only 11 eggs were fertilized and made it to PGD stage. We were adamant about doing PGD even though we were using a donor, because after you go through losing a child to trisomy 21 or any other anomaly, you focus more on having a healthy baby versus the financial cost of PGD. So we had 11 embryos, of which only six were chromosomally normal. That was when we found out that my husband had chromosomal issues too.

We transferred two embryos and within a week I knew I was pregnant! I was so happy! The cost for both cycles came to over $40,000, but to finally be pregnant with two baby boys that we knew were chromosomally normal was worth it! Unfortunately, I lost the pregnancy at five weeks. It ended up being a chemical pregnancy whereby the fertilized eggs never implanted in my uterus properly. I was devastated. We were lucky enough to have two other embryos to freeze, but have since found out that I have immunology issues as well.

We did some fairly extensive testing after the loss of my boys and found that I have a methylenetetrahydrofolate reductase (MTHFR) deficiency, and also have no protection from anti-paternal cytotoxic antibodies. Simply put, I don't metabolize vitamins B_6, B_{12} or folic acid correctly, and my body's own immune system attacks any embryo as if it were a foreign object. My pregnancy with my daughter truly was a miracle! In order to carry a pregnancy, I would have to take mega-doses of vitamins B_6, B_{12} and folic acid, and I would have to go through immunological treatment involving injections with my husband's white blood cells to try to get my body to "accept" his cells.

During the first month of the immunological treatment, my arms swelled up and bruised easily; it took almost four weeks for the injection sites to heal. The next month, only four days after the second treatment, my arms were only very slightly bruised and started to heal very quickly. I was tested in April 2007 to see if the injections had had any effect on my immune system; they hadn't. We decided to move forward with the frozen embryo transfer (FET) though, because I felt that the real reason behind my loss must have been the MTHFR disorder. I remembered that I had been taking high doses of B_6 and B_{12} when I conceived Lillie. I had been working long days and was under a tight deadline, so I was taking those vitamins to help with stress, never realizing that it would help me carry a pregnancy.

We went through the FET process in June 2007, and, unfortunately, it failed. I was heartbroken. Even three years after letting Lillie go, I still have moments of extreme sadness. I still struggle with the loss of Lillie and with the loss of possibly never being able to have children. So here I am, more than three years later, without children and without the hope of having any naturally. While my story has come to a close for having children, going through terminating a much wanted pregnancy, the subsequent infertility, and miscarriage has taught me a lot about myself.

One thing I have learned is that I am stronger than I ever thought I would have to be. I have learned to try to be content with who I am and what I have become. I hope that through my experiences I can help others to cope with their losses. Whether it is the loss of a much-wanted child through termination for medical reasons, or the loss of fertility, or of a subsequent pregnancy, I have been there and I know how painful it is. I now administer to the private discussion forum for *A Heartbreaking Choice* and help to maintain the web site at *aheartbreakingchoice.com*.

I also know the joy of life. The many losses have taught me to never take life for granted. Life is precious, but so is quality of life. We who are so humane to our pets are judged for being humane for our children. Isn't that what makes us good parents? We have the ability to know that instead of giving our children a life of suffering, we have given them an eternity of peace. I am currently looking into adoption, and am hoping to adopt a child from Central America.

6

Barbara's Story **"A Letter to Julian"**

Dear Julian,

July 29th, 2007 was the best day of my life. That was the day we found out that you were coming to see us in nine months. Daddy and I were so scared but more excited than we had ever been for anything in our lives. I immediately started thinking about our future together; watching you grow, teaching you new things, and getting to know my perfect little baby.

Our doctor thought you might have been an ectopic pregnancy when I was only four weeks pregnant with you. That meant that you would have been growing somewhere inside my body other than my uterus, where you should have been. After two terrifying weeks where we thought we lost you, we received confirmation that it was just a mistake everything was just fine. At six weeks and three days, Daddy and I went to see you on an ultrasound for the first time. I was even more in love with you! You were only the size of a grain of rice, but you were *my* little grain of rice. We put your picture up in our bedroom and hung it on the refrigerator so we could see you all the time.

As the weeks went by I got more and more excited as my belly started to grow fat and I could feel the pains of pregnancy. As hard as it was at times, I would have never traded it. I know I was sick a lot and it may have scared you, but I was just fine. When I was 10 weeks pregnant with you, I couldn't even fit into my regular jeans anymore; time for maternity clothes! It was so exciting to see the proof that my little baby was in there. At that point, I had pretty much decided you were a boy. There was no doubt in my mind; so much so, that Daddy and I never even settled on a girl's name although we had your name picked out pretty fast. Your name was to be Julian Joseph.

Daddy and I had planned a trip to Boston in October. At that time, I was about 14 weeks pregnant with you. That was when you went to your first Red Sox game! In case you don't remember, Manny Ramirez hit a walk-off homerun to win the game for Boston. We were so excited that our little unborn Julian was able to go to a Red Sox game. We even took a picture of you in my belly and planned to give it to you later. The rest of our trip, we did a lot of resting, relaxing, and shopping for maternity clothes. By that point, I felt like you must have been 10 pounds already. My belly was getting bigger day by day.

When we got home, I had an appointment to see the doctor. I was 15 weeks and five days pregnant with you. Everything was going great. I had gained three pounds, finally! The doctor measured my belly to see how big you had grown and he said we were doing great. Then he took out a little device called a Doppler that would be able to hear your heartbeat. Daddy wasn't there because he was at work. I felt so bad that I'd hear your heartbeat before him. The doctor put the cold Doppler on my belly and rolled it around. It went on forever. He couldn't hear much of anything so he thought the battery was dead. He changed the batteries, and then tried again; still nothing. Then the doctor told me to go have an ultrasound done, just in case. I wasn't scared or anything; I was just excited I'd get to see you now that you were a lot bigger.

The familiar face that performed my last ultrasound greeted me. I lay on the table and she began looking at the images of you. She told me that because she was not a doctor, she could not tell me where the heartbeat was, if there was one. However, as you showed up on the screen, she motioned toward a tiny little spot on the screen that was flashing back and forth. There was your heartbeat! I was so relieved. I watched as she continued the ultrasound. Every time she'd press down on my belly, I would see you move away from the pressure and flap your arms like a bird; like you were waving. I laughed every time and it made the picture go blurry. The first time I had had an ultrasound; it was so fast…maybe 15 minutes. This time, I lay on the table for nearly an hour.

The technician was taking hundreds of pictures of you. I asked her to make sure she got a good picture I could take home and she said, "Sure." She measured your head, spine, legs, arms, and almost every part of your body. When she was done, I saw a very worried look on her face. She told me she had to go and get the on-duty doctor and talk to him. I still wasn't worried. I waited and waited and finally she came to tell me to go home and to wait for my regular doctor to call me. I thought that was odd. I asked if I could go back to work. She told me no; to go home and wait by the phone. I was a little bit worried at that point. I left and called Daddy as soon as I got in the car. I told him everything that had happened and he got very scared too. He left work to come home and be with you and me.

When Daddy got home, we started to go over all the bad things that could be happening. We knew you were alive, though, so that was good. We knew if there was something wrong with you it wouldn't matter. We'd love you just the same. You were our perfect little baby and nothing could change that. The doctor called late that afternoon. Daddy answered the phone and looked so scared. I could see tears welling up in his eyes. He talked to the doctor for a couple of minutes then hung up and just started crying. I asked him "What? What?!" The doctor had told him you had "multiple congenital defects" and that we would need to wait until the next day to come in and talk to him. Our hearts dropped to the ground. We still had hope, though, that it was something we could work through. That night dragged; we couldn't eat or sleep, all we did was think about you.

The next morning, we tried our best to stay positive, as we got ready to go see the doctor to talk about you. My heart raced as we sat in the waiting room. I barely had enough strength in my legs to walk to the doctor's office when he came to get us. We sat down and he simply pushed the report from the ultrasound in front of us. We read it in fear. There was a list of all of the major body parts with checkboxes beside each one: YES or NO. In the "no" column was stomach and liver. There was no check next to the word heart, it just said "uncommon" beside it. The doctor told us there was also what looked like a cyst containing spinal fluid on the back of your neck. As bad as it all looked, we still had hope. We were willing to do anything to fix the problems. The doctor suggested we go see a specialist who could tell us more about what was going on inside your body. As we left the doctor's office, we were calmer than when we went in. We thought that the news we received was so much better than what we had imagined in our heads.

The next day, we went to see the specialist. He performed another ultrasound. We watched on the screen as you flapped your arms again. The doctor took a lot of measurements. When he was done with the ultrasound, he asked us what we already knew about your condition. We asked him to tell us everything he saw. He saw many cysts around your neck; the largest was twice the size of your head. This is a condition called cystic hygroma. Then he told us there was swelling in your abdomen where water was collecting under your skin. We later learned this condition is hydrops fetalis. We asked him if you could live with these problems or if there were any chance that they would get better. We saw tears in his eyes as he tried, in the nicest way possible, to tell us that you were in very bad health. He told us these problems could come from Down syndrome, Turner syndrome, or that they just formed on their own for no particular reason. To us, the news still didn't seem all that bad. Daddy's cousin has Down syndrome and we figured you might turn out like her. I don't think we cried in that doctor's office. We felt there was hope for you still!

When we got home we did some research on cystic hygroma and hydrops. We learned something very scary; that the two conditions together have a near 100 percent mortality rate. I could not find a single case of a fetus being diagnosed with these problems and making it to birth. That terrified us. The thought of making the choice to let you go started playing in our minds. It was not because we were scared of having an imperfect baby (remember, you were our perfect little baby no matter what the doctors said), but that the longer you lived, the greater chance there was that you would start to feel pain in your tiny body. Neurologists all have different opinions on when unborn babies can feel pain and sensations, but a lot of them agree that it can happen as early as the twentieth week of pregnancy. That day, I was 16 weeks pregnant; just about four months and almost halfway there.

We wanted so much to be selfish and continue the pregnancy. We felt that if you were going to leave us, God would take you away. It wasn't my choice to take you away. Daddy and I aren't very religious but we do believe in God. We don't believe he did this to you; we believe that nature happens. We fought with our hearts and minds for what seemed like years. We wanted to do the right thing for you, not for us. As the days went on, we knew what we had to do, but that didn't make it easier by any means. We searched for approval from somewhere that we were making the right choice. None of the doctors would give us an honest opinion on the choice we were making. That made it so much harder. Your grandmas, grandpa, and aunts agreed with us, but it wasn't enough. Grandma B (Daddy's mom) called your Daddy's grandma—your great-grandma. She was a pediatric nurse for more than 40 years. Great-grandma is a very religious woman. She lives by the light of God and no other way. She told Grandma B that she had seen your situation many, many times and never once had it turned out well. This made us feel like we were making the right choice. We knew what we had to do.

We tried to find a hospital that would help us let you go. Our doctor told us there was not a single one in our town. There was a clinic, but I didn't want to let you go in a place surrounded mostly by women who did not want their babies. I have always been pro-choice, but I did not feel like I was making a choice to let you go. I believe the choice was made for me and that I just had to follow through with it. We had to call UCLA Medical Center to schedule an appointment to let you go. We made an appointment for the following Tuesday. The process was to take two days and you would be gone from us by Wednesday afternoon.

Over the weekend, I was too scared to talk to you and show you love. It was already going to be so hard to say goodbye. Daddy and I were afraid and just pretended like you were not there. I regret that so much, Julian. I wish I would have talked to you and told you a thousand times how much I love you.

My mommy flew all the way out from South Carolina on Tuesday to say goodbye with us. Daddy, Grandma B and I drove to Los Angeles on Tuesday morning. My mommy met us there. I was scared, but at the same time relieved. I knew we were going to release you to a much better place where your problems wouldn't matter anymore. When we got to the hospital, they started the preparation for the procedure, which would happen the following day. We met a very nice doctor who was very compassionate and understanding. The doctors and nurses began giving me drugs to relax me and to get my body ready for what was to happen the next day. I didn't feel very well after all of the medications. I remember laying on the table and my mommy waving alcohol swabs in front of my face. I think I lost consciousness. She kept telling the doctors how white I was and that my lips were even white. Grandma is a nurse, so she knows what she is talking about!

The preparation was almost over; I signed a lot of papers and it was time to go to the hotel and let the drugs get my body ready. As we left, I became very sick in the car. We didn't make it more than two miles on the freeway when we had to turn around. I was very weak and throwing up. We went back to the hospital to talk to the doctor. I was going to have to be admitted to the hospital, so the doctor offered us an option. She gave me the choice of being induced into labor rather than have the procedure we were originally going to have. The original procedure scared me, but I was sure I had no other choice given how old you were. I decided right away to have labor induced. They would give me medications that would cause my body to think it was time for you to be born and when you came, because you were so young, you just wouldn't be able to breathe as soon as you left my body. I knew that was what I had to do.

Grandma B left to go home, but Daddy and my mommy were right by my side the whole time. Daddy was so tired and sad, but he kept going for you and me. I was so proud of him for being so strong. We just couldn't believe that by that time the next day, you would be gone. I went into the hospital and they started the induction just around midnight on Tuesday. About an hour later, I started to feel really strong cramps in my tummy. I am sure you felt them, too. At 6:00 AM that morning, my water broke. I was officially going into labor.

I went through the whole day without crying. I was hurting so much physically and emotionally to let you go, but I had the greatest sense of peace. Daddy must have only slept two hours all night, but stayed up all day and took care of me. As the day turned into evening, the cramps in my tummy got very strong. There was nothing to do in that hospital room other than think about you. The World Series was on television and, in case you don't remember, the Red Sox were playing. I watched little bits and pieces here and there to pass the time.

At 11:00 PM I started bleeding; I called the nurse and she told me that meant you would be coming soon. The pain in my tummy became intense, but still I didn't care. I was so happy for you even though I was sad for myself, Daddy, and everyone who loved you. I told Daddy to go down to my belly, tell you goodbye, and let you know how much we loved you. He went to where you were, put his face to my belly, and said "Goodbye, Julian. Mommy and Daddy love you and we're going to miss you so much." Just before midnight, I could feel you getting ready to be born. I felt your tiny body move through my body and leave me. You were born at 11:54 PM on October 24, 2007.

Being able to give birth to you was the biggest blessing I have ever had in my life. I am so glad I got sick from all the medication and had the opportunity to deliver you. You laid with me for a minute or two, but I was too scared to hold you. I knew there were things very wrong with you, and I didn't want to know. To me, you were and still are, my perfect baby. I regret not holding you and I hope you can forgive me, but by that point, you were already with God. I held Daddy's hand as we thought about you and said goodbye. The doctor took you away. I was so exhausted. I prayed to God, talked to you for a minute, and then fell asleep. I woke up the next morning and my big belly was gone, along with my heart.

It was so hard to come home without you. We felt so empty. I cried and cried because I missed you so much. Daddy cried a lot, too. I want you to know that Daddy is a very strong man, but ever since you came into our lives, he melted. You were his kryptonite. You still are. We talked to you as much as we could in the following days. I needed you to know that I didn't want to let you go. I took on all of this pain and sadness to keep you safe and happy. I would do it over a thousand times if I had to. Julian, I was so scared that you didn't understand. I was afraid that you thought Daddy and I didn't want you.

As I write this, it's been only six days since you left us. We think about you every minute and we dream about what you're doing, but it's not sad.

I get sad for us; that we will have to spend our whole lives without you. We won't be able to hold you, kiss you, and cherish you. When I think about how you feel, I get a great joy in my heart. I know you are just fine, that you are much happier, and that you are the perfect little boy I always imagined. I can see you in my mind when I think about you. I know just what you look like. Every time we talk to you and we talk to God, it gets easier for us. I don't cry all the time now. As time goes by, I know it will get easier and easier but you will always be in our hearts. When we go on to have another child, it will only remind us more of you.

We will love and cherish your brother or sister like they never imagined. We will give them all of the love that we know you would have given them. We will never stop loving you or missing you. Little things will always remind us of you, even when we are old and have grandchildren. We have so many happy memories from when you were with us, and believe it or not, from when you were born. When the holidays come, we will always wish you were here with us. It will always hurt to put up a Christmas tree without you putting candy canes all over the bottom of it. Nevertheless, we know you are right here with us. I have never felt so loved in my life. I know, now, that you understand what happened and why we let you go. I feel it every single day. Before now, I never put a lot of weight into prayer. Julian, I really do feel you all around us, helping us heal.

Daddy and I went to the supermarket this weekend. We went to the florist department in search of flowers to have in the house. We looked all around and couldn't find any we liked. As we were walking away, the last flowers we saw were orchids. We have beautiful pictures that Daddy took of orchids hanging in our kitchen. We picked up the flowers to see how much they cost. On the tag, Daddy pointed out the name of the kind of orchid. It read "Julian." I wore an orchid in my hair on the day Daddy and I got married. We know that it was you letting us know that you were okay and that you weren't mad at us. We felt so at peace.

I am so happy when I think of you, Julian. I was blessed by the grace of God to have you in my life the past four months. If I had the choice for none of this to ever have happened, I would not take it. You were our little miracle. You came to us only three weeks after we decided we were ready to have a child. Daddy and I will always be closer than before because of you. You made us a family, not just husband and wife.

Julian, I love you so much. You fill me with as much joy as if you were here in my arms. I know someday we will all be together again. I am going to miss you every day of my life, even if I don't talk to you every day. I am afraid of the day when I stop talking to you daily. Please know that doesn't mean I have moved on or stopped loving you, but that time has healed us and made us stronger. We won't always need to talk to you to feel better. I love you my little boy.

7

Briar's Story "Rethinking Choice"

For as long as I've been old enough to be aware of the issue, I've been a supporter of a woman's right to choose. Whether a pregnancy was the result of carelessness, an accident, or a crime, I thought that no woman should have to bear a baby that she didn't want, and that only the woman facing an unwanted pregnancy should have the right to decide what to do. I attended annual Planned Parenthood galas, fully in support of protecting reproductive choice for all women, but, really, I wanted to protect this right for other women: women who weren't ready to—or didn't want to—have babies. I knew that having an abortion was not a decision that I could make for myself. At last fall's gala, I was 33 years old, married, and trying for my first baby. I cheered for choice, but was glad to know that it was not a choice I would face.

But then it was. My husband and I found out we were pregnant the day after Christmas, and we were thrilled. I was nervous, knowing that first trimester miscarriages are not unusual. Mostly, though, I was excited, and I started a series of happy visits to my obstetrician, submitting to the recommended screening tests and paying very little attention to what those tests were for. To me, they were chances to check in with the doctor, hear what to expect next, and—most wonderfully—see or hear my baby. Our first ultrasound was amazing; already I could see the tiny little life growing inside me, with the little heart beating away.

At our next ultrasound, we watched our little one wiggle and jump on the screen, and we were fully in love. At my 12-week visit, I heard the wonderful sound of my baby's heartbeat, and I knew that we were in the clear. Four days later, my obstetrician called. My blood work from one of the screening tests to which I had given so little thought came back from the lab showing an elevated risk for Down syndrome. "There's only a three percent chance that anything is wrong," my doctor told me, "so that's a 97 percent chance that everything is fine." She then asked if I wanted to undergo the diagnostic test that would let us know for sure.

With that telephone call, everything I "knew" changed. My husband and I had never even talked about the diagnostic tests (which, unlike the screening tests, could definitively diagnose chromosome abnormalities, including Down syndrome). We barely knew that those tests existed, having skipped the "problem" chapters in our pregnancy books. We considered our options, and had our first halting conversation about how we might deal with a poor diagnosis. We decided that we needed to know for sure; I would have the additional testing. Two days after the diagnostic test, we received the preliminary results showing that our baby almost certainly had Down syndrome. We would have to wait another week for the final results, but we were told that the initial results were 98 percent accurate, and we knew we had to think about what to do next. We cried, talked, researched, and cried some more. We decided that if the diagnostic test confirmed a Down syndrome diagnosis, we would end our pregnancy.

During the week of waiting for final results, I went to work, but didn't function. I could barely have a conversation without breaking down. I couldn't eat, and didn't sleep until total exhaustion finally set in. Meanwhile, my husband and I made arrangements, assuming the worst. We went to a clinic to receive the state-mandated information on abortion, met with a counselor there, and scheduled our procedure—hoping against hope that the preliminary results were wrong, that we would get the final results back and cancel the procedure if we were on the right side of the improbable odds. Exactly one week after the diagnostic test, we got the telephone call from our genetic counselor with the results. She confirmed that the initial test results were correct: our baby—a boy, she told us—had Down syndrome. The next day, we went back to the clinic and said goodbye to the baby that we already loved. I was 13 weeks and six days along.

The day my OB called with our bad screening test results, I started searching the Internet for information about Down syndrome. I also searched for information about pregnancy termination, and questioned what kind of horrible person I was for considering ending the life of my baby. I knew that my baby was sick, and possibly very sick. I knew that some cases of Down syndrome are more minor, with milder retardation and less affected body systems. But I also learned that some cases are very severe, with major heart defects, significant mental retardation, and other debilitating developmental problems. A high percentage of Down syndrome babies miscarry. The spectrum of problems is wide, with the negative end of the spectrum quite devastating, and no test could tell us where our baby might fall on that spectrum. Ultimately, the uncertainty of our baby's condition, the knowledge that if he survived the pregnancy he would not lead a "normal" life, and the very real possibility that he could suffer significantly in an abbreviated life all led us to our decision to end our pregnancy.

Though I believed in my head that our decision to terminate was the right one—for my husband and me, for our future family, and for our baby—I felt incredibly guilty and very isolated, and my heart ached. Even though we had very supportive family and friends (at least among the limited circle that knew the true story of our loss), I didn't want to talk about our situation with any of them. How could they possibly understand our decision when I could barely comprehend it myself? But I discovered in my Internet research about Down syndrome that, both fortunately and unfortunately, I was not nearly as alone as I had felt. That research led me to stumble across an Internet message board for women who have ended a pregnancy for medical reasons…a cyber-sisterhood of heartbroken women, posting messages of pain, sympathy, despair, support, and love for their lost babies.

> *"She was our first baby, our miracle. We tried for over a year, went through a hysteroscopy, laparoscopy, four months of Lupron to treat endometriosis, and lots of heartbreak. We thought our prayers were answered when we got pregnant. Now our hearts are broken."*
>
> —Laurie

The women on that web site described a staggering variety of devastating diagnoses. In my naiveté—thinking that a miscarriage was the worst I might face—I had never known how much could go wrong with a pregnancy. Some of the women on the board also terminated after receiving a Down syndrome diagnosis, but the majority of the conditions these women described were foreign to me: Turner syndrome, trisomy 13, trisomy 18, hypoplastic left heart syndrome, hydranencephaly, acrania, and fetal hydrops… a seemingly unending list of awful diagnoses. Some conditions were incompatible with life. In other cases, a baby might have survived to term, only to face an abbreviated life with severe difficulties, multiple surgeries, and a great deal of pain. Some babies had conditions so severe that their mothers were left with the "choice" of ending the pregnancy or waiting for the inevitable miscarriage.

> *"I hadn't even heard of it before our diagnosis, and remember being completely shocked, heartbroken and horrified by the external symptoms our little boy was showing. He had a cleft*

lip/palate; six fingers on both hands and his intestines were outside his body. But I remember thinking, "It doesn't matter; now you're going to tell me what can be done for him." What I wasn't ready for, and what took me a moment to realize, was that the consultant was saying they were only symptoms of something far more serious. He then listed the "difficulties" associated with T13, and with every one my heart just broke a little bit more. I spent far too long trawling through T13 web sites and just felt I could not bring a child into this world just to suffer, and that was all I saw. While I respect the opinions of those who continue, I'm glad I had the courage to terminate and restrict the suffering. My little boy only ever existed in the one place I could protect him."

—MJ

Some diagnoses, like mine, fell into a "gray" area. I read those messages and cried for them, for me, and for all of our babies. And there were tears of relief, too, because I knew that there were others out there like me, who had faced this awful choice and come to the same conclusion that I had. Before I ever posted a message of my own, those women seemed to be responding to my own thoughts.

"I cried, all of us on this board did and we still do. But none of us who ever decide to terminate loved our children any less than anyone else. We let them go BECAUSE we loved them and we didn't want them to suffer. You are not a horrible person, you are a compassionate person."

—TJ

Eventually, I did post messages of my own, weeping as I typed out my feelings of guilt and emptiness and loss. In response, I received limitless support, kindness, typewritten "hugs," and reassurance that my feelings were normal and that, in time, the emptiness, the desire to shut myself away from the world, the breakdowns, the hopelessness, and the deep, deep sadness would slowly, slowly start to get better. They reminded me of the reasons that we had all decided to terminate: not because we were bad people, or to make our lives simpler; but because we loved our babies and wanted to protect them. I've never met those women, and in some cases, I don't even know their real names. Yet they have been among the most kind, gentle, and loving people I have known in my life, and they've done more for me than offer their kindness and support through my darkest days; they have forever changed my thinking about the "right to choose."

> *"I never imagined I would make the decision to terminate either, but love is a very powerful motivator and will make us bring great heartache upon ourselves to spare our loved ones from suffering."*
>
> —Mollie

I quickly discovered, through the microcosm of that message board, that there is no "type" of woman to face this choice and make the decision to terminate. We are teachers, scientists, therapists, nurses, stay-at-home moms, doctors, restaurant managers, and lawyers. We live in all parts of the country, in Canada, and overseas. Some are not at all religious, but many hold a deep religious faith, and some postings shared Bible verses, or discussed struggles with God and faith in the face of so much heartbreak and pain. Prayers were offered every day, and lost babies were referred to as "angels." Some of the women were not necessarily "pro-choice" before being faced with their baby's terrible diagnosis. Many, pro-choice or not, admitted having said—pre-diagnosis—that they would never consider an abortion for themselves. Some had gotten pregnant easily, while others had struggled, sometimes for years.

Most of the women received their baby's diagnosis sometime in the second trimester of their pregnancy, though several were in their third trimester. (A few, like me, were "lucky" enough to be diagnosed late in the first trimester.) My own termination was a surgical one, a dilation and evacuation (D&E)—the only option I was given at my stage of pregnancy, and really the only procedure I knew about. But I learned that many women, particularly those later in their second trimester, ended their pregnancies by being induced, going through labor, and delivering tiny babies that, in some cases, they saw, held, and kissed. Some of these women were able to receive pictures of their babies. Regardless of the type of termination procedure, some women were able to receive a tiny footprint or handprint from the hospital or clinic. Some created memory gardens, or planted trees, or assembled memory boxes to honor their little one. Some of us have only an ultrasound photo as a tangible reminder of our lost babies.

> *"At the 20-week ultrasound they found a heart defect—HLHS. We had 10 days of frantic research and as you all know, it was an incredibly painful decision to terminate. I have no regrets and am entirely at peace, but I just ache for my baby. We chose labor and delivery, and our son was born 2/18/07. He came in*

the middle of the night, so I had 10 precious hours to hold him and sleep with him. His brother named him David."

—Lisa

I've heard women who have not faced this situation say "I would never get rid of my baby," or "I would love my baby no matter what"—the implication being, of course, that those of us who have made the decision to terminate did not love our babies. I know that some women who face a terrible prenatal diagnosis continue on with their pregnancies, and I know that that is the right decision for those women. I also know that, for the women who end their pregnancies for medical reasons, and for the women who continue, each decision is made out of love.

"Angelia was our first baby and she taught us so much during her short existence. I miss knowing she is with me and I miss feeling her move inside of me. I am blessed to have had her with me as long as I did. I'm glad I got to hold her and tell her that I loved her after delivery. I will love her forever and will miss her every day of my life."

—Jodi

So much of the rhetoric around abortion ignores the real-life tragedy for each woman who faces a bad prenatal diagnosis. Maybe in some cases women decide to end these pregnancies for "convenience" or because their babies are "imperfect." But what I saw on that message board, time after time, was a rapid, intense, and terrifying post-diagnosis learning process, an incredibly difficult, heartbreaking decision, and—even with babies with indisputably fatal conditions—a terrible and consuming sadness in deciding to let those babies go.

"My angel had a brainstem. My doctors told me that she would probably have lived at birth, breathed on her own and had a heartbeat…but that she may not have sustained it on her own for very long and would have been subject to all sorts of life support. My baby didn't have any other brain tissue…this would have resulted in endless medical problem as she grew… seizures, dysphagia, aspiration, pneumonias, skin breakdown (bedsores), she would have needed a shunt to release the fluid from her head, multiple surgeries. She wouldn't have been able to see or hear, she may have had sensory issues that made our

touch painful to her...and most of those children don't live to be three."

—J

I know that my own baby might not have suffered excessively; he might have made it to term and he might not have had serious heart problems. His retardation might have been mild, and he might not have needed significant and repeated medical intervention. I know that some of the women on the message board who terminated for other fetal anomalies would not have terminated for Down syndrome. I still struggle with the what ifs and I imagine that I always will. But more than ever before, I believe that a woman faced with a terrible prenatal diagnosis must be able to do what she believes is best for her baby, even when that means letting her baby go. No legislator should be able to tell any woman that she must carry to term a baby with no brain matter. No woman should be forced to continue a pregnancy to term while her baby struggles to survive in a womb with no amniotic fluid. Would any legislator tell his or her own daughter that she must go on with a pregnancy, knowing that there is no chance that her baby's heart will continue to beat outside the womb? Or when her baby's abbreviated life will consist of round-the-clock medical care, invasive procedures, and pain? And even in a "gray area" like Down syndrome, should someone else have the right to decide for me how difficult a life my baby should endure?

I know that some people will think I am a horrible person because of the choice I made. I also know that my husband and I made the heartbreaking decision that was right for us. And despite the doubts I will always face, and sadness that I will always carry with me for my lost baby, in my heart I know that my decision doesn't make me a horrible person. I know this because some of most wonderful and caring women that I have ever "met" have made the same choice. These are the women I will think about when I cheer for choice at my next Planned Parenthood gala—these women who wanted nothing more than a healthy baby, who loved their babies so much, and who made the choice they never, ever wanted to make.

8

Carrie's Story "Our Warrior Princess"

I had just turned 40 years old in the late summer of 2005, and had unsuccessfully tried to get pregnant for 22 months. With only one ovary left and what we thought was a problematic fibroid, my husband and I decided it was time to schedule the surgery to have the fibroid removed.

A week before the surgery was to occur, I most happily discovered I was pregnant. We were stunned at first, and then we joyfully began to get ready for our baby.

I elected to have a chorionic villus sampling (CVS) test, due to my advanced maternal age. My husband and I felt like we were being grilled by the nurse as to why we asked for the CVS in the first place. *Well, what would you do? Do about what? If the CVS came back with poor results?* What kind of poor results? *Well, they can vary.* Yes, I would imagine. *So? So… So, why do you want a CVS?* There was an uncomfortable silence and oddly worded questions for another 10 minutes or so.

They seemed to need to hear me say (and my husband as well) that we would terminate the pregnancy if the news was bad enough, but they didn't ask directly. We had to say it without being prompted, like it was a box to be checked on a list. It was a very strange conversation.

I was still bleeding days after the CVS, so I went in for a sonogram and discovered I had a torn placenta. I was put on bed rest for three weeks. I followed the doctor's instructions to the letter—I didn't pick up anything heavier than a coffee cup. I prayed, meditated, I did everything I could emotionally, spiritually and physically. I tried to focus on healing my placenta abrupta. I had a picture in my mind of our little family on a far-off Christmas morning, and how this terrifying time would be a distant memory. We even called our baby "Zena" for awhile, our little warrior princess (a combination of the name of the television character "Xena" and the Arabic name "Zenat"). I talked to her and asked her to please not go—we would have a wonderful time when she got here. I remember eagerly watching the baby shows on television at first, but then I slowly stopped watching them. A bone-chilling fear had crept in that the pregnancy was not meant to be. I tried so hard not to feel that way. I look back at that time and I weep. I often think she stayed only because I asked her to.

The call came three days before Thanksgiving, a Monday night at 6:15 PM. Dr. A was calling with the initial verbal report from the lab. "The test results show your baby has a 14/22 marker chromosome," he said. "We need you to come in right away this week so we can determine if you or your husband carries the marker, so you won't need to worry."

I wasn't even sure of what I had just been told—it felt like someone had torn my soul open, and a cold wind was blowing through it. Dr. A attempted to comfort me, told me not to panic, and whatever I did, under *any* circumstances, do not research it on the Internet. Although he never said there wasn't a problem, he really downplayed the CVS results. I consider myself to be a bright, resourceful, independent thinker. But at that moment, as my universe was collapsing, I viewed him as the expert, and trusted his advice. And honestly, I wanted to believe him. I had not met him in person, as it was a big practice, and the doctors varied depending on who was in the office that day.

He called me back the next evening just to see how I was and make sure I had not gotten online.

The following week, Dr. A called to say he had called the lab back to clarify our test results. He told me the lab confirmed that we had a 95 percent chance that everything would be okay, and our baby would not be affected. We did not carry the marker. He said the chances were excellent that everything would be all right. Again, I chose to believe him. After all, it was what I wanted to hear. So, my husband and I actually allowed ourselves to go look at strollers and baby clothes, and begin to have hope again.

We had yet another follow-up, with yet another doctor, later that week. We were all smiles, as my bleeding had stopped, and we believed that statistically our chances were excellent that the baby was fine. This doctor, a fetal cardiac surgeon, greeted us somberly, and asked how we were doing after news of, in his words, "being hit by lightning." "Well, that was scary, but it looks like things are going to be fine," we answered. This doctor stared at us, and asked if we understood the news. We said we did, and how Dr. A told us of our 95 percent chance that everything would be fine. This doctor said that we really needed to follow up with the genetic counselor as soon as possible.

When we met with the genetic counselor about a week later, she was outraged that Dr. A had misled us into believing that our baby was fine. I was confused and asked her to call back the lab for clarification of the results. Why did the lab tell Dr. A what they did? How did they come to the "95 percent chance everything was okay" conclusion? Of course, they didn't. It was the spin Dr. A put on the information. The genetic counselor, while initially quite cool with us, began to truly partner with us in our quest to find out about this very rare disease. She told us that no matter what "odds" she gave us, no one could promise us anything—ever. That was when we dived into the Internet, despite Dr. A's warning. We sent the genetic counselor articles we found online to see if they were applicable to our baby's disease. We were frustrated by the lack of access to articles, sometimes costing $75.00 each, when they most likely wouldn't even apply to our case. This was when we took the "wait and see" approach, to see if any obvious, troublesome signs appeared in our girl.

Finally, the complete and final written report from the CVS test came in after a delay due to slow-growing samples. Our baby had a marker chromosome 14/22 in 100 percent of her cells, but they couldn't tell if the marker chromosome had genetic material on it. While we already knew it was not inherited, not even our genetic counselor (who had never seen an actual case before) could give us a true indication of the marker's impact on our baby. It might have been benign, or not. No one could give us any more information than that. We learned the extra chromosome 22 could mean our baby had cat eye syndrome. Both my husband and I wanted the baby very much, and neither one of us was willing to end the pregnancy on a "maybe."

It was Christmas Eve morning when our genetic counselor called us with news of a possible test that could tell us if the marker chromosomes of our little girl, Emma, had active genetic material on them. I had an amniocentesis done two days later, and the results came in on January 13, 2006. It confirmed without a doubt–that our Emma had two extra copies of chromosome 22 in every cell of her body. She had cat eye syndrome. The occurrence of this disorder is approximately one in 150,000. The last three weekly sonograms showed she had a tiny stomach and very low amniotic fluid, which indicated her kidneys were beginning to malfunction, a hallmark of chromosome 22 disorders. My amniotic fluid level was at less than five percent of the expected volume for that stage in my pregnancy.

We consulted with at least 10 doctors in three countries, including the only specialist in the world doing research on 14/22, located in Germany. No one gave us any hope. My husband and I chose to end our pregnancy to spare out little girl what would most likely be a short, painful life, filled with many surgeries to correct the many malformations.

We let Emma go on January 20, 2006.

My doctors told us a dilation and evacuation (D&E) procedure was our only option, and that the anesthesia would make it painless for both of us. The doctor who performed the procedure tried to reassure me that we made the best choice, and added that he thought I was just days away from miscarrying anyhow.

The first couple of days afterward went as well as could be expected in such a sad circumstance. Then, something began to feel wrong. I went to the doctor, and was thoroughly examined. Everything looked okay, so they sent me home. Over the next 16 hours, my health plummeted. I took the rest of the night minute by minute. Looking back now, I should have called my doctor, but I didn't. I wasn't even sure at that point that I wanted to live.

When I saw the doctors the next morning, I learned that a large blood clot had developed overnight in my uterus. I was in grave danger, and I needed another D&E immediately. They preserved my uterus, but not for long.

We rescheduled the fibroid surgery three months later, as my menstrual flow and pain had become unbearable. I woke up from the surgery, sadly, with a hysterectomy. The surgeon explained that my uterus would not stop bleeding during the surgery, and that a hysterectomy was his only option.

Three weeks later, with the pathology report in hand, my surgeon informed us that the fibroid had been misdiagnosed. It was actually a large adenomyosis, whose only treatment was a hysterectomy. I also learned that the placenta had attached itself to the adenomyosis. That explained why I had so much trouble and pain after the termination. He told me that had I waited to miscarry, I might have bled to death.

As I look back at this transformative experience now, I can say I am a different person, I believe, for the better. Emma taught me so much. I think I have a measure of compassion for others that I did not have before. I have a difficult time being apathetic now, and feel almost compelled, in her honor, to actively strive to make the world a better place and to make myself a better person.

In her honor, we chose to go public and tell her story, so that other families would not feel alone in their difficult choices about the health care decisions for their children. Our dear Emma is never far from our thoughts or hearts.

9

Catherine's Story "The Blue Marble"

When I became pregnant for the third time (after a miscarriage and a beautiful baby girl) I was 37 years old. When I was pregnant with our first child (Alice) the screening test for genetic defects such as Down syndrome (trisomy 21), trisomy 18 and trisomy 13 was given in the second trimester. For my third pregnancy we were offered a first trimester test, to include blood work, an ultrasound and genetic counseling. Of course, my husband and I wanted the test. We wanted to know there were no serious problems. Neither of us had really considered at that time what we would do with an undesirable test result.

I vaguely remember the day of the first trimester test, but I do remember having to bring our daughter along with me and corral her the entire time. She is usually a good kid, but still a challenge at times, especially with long waits (and what nearly two-year-old is that patient?). I remember meeting with the genetic counselor, staring at the diagrams of abnormal chromosomes and thinking, "That will never happen to me." I was nodding and smiling because I understood what she was talking about, I understood the odds, and I understood the chromosomes—I got it. But it wasn't going to happen to me, so as far as I was concerned, it was a review of a genetics lesson I had in college and a lot of waiting around for a blood draw and an ultrasound. But it wasn't anything else. My results were going to be just fine. It was a formality, a "just to be sure."

During the ultrasound I saw my baby for the first time. None of the medical professionals gave any indication of a problem, even when I directly asked. "Everything looks fine so far," they said. I left for the blood work portion of the test feeling warm and fuzzy. Even my daughter's impatience while waiting 45 minutes for the blood draw did not faze me. I was really excited. And for some reason, I was absolutely convinced I was having a girl.

I had my testing done around 10 and a half weeks gestation. When the genetic counselor called me several days later to tell me there was an elevated risk for a chromosomal anomaly, I was surprised. But then she told me, "Catherine, your odds for Down syndrome are 1:49, and 1:50 for any other trisomy at this point in your pregnancy." She asked me if John, my husband, and I wanted to do a chorionic villus sampling (CVS) test. CVS is a genetic test where placental tissue is tested for chromosomal anomalies. I told her I would talk to John and get back to her. But as far as I knew, because I was not told otherwise, the ultrasound did not pick up anything abnormal. I assumed the increased odds for a chromosomal anomaly were due to the blood work. And I knew there was a decent margin of error there.

I called my husband at work immediately. The CVS test was only performed at the hospital on Wednesdays. On Tuesday I was to leave for my "Mom's last hurrah" trip with my daughter to visit friends in Chicago and St. Louis. John and I talked about the odds of a chromosomal anomaly, the odds of miscarriage the test carried, the plane fare, the likelihood of rescheduling the trip, and about what kind of testing we were comfortable with. CVS must be completed at our hospital by 12–13 weeks gestation. We decided we were okay with the odds given to us, and we'd wait until we could get an amniocentesis at 16 weeks gestation.

I left for my trip as planned on Tuesday. I had a good time with my friends, but the first trimester screening test results nagged at me. One night I went to eat dinner and hang out with my friend Maria at her house. I had not seen her in a year or so and it was fun to catch up. After dinner, Maria asked if Alice would like to watch a video, so we decided to watch a Charlie Brown one. As I waited for Maria to come over to the television from doing the dishes, a photograph caught my eye. The photograph was of her husband, his parents, and a boy with Down syndrome. "Is this Sam's brother?" I asked. "Yes," she said. I guess I knew then. I knew then that my world was about to change. But how and to what extent it would change I did not know.

So I came home and waited for the amniocentesis, and thought about Sam's brother.

At the amniocentesis appointment an ultrasound was done. The ultrasound technician and the doctor performing it were both upbeat. No one ever gave any indication that there was a problem, although the doctor reading the results said that he was not able to see the heart very clearly. Nancy, my friend who had volunteered to come along since John was busy, was there to hear the news, "Catherine, you're having a boy!" No dire looks. No getting other doctors for second opinions. No indication whatsoever there was a problem. So, maybe there wasn't? Maybe I was wrong about that sinking feeling, and about that gut instinct I had about our baby when I saw that photograph of my friend's brother-in-law?

It had been during one of those phases when our daughter was refusing to nap that the telephone rang. I was pregnant, exhausted, and desperately trying to take a nap myself. I needed a break. But unlike on most days when I tried to rest, I had not taken the telephone off the hook. So I answered it.

"Catherine, it's Dr. T. Catherine, I am sorry to tell you your baby has Down syndrome."

And with those words, my world felt like it ended.

I cannot describe the sound that emanated deep from my soul with those words—it was a deafening howl of grief I hope to never hear from myself or anyone else ever again. And then I cried. I don't even know for how long. And that was when the veil of black came over my eyes, and over my soul. And the doctor was still on the telephone.

"Catherine, are you alone?"

"Yes. My husband is at work. He's teaching right now," I sobbed.

"Do you want to come to the office?"

"My daughter…"

Alice was in the other room. She never went to sleep that afternoon. I think now of how scary that day must have been for her. Thank God kids don't remember anything at her age. Mommy's cries of anguish must have ripped her up as well, as when I started screaming in my anguish, she did as well.

"You can bring her."

"I don't think so, I don't know, I don't know what to do." I was shaking. My baby. There was nothing I could do. Nothing.

"Catherine, are you going to be okay? Can you call a friend?"

"I'll find my husband."

I know him. I know my husband. I love him to pieces, but he does not handle severe crises in the best way, well, not the best way for me at any rate. He folds in on himself. I so badly needed him to not do that.

I called his office, the main number. I tried so hard to remain composed as I asked the administrative assistant when he'd be out of class. I told her it was his wife calling. But then I started to cry. "It's an emergency."

"Hold on."

"Catherine? It's Leslie. Are you okay?" (The assistant had transferred my call to John's boss Leslie.)

"I need John. Send him home." I had totally lost it by that point.

"He should be on his way back from class now. I'll send him home. Are you okay?"

"No. I need John."

I have no idea how I got through the next half-hour before John came home. I don't know what I did. I can only guess that I held on to Alice as tight as I could. I can only guess that the baby kicked me and stirred up feelings I did not want to face. I can only guess that Alice just looked at me crying and started to cry herself, sensitive little thing that she is. I honestly just don't remember. And while I remember a lot of what happened to us, a lot of it seems to be completely erased from my memory.

I do remember that when John came home, I was sitting on one of the stools at the kitchen counter. I remember him walking through the door, and looking at me, searching my face for what was wrong. I said, "Honey, I need you to stay with me. Do not shut down right now. I need you. Our son has Down syndrome." John took hold of me and held on tight. We clung on to each other so tightly, as if in letting go one of us would drown.

I still cannot remember what Alice was doing or where she even was at the time. Later, John and I sat down on the couch. He didn't shut down, but he didn't talk either. But he did go to sleep, which was another one of his extreme stress responses. I knew that, but I was so angry he was not consciously with me. I did not even know what to say to him. I did not know what he was thinking, not at all. I wanted to scream at him, yet nothing would come out of my mouth, and it would have been pointless, anyway. I knew he was in pain, too.

Suddenly I felt I had to go back to my OB's office. I had to see her. I physically had to see her say that there was a problem. I had to see the test results to make sure there was no mistake. It was already 4:45 PM. The office closed at 4:30 PM. But we lived close by, and I did not care. I jumped into the car and sped off. I knew the staff would still be there, finishing appointments. I don't know what I looked like when I streamed through those office doors. It must have been awful. I almost ran smack into one of John's co-workers on the way in. "Hi Catherine! Catherine?" I flew past her, and to the receptionist. Tears streaming down my face, I told her I was Dr. T's patient and gave her my name. Literally within 30 seconds Dr. T was there, pulling me out of the waiting room and into her office. She hugged me. I sobbed. I sat down and she showed me the lab results. I couldn't believe what I was looking at. "Honestly, Catherine, nobody really knows what they would do unless they are faced with this. Nobody." She apologized again and again, and hugged me again. I knew I had to leave and go home. The office was closing. Going home was facing the truth, and facing our decision square on. I just wanted to run, all the while knowing I could not. I honestly don't remember the rest of that day.

That night the genetic counselor called us at home. She had not been the one to deliver the news; and she wanted to see how we were doing. She stated that there was a lot of misinformation on the Internet, and pointed me toward a few web sites. She told me that when I was ready, she had lots of information about schools. She appeared to assume we'd carry the pregnancy to term—or at least wanted me to think that was what we should do. I was so stunned that she was clearly trying to coerce our decision, that I could say nothing to her. I thanked her and hung up.

John was raised in a strict Catholic family. Since I first met him so many years ago, his conservative beliefs had changed a lot. He became much more liberal. I have considered myself to be pro-choice my entire life, but always felt like I would never be able to have an abortion myself. (Besides, I didn't think I'd ever even need to consider it.) This was one situation where I did not even have an inkling of an idea as to how he was feeling, or what he was thinking. I was sure he was as conflicted as I was.

We so wanted this baby. We made him. And now what? Would this change anything? My first reaction was that we had to continue the pregnancy. I had started feeling his kicks a couple of weeks prior and I was so enjoying the tiny kicks and flip-flops in my belly—the ones too imperceptible for me to have noticed early on in my previous pregnancy. I had that connection with him. Feeling the kicks was the one and only thing I enjoyed about being pregnant with Alice.

Over the next several days John and I retreated to our own little corners, both doing as much research as we could. The more I learned, the more I started to feel that what I saw was not what I wanted for our son. I worried about what would happen to him after John and I were gone, and how it would affect not only him, but his sister. The laundry list of health problems scared the pants off of me. The more I learned, the more I felt like we had to let him go.

Quietly, John was coming to the same conclusion.

It was not an easy decision for me or my husband as to what to do next. But there we were. Ultimately, my husband and I took a week to figure out what to do. We talked, cried, and did a lot of soul-searching. In the meantime, we had another ultrasound so they could look at the baby's heart. What they saw confirmed our fears—our son also had a heart defect, which is common in people with Down syndrome.

We knew time was running out to decide, as the cut-off for pregnancy termination is 24 weeks in our state. By the time I was 18 weeks, we had decided. But it was a Friday night. So we waited until Monday to call to make the appointment to end the pregnancy.

Neither of us had ever had to struggle with such a horrible choice. By far, it was the worst thing either of us had ever faced. I had never cried so much in my life. Or felt so alone. Our society does nothing for people in this position. It was just the two of us. And we felt awful, alone, scared, and horribly guilty. I was just thankful that we agreed in our decision.

However, the next day, Saturday, we both did a complete 180 degree turn in our thinking, after having presumably already decided to end the pregnancy. We both seemed to travel the same route that day.

That day I drove to the post office to mail some Christmas packages. I had to get that done before everything else going on would make it too hard to spread any Christmas cheer, or to even care about it. I remember driving down the road thinking, "Maybe this is okay. Maybe we can handle it. Maybe it won't be so bad." As I turned to get on to the highway, Elton John's song "Daniel" came on the radio. John had made a comment earlier that if we did not end the pregnancy he'd want to pick an easy name for our son. Hearing "Your eyes are blind, but you see more than I" hit home to me—I don't even know why, really. His name should be Daniel. I thought we'd keep him. And that would be his name.

My husband and I didn't talk about it anymore until later that night. I took the dog for a walk. As I was rounding the corner back onto our street, I had an epiphany—or at least a vision of things to come. I love my John—I think we have a great marriage and so far, to this day, we have managed to weather this storm all the stronger. I know that is not always the case. This can rip people apart. But that has not happened to us. In any case, I suddenly became very worried about how this would affect our marriage, and by consequence, our daughter. There were so many medical reasons for us to not continue the pregnancy. There were so many issues of affliction—ours, our daughter's, and our baby's—to consider. But the effect that it was likely to have on our marriage (and ultimately, our children) had not really sunk in, until then.

So I went home and talked to John. And sometime that afternoon he had also reversed back to his original decision to end the pregnancy. I was really frank with him about what I was thinking while I was walking the dog. He agreed, and we both ended up back where we had started. Back to what we thought at the beginning of that day was our final decision.

When I called to make the appointment I was told I could not get in for another week. Having to wait another week, knowing that the life I could feel moving inside of me—the baby that we conceived purposely and in love—was not going to be there much longer was agonizing to a degree I cannot describe. I prayed every night to God to please take my baby boy peacefully, please don't make us go through this, and please don't let it be us ending his life. When he wouldn't move for a few hours I hoped God had answered my prayers. That is an awful kind of hope to have. Then he'd kick me again and my heart would sink back into the abyss. I didn't want to go through with it, even though we felt we had to and that it was the best choice for our entire family, including our unborn son.

I went in for the laminaria insertion—a procedure which begins cervical dilation—on a Monday. My husband and I just froze when we had to sign our son's death certificate while he was still kicking inside of me. After all the paperwork was done the doctor left the room for a little bit to let me undress and to give us a few minutes alone. We both just stared at each other and hugged, and I cried. When I had to lie on the table and put my feet up in the stirrups the tears were just running down my face. John was sitting next to me, holding my hand, looking into my eyes. I have only seen my husband cry a handful of times, so when I saw the tears streaming down his face as well my heart broke twice over.

The laminaria insertion was a lot more painful than I expected, both physically and emotionally. I had only mild cramping after the laminaria insertion, but nothing ibuprofen couldn't handle. But physical pain was really not my concern at that point. The day of waiting in between the laminaria insertion and the termination was hell. I could still feel my baby moving. I kept praying. "God, please take my boy. Let him be with you. Please give him peace." How awful that felt. There is very little I remember about the rest of Monday, or Tuesday for that matter.

On Wednesday I took the pills I had been prescribed to take that morning. By the time we got to the hospital the pain was almost as bad as labor. I was in agony. I could barely walk.

We finally got taken back to the outpatient area behind the waiting room. So many people were there for all kinds of things. I wanted to be alone, but all that separated us from the other patients and their chit-chat was a curtain. The nurse gave me some morphine for the pain. I have to think that my little boy just went to sleep then. By that point I was just trying to block out of my mind what we were about to do. I almost succeeded, at least for a few minutes.

After what seemed an endless wait they finally came to get me, and I had to walk to the operating room by myself, without my husband. To me it just seemed cruel to have to walk alone, without him. When they opened the door and I saw the table and the stirrups I started to shake. And bawl. I knew I couldn't turn back, but the finality of it was hitting me like a load of concrete. It's one thing to decide to end a pregnancy; it's another thing entirely to do it. The doctor held my hand as I went under anesthesia.

After the procedure I was taken to a post-op room. I was alone. I woke up crying. All that came out of my mouth was "I just wanted a baby!" crying and sobbing. I felt so out of control. There were two nurses, and one of them came up to me and told me that she had ended a pregnancy due to severe birth defects. I was still really out of it from the anesthesia. I wish now that I could have talked to her then. She was so sweet and I needed to hear that more than I needed to hear anything at that point. I needed to know I was not the only one. I needed to know there was a life afterwards—that somehow she had picked up the pieces and carried on.

I was in recovery for five or six hours. I had asked the doctor for a private room on Monday; she was able to give me that. Thank God. After my time in recovery I went home and slept. I felt okay the rest of that day, but the next day I was very sore in every muscle in my body. Again, I don't remember what Alice was doing, or what I did. Nothing. It's blank.

I went through two weeks of feeling numb—I couldn't feel anything—nothing at all. But I had a hard time looking at my husband, or even my own reflection in the mirror. Honestly, my daughter was my lifeline. Because of her I got up in the morning. Because of her I was forced to get on with life. While I do not believe in not confronting problems, to have to put on a mask for her sake every day probably saved me. Otherwise I'm not sure I would ever have made it out of bed.

The memories of that day are fuzzy now, but they were very vivid to me for several weeks immediately afterward. For awhile it was really hard to shake the memories, especially of the first sight of the operating room. That haunted me. I know the doctor does these procedures on a Monday/Wednesday schedule. I don't think about it every week any more, but some Mondays and Wednesdays I wonder what poor soul is suffering through this now. My heart goes out to them.

Danny has made it plain as day to me that he is okay, that he loves his mommy and daddy, and that he understands why we made the decision we did. I have found my faith again. And while some people would not agree with me, I know that God understands, too.

After a time I felt like my our needed to be remembered and honored in some way. I felt that to not do anything was to not acknowledge what had happened, that he existed, and that, in albeit an unconventional way, he was loved. It had been eating at me, so I finally got up the courage and talked to my husband about it. John did not like to talk about what we had been through; it was too painful for him. I hated to bring it up but it was so very important to me. I told him I wanted to plant a tree to remember our boy, and to give some life back to the world as well. John agreed. I told him I wanted to say a prayer for him when we planted the tree. John agreed. I told him I wanted our boy to have a name. John freaked out. "Absolutely not," he said. So I told him our baby had a name in my mind, but I didn't have to share it with him. While he never said as much, I can only imagine that naming the baby whose life we ended made it too real for John. I can understand that, so I did not push the issue.

We decided to plant a redbud tree around the time he would have been born. I love its little reddish-purple flowers and heart-shaped leaves. We would have to move a Rose of Sharon bush to put it where we wanted, but it would be worth it. Two days before what would have been his due date, I went to the nursery with Alice to pick out a redbud tree.

I picked out the tree, and drove to the pickup area to have it loaded into our van. The nursery worker loaded it into our van, and I shut the doors. I turned the key in the ignition. The instrumental opening to the song "Daniel" was just starting on the radio. I could not believe that it was a coincidence. I cried the whole way home. I was so sad to not be bringing my baby home, but this tree instead. But again, I just knew Danny understood, and he knew what we were doing for him with the tree we were planting—it was so clear to me.

When I dug the hole to plant the tree, I found a blue cat's eye marble. It was as if Danny had left it there for us—the perfect memento of the little boy we loved and let go.

As time progressed that spring, the Rose of Sharon's leaves opened up. The redbud's leaves opened up. Not a single branch on either showed signs of dying. The rest of that spring, every time I went to check on Danny's tree, I could feel him in my heart. It is not a feeling I can easily describe other than just feeling full to the brim with love, happiness, and sadness all at the same time.

I still feel like our little boy is back there playing around that redbud tree, and he is at peace. And finally, so am I.

The road to recovery has been long and hard. I honestly can't remember much of my journey back from that dark place—I guess self-preservation has blocked a lot of it out. I remember details, but emotions are hard to pin down. And what I do remember I cannot find words for. But what I do know and what I do remember is that at some point I was able to look in the mirror again. At some point I realized that I was not selfish—we took the pain so that Danny would be free. Along the way I have met some wonderful women who have had made the same difficult choice as me and my husband. I have rediscovered my faith in God. I know people can be horribly judgmental and have a hard time seeing the world in shades of gray—more personally than

I ever thought possible. I have learned to be less judgmental myself. I know which friends I can count on and which I cannot. I have more patience to handle the little irritations in life that get to a lot of people—I know how little they matter. I know all too well how important it is to protect reproductive rights. I know I can depend on my husband for anything. I know what true love is.

10

Christie's Story "Even the Darkest Cloud Has a Silver Lining"

It was October of 2002; I was 31 years old and was married with a 20-month-old daughter named Miranda. My husband and I had decided it was time to give Miranda a baby brother or sister. I didn't want the age gap between Miranda and her future sibling to be any more than two or three years. I wanted her to grow up as close to her siblings as I had been with my sisters. I finished up my pack of birth control pills early that month and was planning to chart my cycles (using basal body temperature and cervical mucus as my guide) for a couple of months before actively trying to conceive in January. I had it all figured out—or so I thought.

By mid-November I had completed one normal cycle and had begun charting my second and final cycle before gearing up to begin actively trying to conceive in January. During the latter part of that second cycle I felt a strange tightening feeling in my stomach one day while exercising. Since I had been charting my cycle, I knew that if I took a home pregnancy test I would know with some certainty whether I was pregnant or not. I took the test. It was positive! I was so shocked since we weren't even *actively* trying to get pregnant yet. I was also surprised that it had happened so soon since it had taken five months to get pregnant with Miranda, but I was so happy to have avoided the months and months of trying to conceive. Our second baby was coming!

The happiness didn't last very long. I started spotting brownish blood about a week later at just five weeks gestation. I had never spotted during my pregnancy with Miranda so the spotting scared me terribly. I was almost certain that I was miscarrying. I had never had a miscarriage before and often wondered what it felt like to lose a pregnancy. I felt such sympathy for other people who miscarried—how terrible, I thought.

I went to see my OB/GYN two days after the spotting began and she performed an ultrasound. At only five and a half weeks along, not much could be seen. My OB/GYN warned me that I had a 50 percent chance of miscarrying the pregnancy. There was nothing that could be done—we would have to wait and see. The spotting continued for two and a half more weeks. Each day I would wake up and wonder, "Is my dear little bean okay, or will the spotting turn from brown to red and I will miscarry?" Our bean was so dearly wanted. I was scared to death.

I was scheduled for another ultrasound at seven and a half weeks because the spotting hadn't ceased. The morning of my appointment there was a small snowstorm. Although most of the local schools and businesses were closed, I was determined to make it to my ultrasound appointment. I just HAD to know if the baby was okay or not. Much to my delight a fetal heartbeat was seen flickering away on the ultrasound screen. The spotting finally stopped a couple of days later.

As I had the viability ultrasound at seven weeks, my OB/GYN decided that I didn't need another ultrasound until the routine mid-pregnancy ultrasound at 20 weeks. I was sad that I would have to wait so long for another peek at my baby, but I trusted my OB/GYN's judgment that everything would be fine. The alpha-fetoprotein (AFP) test at 16 weeks came back normal. I started feeling the baby kick at 18 weeks. What a wonderful feeling. Knowing that the baby was alive and moving around kept my mind at ease. Right around the time I started to feel the baby kick, my husband and I had signed the paperwork to start building our first home. We were so *thrilled* about our future. A new home, a new baby—what could be more perfect, right?

The morning of my 20-week ultrasound was filled with excitement and anticipation. My husband had taken the day off from work so he could come with me to see if we were going to be giving Miranda a baby brother or a baby sister. Like most parents-to-be, we believed the whole purpose of the mid-pregnancy ultrasound was to determine the gender. As he and I sat in the waiting room, he teased me about the fact that females tended to run in my family (I had two sisters, two step-sisters, three nieces, two step-nieces, and one daughter). He was so convinced that this baby would be another girl, so we started tossing around possible names for a baby girl. We had decided then and there on the name "Madison" if it was a girl.

We were called back to the ultrasound room where, for the most part, everything seemed to be fine. The ultrasound technician asked us if we wanted to know the gender of the baby, and we enthusiastically said "yes." It was another GIRL! We were so excited to be giving Miranda a baby sister.

I was very close to my sisters growing up, and I was over the moon with joy that Miranda would have a sister as well.

I assumed that the technician was wrapping things up and taking some final pictures when she asked us to remain in the room for a minute, and then walked out. Five minutes later she returned with one of the other OB/GYNs from the practice who explained to us that the technician couldn't get a clear enough picture of the baby's heart. They would need to try to get a picture showing the four separate chambers before they would let us go home. The OB/GYN tried for about 10 minutes but still wasn't happy with the images she captured of the heart. She explained to us that we would need to go to a maternal-fetal medicine specialist (perinatologist) the following day for a level II ultrasound to look at the baby's heart and also to look at the baby's spine which appeared a bit abnormal. We were shocked and bewildered that anything was potentially wrong with our baby. We left with a script in hand for an appointment the next day to "Evaluate fetal heart and spine."

I called my mom (who lived in a different state) as soon as we got home from the ultrasound appointment. I mustered all of the enthusiasm I could to tell her that the all-female streak in our family was being continued, but then I broke down and sobbed that something might be wrong with the baby's heart.

The following day was Good Friday. Our appointment with the perinatologist was at 11:00 AM. My husband and I dropped Miranda off at a babysitter and proceeded to the perinatologist's office. As we sat in the waiting room, I was still naively unaware of the significance of Madison's health problems. I knew that something might be wrong with her heart, and possibly her spine, but assumed they could be fixed.

As the technician performed the level II ultrasound, the room was tense, dark, and eerily quiet. She took numerous pictures of Madison from the top of her head to the tips of her toes. At one point during the ultrasound the technician typed onto the screen "diaphrag hernia." I had no idea what that meant, but assumed that if the baby had a hernia it could also be fixed easily. After about 45 minutes of taking pictures of our baby, the technician very quietly left the room. As I remained lying on the exam table, my husband tried his best to ease some of the tension in the room. My mind was telling me to remain upbeat and positive, but my heart knew that something wasn't right. The perinatologist came in about 10 minutes later. He introduced himself, shook our hands, and then immediately said, "Your baby is very sick." Those five words would change everything.

He proceeded to tell us that Madison had what is called a left-sided congenital diaphragmatic hernia (CDH). For some unknown reason, her diaphragm never closed properly at around eight weeks gestation, and as a result her stomach and intestines had migrated up into her chest cavity. The extra organs in her chest had prevented her lungs from growing. Her trachea and esophagus were pushed out of their normal position and her heart was pushed over into her right armpit. I was already showing signs of polyhydramnios (excess amniotic fluid), which is common in situations where the baby can't swallow. Her heart seemed to be okay for the most part, though it was in the wrong place in her chest, was twisted around almost backward, and I would later read in a formal report that her heart did have possible outflow abnormalities. But her heart wasn't the primary area of concern. It was the lack of lungs that was the critical factor. As long as Madison was inside of me and her blood was getting oxygenated from the placenta she would be okay. However, once she was born and the umbilical cord was cut, she wouldn't be able to breathe on her own. Even a ventilator couldn't help her if there wasn't enough lung tissue to inflate.

We were devastated by all of the things the perinatologist was telling us. I'm sure that some things he said to us that day went right over my head. I was in a total fog once he told us how sick Madison was. I couldn't believe that this was happening to me. To me! I took excellent care of myself while pregnant—didn't smoke, didn't consume alcohol, exercised regularly, even ate vegetables (which I don't normally eat), and I had no family history of birth defects of any kind. It all seemed like a bad, bad dream, and I wanted desperately to wake up.

As I lay there on the exam table, something in my gut was telling me that this little baby just wasn't meant to live with us. I can only assume that it was my mother's intuition telling me that Madison would never come home with us, she would never sleep in the bedroom of the new house we had picked out to be hers, she would never play in our new back yard, she would never eat popsicles on our new front porch in the summertime, and she would never wear the mountains of hand-me-down clothes I had left over from her big sister.

The perinatologist asked me to get dressed and to come into his office so that we could talk some more. Once my husband and I were in his office he told us that Madison's hernia was one of the worst he had ever seen. He showed us a medical reference book that included a diagram of a diaphragmatic hernia. He then mentioned the option of termination to us (I believe he called it "interruption"), but I was not fully convinced yet that our situation would warrant that. I still had an iota of faith that Madison's problems could somehow be fixed. It was a combination of denial and naivety. I asked him if most parents with a CDH diagnosis terminate the pregnancy, and he said that many of them do. At that point we were 20 weeks and five days along. Given the laws in our state, we would have three weeks and one day to decide whether we wanted to interrupt the pregnancy or not. The perinatologist told us that if we wanted a surgical termination (a dilation and extraction, or D&E), he could refer us to someone, and if I wanted an induced labor termination, my own OB could perform it. It was a Friday afternoon, so the perinatologist told us to think about everything over the weekend and to call him back on Monday.

We left the perinatologist's office that day unsure of what would happen next. It was Easter weekend, and I tried my best to remain cheerful and upbeat for Miranda. But inside I was dying. My baby was sick, and it seemed that nothing I could do would make her better. I spent endless hours on our home computer researching CDH, researching lung development, and researching experimental procedures of in utero repairs. I started posting on an Internet message board for families of children with CDH. I talked online to many moms of kids with CDH. Some of them had children who survived; some of them had children who didn't survive. Over that weekend I would wake up several times in the middle of the night to get back on the computer to do more researching. I was looking for anything to give me hope that my Madison might be okay. I was clinging to the overall 50 percent survival rate for CDH and hoping that my Madison would be one of the survivors.

My husband and I had talked to several family members over the phone that weekend (they all lived out of state). We also talked to my husband's uncle who worked as an OB/GYN. We asked him for not only his medical opinion but for his personal opinion on our situation. His opinion would be very influential in our decision making process. Everyone in our families was supportive and tried their best to be there for us to bounce ideas off of, to cry to, and to just listen as we tried to make sense of it all. No one could tell us what they would presume to do if they were in our situation. It would be squarely up to us.

Over that weekend, my husband and I repeatedly discussed the options of termination versus carrying to term. We literally went back and forth about 20 times as to whether we would continue the pregnancy or not. We finally decided that we needed more information in order to feel comfortable making a decision either way.

Monday morning came and my husband and I called the perinatologist we had met with on Friday and asked him to set up a second opinion level II ultrasound for us. We were scheduled for one the next day. We went to the scan and found this perinatologist to be very kind and accommodating toward us. He was very helpful and very considerate, taking his time with the scan and making sure that we understood everything that he was explaining. Unfortunately, his medical opinion concurred with the opinion of the first perinatologist, that our Madison had a very bad case of CDH. He explained to us that, although the overall survival rate for CDH was 50 percent, the survival rate drops significantly if the CDH is found before 24 weeks (which ours was). He told us that Madison's chances of making it to term were 10–25 percent. He told us that if she lived through childbirth she would need to immediately be put on an extracorporeal membrane oxygenation (ECMO) heart and a lung bypass machine, and that she would need to be on it for quite some time. I had learned about ECMO from my Internet research and knew that extended use of it could lead to blindness, hearing loss, and potential brain damage from brain bleeds.

We walked out of the second opinion ultrasound knowing what we had to do. We didn't want Madison to suffer for even one second. And we didn't want Miranda to see her baby sister suffer in a body that was too sick to perform the most basic bodily function—breathing. We didn't have any family in the area to help out if we had chosen to continue the pregnancy, and I was certain that all of the technology in the world couldn't help my Madison anyway. Lung transplants are not done with newborns. I also felt there was a reason that we found out about her CDH so early instead of at birth, when many parents do. I knew that I needed to trust my instincts and follow my heart. As much as I didn't want to say goodbye to my baby, I knew that I had to. For the previous five months every piece of food that I ate, every bit of exercise that I trudged through, and every wink of sleep that I got were to nurture her to grow and develop. I had bonded with this little baby and had so many hopes and dreams for her. She was to complete our family. Now I would have to let her go.

We called my OB when we got home that day and asked her to schedule us for a labor and delivery (L&D) termination. I chose L&D because I desperately needed to see my baby girl. I needed to kiss her sweet face and hold her tiny hands in mine. I had to see her just one time.

My induction was scheduled to begin two days later, on Thursday evening. I was to deliver Madison in the exact same hospital where two years earlier I had delivered my daughter Miranda. Thursday afternoon I had to leave Miranda in the care of a neighbor so that my husband could come with me to the hospital to get checked in. My mom and sister were set to fly into town later that evening to help us with Miranda and to provide us with much needed emotional support. Once I got to the hospital, I was walked to a labor and delivery room at the very end of the hallway. I'm assuming that was for *my* benefit so that I wouldn't have to hear all of the other laboring moms-to-be and their newborns. I was immediately hooked up to an IV drip of Pitocin. My OB came and inserted eight or so laminaria sticks into my cervix to begin the dilation process. I didn't find the insertion of the laminaria to be especially painful, just uncomfortable. I had asked my OB and the nurse if it would be possible to check for Madison's heartbeat periodically with a Doppler so that I would have some idea of when she passed, and they agreed.

My mom arrived at the hospital about 8:00 PM, just in time to say hello and to hear her newest granddaughter's heartbeat for the first and last time. Visiting hours were ending so I sent my mom and my husband home to help my sister, who was looking after Miranda. I didn't think that anything was going to happen with my labor during the nighttime anyway, so I figured that they might as well go home and get some rest. I sat in my hospital room alone and watched television until about 10:00 PM, then I tried to get some sleep.

The laminaria didn't do much to dilate my cervix. Thankfully, I didn't have much cramping either. When my OB returned at midnight she removed the laminaria and placed a prostaglandin suppository in my cervix. At that point she said that I was about one to two centimeters dilated. She had warned me before I entered the hospital that the labor could take anywhere from 12–36 hours. After inserting the prostaglandin she told me that it would need to be replaced every four to six hours, or as needed, until I dilated adequately. For a tiny baby like mine that would mean to only six centimeters or so. The prostaglandin made me pretty ill. I had persistent vomiting and diarrhea for the next four to five hours. I thank God for the wonderful night-shift nurse who took care of me because I know that I was no fun to care for during those hours. It was not a pleasant night, and I got very little, if any, sleep.

My OB returned at about 8:00AM and inserted another prostaglandin suppository, along with an order for anti-nausea and anti-diarrhea medicine to be put into my IV. At that point I was still only about two centimeters dilated. I had the nurse check again for Madison's heartbeat, and it was still there, as strong as ever. The second suppository that my OB inserted seemed to do the trick. I started getting very painful and very strong contractions about 20 minutes after the insertion. I asked the nurse for an epidural at that time (about 8:20 AM), but unfortunately the anesthesiologist was tied up in a c-section delivery and couldn't break away to help me. When my mom and husband arrived at the hospital about 8:40 AM, I was in agonizing pain. The nurse tried to alleviate it with some morphine shots into my hips but it didn't help. The only relief I felt was after my water broke about 8:45 AM.

The nurse checked me and said that I was about seven centimeters dilated and that Madison's head was crowning. My OB was immediately paged, quickly arrived to my room, and after two short pushes my Madison was born, at 9:04 AM on April 25, 2003. My second daughter Madison was born exactly two years, two months, two weeks, and two days after my first daughter Miranda.

My OB checked for a heartbeat on Madison but couldn't find one. She then placed Madison on my chest and cut the umbilical cord. I could feel my sweet baby's skin against my own; she was so warm and moist. Just the way a new baby should feel. The nurse wiped her off a bit, wrapped her in a receiving blanket and gave her back to me. Here was my sweet baby girl! Holding her in my arms was a bit surreal. She was so very tiny, but seemingly perfect. She looked like a peacefully sleeping angel, with her hands crossed over her chest. I examined every inch of her little body, from the top of her head to her tippy toes. She was absolutely beautiful. She had whispery soft blonde eyelashes and eyebrows. My mother and husband also took turns holding Madison. We took some photos of Madison by herself, of me holding her, and of my husband holding her. About 30 minutes after her birth the hospital chaplain came to my room and said a prayer over Madison. He offered comforting words to us to ensure that we knew our sweet angel was in Heaven with Jesus. We had the nurse make two sets of Madison's hand and footprints.

We kept Madison with us for a little over two hours. In that time I experienced a strange sense of calm. I didn't even cry very much while she was with me. I was so focused on her and cherishing the limited time that I had with her that I didn't want it clouded with tears and sorrow. At the same time, I was so exhausted from my horrible evening before her birth that I was afraid I might doze off while holding her and accidentally drop her. So after some time, I let the nurse take her away from me. The nurse informed me that I could have Madison brought to me again if I wanted, but I never did. After two hours had passed I had noticed the change in the color of Madison's skin from pinkish to purplish to bluish. I didn't want to remember her that way. I wanted to remember her as she looked when she was first born—pink and warm and beautiful.

The nurse gave us a list of funeral homes and crematoriums in the area that we could contact if we wanted a private burial or cremation. Since my husband and I had no family in the area and since we weren't sure if we would remain living there forever, we decided against a funeral or burial. We decided on a cremation. My husband called the crematorium and arranged everything with them over the phone from my hospital room.

After Madison was taken away I was transferred to a room on the gynecological floor to recover, away from the other new moms. Physically I felt okay within hours of delivering. Emotionally I felt lost and alone. It was in my recovery room that I finally allowed myself to start grieving. The tears started and they didn't stop. There was a bereavement nurse who came into my recovery room and tried to "assess" my needs, but I just wasn't in the mood for talking. My husband brought Miranda in to visit me later that day. It was so hard to look into her eyes. Here was a two-year-old, so full of life and happy to see her mommy. Not a care in the world. But what she didn't know was that she had just lost her baby sister. I spent Friday night in the hospital and was released Saturday morning.

My milk came in about a day or two later. It felt like another cruel joke of nature to provide me with an abundance of milk, yet no baby to drink it. For several weeks after Madison's birth my stomach still felt distended and firm. I avoided going out in public for fear that someone would ask me if I was pregnant. For two weeks I remained indoors and only ventured out for short trips as necessary. The crematorium called us a week after her birth to tell us that Madison's ashes were ready. I drove with my husband to pick them up. It was very difficult walking in the door to the crematorium, knowing that wasn't the way we were SUPPOSED to be bringing our baby girl home. It wasn't fair. But once I had her urn in my arms, it felt good to be able to have her with me again, so physically close to my heart. I clung to her urn the entire car ride home. And it felt good. We were finally taking our baby girl home to be with us forever.

My post-partum check up with my OB was scheduled for two weeks after the delivery. Most vaginal delivery post-partum check-ups are done at four weeks post delivery. But since I wanted to try to conceive again as soon as possible, my OB told me to come in at two weeks post delivery. The appointment was grueling for me emotionally. Not only did I have to confront being in that office again, knowing that the last time I was there I was still pregnant, but I had to sit in a waiting room full of blissfully happy pregnant women. Then I had to explain my situation, with my voice uncontrollably quivering, to the receptionist who was understandably confused as to why I was there and wanting to try to conceive again only two weeks after delivery. My OB was able to tell me that my physical recovery looked great and that I could try to get pregnant again after my first menstrual cycle.

I never felt the need for any kind of individual counseling or medication to help me through my emotional recovery. I did attend a few local M.I.S.S. (Mothers in Sympathy and Support) group meetings, but I found most of my solace and support from online support boards where I was able to connect with other women who had terminated pregnancies for medical reasons. By talking to others who truly understood what I was feeling, I was able to move forward in my healing and not get stuck on the unfairness of it all. On *BabyCenter* and *A Heartbreaking Choice* I was able to read stories of women who had terminated before me, and how they had put their lives back together and even went on to have perfectly healthy babies after suffering such a loss. They provided me with the inspiration and the empowerment to try again to give Miranda a sibling.

Spiritually, my beliefs didn't change much after my termination. I have always believed in God and Jesus, and I know that they helped carry me through my grief. Fairly early on, I realized and accepted that what happened to my Madison wasn't some sort of test or punishment by God or an attempt to draw me closer to him. The God that I have faith in would never be so cruel or sadistic. Unfortunately, nature isn't perfect, and sometimes living beings don't form properly. I have accepted that Madison's condition was a mere fluke of nature. There was nothing that I could have done or not done to prevent it. My job was to figure out how to grow as a person because of it and to find the silver lining in the dark clouds.

It has been five years since we said goodbye to Madison. I still think of her daily and cherish the short time we had together. The emotional healing was difficult at times, with setbacks often coming when I least expected them. But I can say with confidence that I have peace in my heart that I chose what was best for *my family*. I know that if I were to be put in the exact same situation today, I wouldn't choose any differently. When given the choice between having a guaranteed clear conscience or being able to prevent my child from suffering—I chose to prevent my child from suffering. The only regrets I have are that I didn't spend more time holding Madison after she was born, that I didn't take more photos of Madison, and that I didn't bring home the blanket from the hospital that she was wrapped in.

I have not tried to hide Madison's existence from anyone close to me (family or friends). I have never felt the need to be less than completely honest about my decision to end my pregnancy, and I have been blessed to be surrounded by supportive and understanding people. Even those people who haven't agreed with my decision still have offered their love and kindness to me.

Madison is, and forever will be, a member of my immediate family. I have on display in my home a large pencil portrait drawn from a photo of her, as well as copies of her hand and footprints. I carry a guardian angel pin in my purse to remind me of her. I have built a special memorial flower garden in my backyard for Madison. Each spring I fill the garden with different varieties of pink and white flowers, angel statues, and a memorial stepping stone engraved with her name, given to me by some online friends. The garden sits just under the window of the bedroom which was to be hers.

I have spoken to Miranda many times over the years about her baby sister Madison. I have tried to explain to her in terms she can understand that her baby sister was simply too sick to live with us. She seems to understand, and every so often she will talk about Madison. Each year on Madison's Angel Day (the day she was born an angel), we release helium-filled balloons and snack on cupcakes. It's our own special way to celebrate Madison as a member of our family.

Over the years since losing Madison I have been searching for the silver lining in the dark clouds that hovered over me. I have been finding ways to turn my loss into something positive to honor Madison's memory. I participate in the March of Dimes *March for Babies* every year to help raise funds and awareness for birth defects. I started my own chapter of a volunteer group which knits or crochets baby blankets to donate to bereaved moms in hospitals and clinics. I am a volunteer host of an Internet message board for women who have terminated a pregnancy for medical reasons. I try my best to make sure that those who choose to terminate for medical reasons never feel alone or unsupported.

I have since gone on to have another healthy baby (yes, a girl). She is my "rainbow baby." Through the clouds and the rain she came and brought light and color back into my life. At a time in my life when I was terrified of being in that vulnerable state of pregnancy again, she came along and helped me to see how truly blessed my life was. I simply adore her and treasure her spunky personality. Watching her play in the backyard with Miranda, eat popsicles on our front porch in the summertime, and sleep in the room that was to be Madison's is bittersweet at times. It is a simple truth that she wouldn't be here if it wasn't for the decision my husband and I made to let her big sister Madison go. I know that Madison watches over her sisters, her dad, and me from above. And I know in my heart that I will be reunited with my middle daughter someday.

11

Christina's Story "My Forgotten Son"

On December 26, 2006, we found out we were pregnant. I stood there and stared at the test as if I could make one of the lines disappear. I was not sure how this could happen, as I had to take fertility medications to conceive my living son. The doctors did not think I could get pregnant on my own, so I thought one month of missed birth control pills was no big deal. This had to be the worst time in our life for a pregnancy. I was on Christmas break from my senior year in college. When I returned for my final semester, I would be completing my internship to receive my teaching degree. Earning this degree over the past four years had been the hardest time of my life. First, I was a wife and mother. Second, I was a student. I did all of this while maintaining a 4.0 GPA.

Aside from the timing, I had not been taking care of myself. Due to my hectic lifestyle, I barely ate and never took a vitamin, much less took folic acid. I also had an old friend who had come to visit for the holidays, and we had a girl's weekend at the Biltmore Estate in Asheville, NC. While there, we toured the winery and sat in the hot tubs of the hotel—all of which you are not supposed to do during pregnancy. My Christmas Eve festivities included two bottles of wine because I still had no idea I was pregnant.

My menses was due to arrive on Christmas day but never came. The day after Christmas, it was still a no show, so I thought I would take a pregnancy test just for kicks. The second line appeared as soon as the test strip became wet. I was in shock. Considering all of my shortcomings in taking care of myself, I felt this pregnancy was doomed from the beginning. As the numbness wore off, I finally managed to call my doctor for a confirmation appointment. At six weeks the pregnancy was confirmed. At eight weeks I had a vitality ultrasound that showed everything was developing normally. The baby was measuring perfectly, there was a heartbeat, and my uterus was great, so we were sent home to come back at 12 weeks. At a routine appointment, we listened to the baby's heart and had a blood test for cystic fibrosis. Because that test came back clear, we were feeling comfortable with things.

At each appointment I would tell my doctor something was not right. I would ask if I drank too much or if not taking the folic acid was vital. My doctor knew my school situation and that this pregnancy was unplanned, but he assured me that everything was fine. He told me that as long as everything I did was before five weeks of pregnancy, things would work out. He said the body would have naturally aborted the pregnancy had I harmed the fetus prior to five weeks. Therefore, with my OB's blessing and making it out of the first trimester, I settled into being pregnant. I began to love my baby and think about how my life would change sooner than I had planned. The baby would have been due at the beginning of the school year, so getting a job would have been tricky. My husband and I developed a plan for me to substitute for a year and go back full time the following year. I pulled out my maternity clothes and enjoyed the good feelings that came with the second trimester. At that time we chose to tell our son, who was four at the time, he was going to be a big brother. He was so excited because he had been asking for a sibling for a while.

When my internship started in January, I was placed in a fourth grade class. Since you cannot hide much from pre-adolescents for long, at 14 weeks I ended up telling them, too. The students were so sweet and understanding. Many of them brought gifts for the baby and asked how I was every day. With the exception of the weight gain and doctors appointments, my life continued as normal. I began eating right, taking vitamins, and not drinking wine.

At 16 weeks, I went for a routine appointment and had my blood drawn for the AFP test. I know many people do not believe in this test because of the high number of false positives, but my doctor really recommended it. If it was a screen positive we would go for a level II ultrasound and move forward from there. If the results were normal, my doctor would see me at 20 weeks for the routine mid-pregnancy ultrasound. He assured me that if it was a screen positive, he would call me with the results.

My nightmare began on March 26, 2007 when my doctor called. I had left school to grab some library books while the students were in a special area. I knew as soon as the telephone number appeared on my phone that it was him. He was calling to tell me that my AFP blood work came back with elevated rates for spinal bifida—one in 126 to be exact. Even though my risk at this time was less than one percent, I knew I was the one. Ironically, I was teaching probability to the students and tried to tell myself that if I had 125 red chips in a bag and one blue one, the chances of pulling a red chip were much greater. I knew in my heart this was the reason I had questioned the pregnancy from the beginning. I was destined to be the 1:10,000. I got back to school before the students returned to class, so I sat in the bathroom and cried until they returned. I then pulled myself together long enough to finish out the day.

My doctor's office set me up with the high risk doctor for a level II ultrasound on Thursday, March 29, 2007. That morning, my husband and I met my mother-in-law to keep our son while we had the ultrasound. I did not want my son present if we received bad news. To start our appointment, we met with a genetic counselor, and she tried to reassure us that these things happen and there may not even be anything to worry about as she took our family history. We were then taken to the ultrasound room where my life would be forever changed. The ultrasound technician had not had the monitor on for 30 seconds when she turned it off, looked at us and said, "I want you to know before I go on I have some concerns." Then she handed me a box of tissue.

She scanned, measured and studied for what seemed like forever. She barely spoke to us, so I knew it was really bad. I remember seeing my baby on the screen, legs crossed and fists clenched. There was a clock on the wall, and I just watched it tick. Each second seemed to last a minute. After she was through with the scan, the doctor came in and went over all of the results with us. They thought our angel had trisomy 18 due to all of the soft markers. The scan showed myelomeningocele spinal bifida, a large omphalocele, hypoplastic heart syndrome, hydrops on the brain…the list went on. I will never forget the words the doctor used, "I am sorry, but your baby is incompatible with life outside the womb." Nothing appeared to be healthy with our baby. We were given three choices: (1) continue with the pregnancy and see what happens, (2) do an amniocentesis to test for a genetic disorder, or (3) interrupt the pregnancy. He went on to explain that if I continued with the pregnancy, the baby would most likely not make it to term. Once the baby was delivered and the umbilical cord was cut, he would only live for a few moments. My husband and I had discussed this prior to the appointment 'just in case', so we knew the answer was to interrupt the pregnancy. This was not a choice we wanted to make, but rather a choice we had to make. It was a choice out of love for our unborn child. We knew we could not bring a baby into this world to suffer. We also had our living child to consider. He would never understand that although Mommy's tummy would continue to grow, he would never have a sibling.

From the maternal specialist I was sent back to my OB/GYN. On the way I called my mother and mother-in-law to tell them the sad news. They were going to be grandparents to an angel instead of a living child. At my doctor's office there were a lot of tears and hugs. Though he agreed with and supported my decision, my regular doctor was Catholic and did not perform interruptions at any stage. Instead he turned me over to the head doctor in the practice whom we met with and he went over what to expect in detail. He did not perform dilation and evacuation (D&E) terminations; he preferred to interrupt by labor and delivery (L&D). He explained the procedure of L&D with us, and set up the appointment for induction. I was to have the laminaria inserted on Monday, April 2, and the induction would be Tuesday, April 3, 2007. I left in shock with a prescription for sedatives to calm my nerves. On the way home we stopped by to pick up our son and had to pretend nothing was wrong.

That night, my mother drove from two hours away to pick up our son. I was hardly functioning enough to take care of myself, much less my child. I walked around in zombie fashion, just existing. He did not need to see his mommy that upset. We did not want him to associate bad things happening with being away, so we decided to give him the news before he left. We explained to him that putting babies together is like a puzzle. If all of the pieces do not go together just right, the baby cannot live. We told him our baby was put together all wrong, and things got really messed up. His stomach was on the outside and his heart was on the wrong side. We told him the doctors had to take the baby out so he could go live in Heaven. For a four-year-old, he seemed to get it. My aunts and uncle also drove in from an hour and a half away to bring dinner and just be with me. My aunt had lost a living child and was the closest person I had who understood my grief.

After everyone was gone, I took a sedative and a sleeping pill and tried to rest. As I was dragging myself out of bed the next morning, we got a call that my brother-in-law's wife had just delivered their healthy twins. This sent me right back to bed with a sedative in hand. I could not figure out why anyone thought I needed to know that piece of information the day after I found out my baby would die. I slept most of the day, only waking long enough to take another sedative. The following day I had to get it together enough to go on a job interview. Since I was no longer going to be pregnant at the beginning of the school year, I felt I had a shot at getting this position. However, I no longer wanted people to think I was pregnant. I did not want to talk about it. I searched my closet for some non-maternity clothes that would fit. I wrapped my belly with an ACE bandage to hold it all in and give the appearance of a flat stomach. I pulled support hose on over that and was able to fit in my clothes. I went to the interview, smiled and pretended everything was fine. After all, teaching is performing. I left the job interview and felt pretty good about my chances. At 12:30 that afternoon, the principal of the school offered me my first teaching position. It was a light in my darkness.

The rest of the weekend was a blur. I spent time on the phone answering hospital questions to get pre-admitted. I could hardly talk through the tears. Many people called to give their condolences, but I had no desire to talk. My husband took the calls and said I was not up for talking. Four days after finding out our baby would not live; I went to the doctor to have the laminaria insertion. My husband held my hand through the tears, although I knew he was about to break down himself. We knew this was the beginning of our baby's end. This would start the softening of my cervix. That night it was impossible to sleep, even with the sleeping pill. All night I apologized to my baby, and told him how much I loved him. I laid awake thinking about what my baby was feeling and what was going to happen in the morning.

The next day we arrived at the hospital by 6:30 AM, and they began all of my preparations. I could not speak without crying. By 7:30 AM, I was having the shot to stop my baby's heart. They did not allow my husband to be with me for this, so I was all alone. I was lucky to have a wonderful nurse who was so compassionate. As I was lying on the hospital bed crying, she touched my hand and said to me, "You are a good mom. Only a good mom would let her baby go and never suffer." I needed to hear those words at that moment and I will never forget those words. Once everything was complete, they started the Pitocin and moved me to the women's floor for delivery.

Labor began about six hours after the induction was started. The pain was fairly intense, so they hooked up a morphine pump. This did not touch the pain of labor, so I was given a shot of Demerol. This lasted a couple of hours but wore off quickly. The hospital I was at did not offer an epidural until 20 weeks gestation, so I labored mostly drug free. After I was so far along, I was no longer allowed to get up to use the restroom and had to use a bedpan. As belittling as it was, my husband volunteered to do help me with this so the nurse would not have to come every time. Just when I thought the pain would be the end of me, our angel was peacefully born at 8:05 PM. Prior to delivery we told the nurses we wanted to hold the baby and have some time alone with our angel. When he was born, they took him out, cleaned him up and wrapped him so we did not have to see all of his defects. Due to all of the birth defects, they could not tell us his gender at that time. We had to wait on the pathology report to find out we had a son. We held him and told him how much we loved him. I took some pictures of him and had the hospital chaplain bless his body. His face was so perfect. It was so hard to believe his body was so malformed. Once he started to get cold, his skin began to peel. At that point I could not handle the pain and sent him to the nurses. I allowed the hospital to dispose of his body, but I wish I would have had him cremated. At the time I could not make anymore decisions, so I did all I could do.

The nurse continued to check on me throughout the night because my afterbirth would not deliver. She checked me every two hours and gave me several shots to help my uterus contract. At 6:00 the next morning, the doctor had to manually remove it. That was the most physical pain I had ever been through in my life. I left the hospital Wednesday, April 4, 2007 with an empty womb, a broken heart, and a memory box of shattered dreams.

Slowly, I reentered my life. My termination fell in line with the school's spring break. I took the week off to recover and rest. My mother still had my son, so I did not do much but lay on the sofa and sulk. The question of '*why me*' never seemed to end. Why me and not someone who did not want their baby anyway? Why me? I have been married for almost 10 years. I have a good job. I am a good mom. Why me? It was the question that ruled my life. At the end of the week, I called my mother and arranged for her to bring my living son home. It was at this time that we realized he did not understand what happened. He thought the doctors were going to fix the baby and put it back to grow. He did not understand we were permanently saying goodbye. My mother had to pull over the car to settle him down and re-explain what had happened. Still today, he talks about his brother who is in Heaven and how he is put back together now.

Physically my body healed, but emotionally I struggled. I did manage, however, to graduate and receive my teaching degree. There were many days in which I could not get off the couch. Sometimes I wonder why I am still alive. I would wash sedatives and sleeping pills down with wine; this went on for weeks. A month after the termination, we took a family vacation to Disney World. The trip had been planned as one last trip as a family of three. Now, it was just a reminder of what would not be. Much to my surprise, I had a great time, but it was coming home that was hard. For me the vacation was a time to forget my problems and pretend nothing was wrong. Once we returned home, all of the pain still existed. I continued my pattern of self-medicating for several more weeks. Finally, in July, I made the decision that I had to live for the son I had, not die with the one I lost.

Even a little over a year later, I still feel incomplete. I know this was the right choice for my family, but I just wish it would have never happened.

This is something I do not wish for anyone to ever experience. I found an online support group that was my saving grace. Everyone in real life wanted to compare my pain to a miscarriage at eight or 10 weeks. No one could understand why I was so upset and why I could not move on. To everyone else, my baby was never real. To me he was, and always will be, my second son. My second son whom no one ever talks about. No one calls on his expected delivery date, or on his angel day. He is my son everyone else has forgotten, but the son I will always remember.

12

Claire's Story "The Three-Year Mark"

My life was going great. I had three wonderful sons and decided to try one more time for a daughter. I stared at the positive pregnancy test and I began to shake. I thought to myself, "Could it be my daughter?" A strange feeling came over me, like something was terribly wrong, but at the time I just brushed the feeling off.

Where I lived, no one was allowed to find out via ultrasound the gender of the baby they were carrying. Since I was desperate to know if I was carrying the daughter I had longed for, I decided to have an amniocentesis done. I was at a routine doctor's appointment after the amniocentesis when the doctor mentioned that he had just gotten my results. "I have some good news and bad news. Which would you like first?" the doctor said. Puzzled, I replied that I would like the good news first. "You're having a girl, but she has a chromosome problem." I was in shock. I had gone to the appointment all alone, not expecting to be given such devastating news. Somehow I managed to walk back to my car where I climbed into the backseat and started to cry.

The genetic counselor from the Medical Genetics department told my husband and me that our baby, who we would name Katie, had a mosaic ring supernumerary marker chromosome (SMC). SMCs are extra genetic materials made up of parts of one or more chromosomes. It is very difficult to determine prenatally from which particular chromosome(s) the extra genetic material comes from. SMCs are different from trisomies in that a trisomy is three full copies of one chromosome. What makes a prenatal determination of an SMC so problematic is that while there is a risk of severe problems for the baby, there is also a chance that the baby could have a normal phenotype (outward appearance and development).

My baby's SMC was a ring, which meant that the ends of the chromosome affected were fused together in the shape of a ring. Mosaic ring SMCs are very rare, and most abnormalities with SMCs happen to those with rings. I was told that my baby had a 67 percent chance of some abnormalities, but we would know more if we could find out which specific chromosome the extra material was from. I struggled with how I could make a decision regarding the future of the pregnancy knowing that she could either be severally affected, not affected, or somewhere in between. We felt that we had to discover which chromosome the SMC was from in order to make the best decision possible for our daughter.

During the pregnancy I had a series of ultrasounds, during which Katie never seemed to move her legs. Her wrists were curled inwards. The doctor told me that those conditions might or might not be anything to worry about.

The genetic counselor had suggested to my husband and I that we should, in order to help make our decision, pick an outcome and for that day pretend that we were living that outcome. One day we pretended that we continued our pregnancy with our daughter and that she had mild to no problems phenotypically. Another day we pretended that we continued the pregnancy and that she had a severe phenotype, but we still managed to care for her in our home. Another day we pretended that she had a severe phenotype but that we institutionalized her. Another day we pretended we carried her to term and gave her up for adoption. Another day we pretended that we had terminated the pregnancy.

We explored our feelings throughout those days and it helped each of us to be able to make a decision. My husband had decided that we should terminate the pregnancy and I had decided that we should continue it.

As if things weren't already stressful enough, they would get a lot worse. We had friends and family who meant well, but made their feelings about what they thought we should do very clear. They were focused on us keeping the baby. What they failed to do was take a step back and realize that our problems were much deeper than just the pregnancy. My husband and I were on the brink of divorce. Instead of supporting us, they thoughtlessly helped drive our marriage apart out of their own needs. Because of them I learned that sometimes in life you need to stand by your loved ones even if you don't agree with what they are doing, because you would want that person to do the same for you.

My husband and I decided to take the middle ground and deferred making a final decision either way. We went for a cordocentesis, a procedure where the perinatologist sticks a needle into the baby's umbilical cord to try to extract blood. The blood retrieved would help us determine which chromosome number, as well as which parts of that chromosome, were affected.

As I lay there on the table waiting for the procedure to begin, I prayed that it would be successful. I had thought that, at most, the perinatologist would try for 20 minutes to get the sample. I had learned that after 20 minutes there was an increased risk of infection, of the uterus becoming too irritated, and of contractions starting which could lead to a miscarriage.

I lay there as still as possible as they inserted the needle through my belly, guided by ultrasound, and tried to get the baby's blood. I lay there still, screaming inside with pain, as needle after needle for almost an hour and a half entered my uterus. The perinatologist desperately tried to latch onto the small umbilical cord. I am forever grateful that the perinatologist tried so hard to get a sample, though his efforts were in vain. Everyone in the room commented on how I was as tough as a soldier throughout the procedure. My uterus then started contracting regularly, the perinatologist was exhausted, and I was sent home expecting to miscarry.

I went home relieved that I was going to miscarry and that we wouldn't have to make a decision either way. But I never did miscarry. My uterus settled down and the pregnancy continued. The perinatologist talked to us again and told us about a very risky type of cordocentesis, where the sample is drawn either directly from the baby's tummy where the umbilical cord attaches to the baby or directly from the baby's heart. This method was only done a handful of times each year where I live and there was no data on the immediate risks of the procedure to the baby, on lifelong complications to the baby, or on the miscarriage rate. I was still in so much pain from the first cordocentesis attempt. Even many days later each place a needle had entered my belly was still stinging with pain. I felt like a failure, but I didn't feel justified in subjecting either my baby or myself to a second cordocentesis procedure.

I contemplated running away at that point. My husband and I were barely talking to each other and we felt sure that we were going our separate ways. I wondered if such a separation was really feasible. I could have moved away with my three boys, but with a possible special needs child, I wasn't sure I would be able to support all four children once the baby arrived. I wondered if I would be able to work or if I would need to be on welfare. I certainly knew that I wouldn't be able to afford to live in the city near the hospital and the other medical services that Katie might have needed. I also knew that my husband would never let me take our three boys. We would have been embattled in a bitter custody dispute. So, in essence, if I kept my daughter, I would be giving up my three sons. I struggled with the question of whether her life was more important than their lives. Unfortunately, keeping my daughter and maintaining my family was not one of the options available to me.

Reluctantly, I agreed to the termination. I take full responsibility for my decision as I think it was the best decision for everyone involved. Although it might not have been the best decision for Katie, it was the best decision for my family.

I went to the hospital and had to be admitted into the maternity ward. There was a very pregnant lady in front of me, laughing and joking away with the admitting nurse. I just stood there waiting for my turn, with each laugh just killing me inside. I finally lost it and ran into the other room and started bawling my eyes out. Another nurse realized what I was there for and came to admit me.

Once I was in the maternity ward I could hear other people laughing and brand new babies crying. I had decided on a labor and delivery termination instead of surgery as it was my lifetime wish to give birth to my daughter and hold her. I thought it would be my only chance. Pills were inserted into my cervix every four hours until labor started. At one point I felt her moving, and wondered if that would be the last time I would feel her inside of me. Ironically it was.

I fell asleep while I was waiting for her to be born and had a dream that my grandfather, who loved children and had passed away years before, had come and scooped her up. She was born after 15 hours of labor. I labored the longest with Katie than any of my other children.

I held her and I cried. My precious little girl. I decided that I did not want a full autopsy done but requested that a chromosome test be done so that I would know what extra chromosome she had. Now that she was born, they would have access to her blood to do the test.

The hardest thing I had ever done in my life was leave the hospital that day without her. I felt so empty when I got home and had to tell my boys that Katie had died.

As I tried to pick up the pieces of my life I kept thinking about how things would get better and how, three years from then, I would hopefully be in a much better place emotionally. I don't know why I focused on three years as the amount of time it would take me to heal, but I did.

In the days following Katie's birth I saw several sets of twin girls. The girls seemed to stare at me, which made me long for my Katie even more. I wondered if they could see my pain and my longing for my own little girl.

I had a very difficult time in the days, weeks, and months that followed. I kept going back down the same path, wondering what I could have done differently. It was awhile before I realized that I was, in essence, digging my own grave. I wondered if things would ever get better.

A few months had passed when I received a call from the hospital that the chromosome report was ready. I needed the closure of finding out which extra chromosome Katie had. I froze when I heard the results. There was a miscommunication that the hospital blamed on me. They never used Katie's blood for the test that would have given us a definitive answer. Instead they used a tissue culture from her which failed to grow in the lab. I felt my world fall apart all over again. I angrily wondered how such an error could have happened. I didn't think I could ever accept the fact that I would never know what chromosome was affected. I fell into a deep, dark pit once again.

I went through so many emotions over time, but I kept focusing on that three-year mark. Other people thought that I should have moved on well before that amount of time, but as a mother you never truly move on from losing a child, ever. The years passed and on each of Katie's birthdays her brothers released balloons in the sky for her to catch. Except on her third birthday, the birthday that I hoped I would be in a much better place emotionally, we couldn't do it.

We couldn't release balloons that day because I was rushed to the hospital. I couldn't help but wonder "Was this how Katie would have wanted this day to be?" It was supposed to be Katie's special day. In the hospital, I screamed like I had never screamed before. I released all of my frustration and pain, and then it happened—Katie was a big sister. As fate would have it, I gave birth to twin girls on Katie's third birthday.

One month later, I laughed for the first time since losing Katie. I *finally* laughed like I meant it. I laughed like I didn't have a care in the world and it felt good, as I was finally truly at peace.

I learned that sometimes in life, things happen that we would never wish upon anyone. We each have a life's plan, and no one on this Earth is privy to that plan regardless of their position on certain social issues. We each follow our own path in life and sometimes we come to a point where we reach a crossroad. Each path leading away from the crossroad has its own trials and neither is right or wrong, but is a journey unto itself. What may be your greatest pain one moment in time may actually set the stage for one of your most special moments in the future.

13

Colette's Story "My Chance at Motherhood"

Infertility—what a dirty word. To me, it meant my existence had no purpose.

My quest for a child began when I was 28 years old and after my first year of marriage. At that point I had heard that we should "get pregnant before you're 30 because your chances reduce dramatically after 30 years old." And so it began. My husband Roger and I tried on our own for about six months, taking my temperature every morning to increase our chances of catching the egg. At first "practicing" was fun, but after a while it became a challenge to keep both of us interested. After six months on our own, my OB suggested we try a common fertility medication called Clomid, which is used to help induce ovulation. We attempted to get pregnant aided by the Clomid, with no success. After a year without conceiving we were finally sent to a fertility specialist. Waiting a whole year would be mistake number one on my journey.

For the next *seven* years I worked together with my doctors, trouble-shooting why I wasn't becoming pregnant. There was no clear reason why I wasn't becoming pregnant. I ovulated properly every month, my fallopian tubes were not blocked, and my hormone levels were fine. My husband's sperm was tested and, while not the greatest in terms of number and motility, we were told it was adequate enough to achieve a pregnancy.

So we decided to try daily injections of hormones, together with ultrasounds to monitor the size of my egg follicles. If my body responded well to the injectable medications I would be inseminated with my husband's sperm. We tried that for several months with no success. I was feeling very discouraged and just needed a break. I waited five months, until the following fall, and then decided to try again. No success. My doctor, still unsure about the quality of my husband's sperm, suggested that we try using donor sperm to help increase our chances of getting pregnant. They would mix the donor's sperm with my husband's sperm and see what happened. I was willing to try anything by that point.

At the beginning of 2004 I *finally* became pregnant. It was unbridled excitement for me to see the beating little heart at my first ultrasound appointment. The nurse, who knew how much I had gone through to get to that point, hugged me on my way out. I was so ecstatically happy, but I did not feel comfortable telling anyone just yet.

At 16 weeks we went in for another ultrasound and were told there was no longer a heartbeat. It was Mother's Day weekend. I spent the next four days in bed. I did not want to talk to anyone. I was utterly devastated. I could not understand why that had happened to me. I felt like the only person left among my circle of friends who had no children, and that my life had no purpose.

After the grief loosened its grip on me, I called my doctor. I was not willing to accept a loss as my final outcome. I wanted children and was going to do whatever I needed to do to become a mommy. Looking back now, that might not have been the best approach. Neglecting my husband and focusing solely on getting pregnant was not the best thing for our relationship. That would turn out to be mistake number two on my journey.

We did another cycle using intrauterine insemination, and again I became pregnant. But that pregnancy was not meant to be either as I miscarried at six weeks. I was starting to think that I might never be a mom. I couldn't stand to listen to other women complain about their pregnancies. I hated them for being moms and I cringed every time another friend had a baby. I was not happy for them, because everyone else had what I wanted—a family.

It took me six months to overcome my grief and to work up the courage to call my doctor again. I was 37 years old and I felt like we were running out of time. My doctor agreed to try one more time, but also suggested that we look into adoption. I had long before decided against adoption. I wanted to carry my own baby.

So we set out to try one more time using the injectable fertility medications and intrauterine insemination. Much to my surprise, everything that cycle worked perfectly. My ovaries produced multiple follicles and my husband's sperm count was so good that I could have opted not to use the donor sperm. But we had already paid for it and figured that if it might help, why not use it.

I got pregnant all right. But this pregnancy was not like the other two pregnancies I had lost to miscarriage. With this pregnancy I felt like I had to eat constantly. I was also very sick from the start. At six weeks I went in for my first ultrasound. I held my breath as I hoped to see my baby's heart beating on the monitor. I noticed my doctor sigh as he showed me a swooshing heartbeat, and then another, and then he moved the probe to the other side of my abdomen where there was another heartbeat, and yet another! He marked them A, B, C, and D. I was both shocked and thrilled. We were victorious, we had finally done it! I could not help but smile as I held my stomach. Wow—quadruplets!

The blissful feeling lasted about 30 seconds, when the cold, harsh reality was thrust in front of me. My doctor did not hesitate to give me his medical opinion. He did not feel it was wise for me to carry quadruplets. He told me that a multiple pregnancy carries with it the risk of miscarriage, birth defects, premature birth for the babies, and the risk of toxemia, diabetes and hemorrhaging for the mother. Then he mentioned something called selective reduction. Selective reduction (or multifetal pregnancy reduction) is the process whereby a multiple pregnancy is reduced in order to increase the chances of survival for the remaining fetuses of the same pregnancy. He told me that if I wanted to pursue that option (assuming that I carried them to all to 12 weeks) I would need to see a specialist. There were only two specialists in the country he would recommend and only one was on the east coast, in Philadelphia, 400 miles away.

I went home and told my husband Roger. I was excited to tell him that we were pregnant—and with four babies. He was not as excited.

For the next couple weeks I contemplated four cribs, four car seats, four highchairs, etc. I was still in la-la land. I thought about names, and whether there were boys *and* girls growing inside of me.

My husband popped my bubble of joy when he said "You know we can't have four babies, right?" He didn't think we could handle four babies, financially or otherwise. But I had tried for so long and had miscarried twice in my journey to become a mom. I wanted these babies! My sister and I would refer to them as the "four little peas."

As we approached 12 weeks and all four peas were doing well, I was sent to another specialist who dealt with multiples. She explained my risks to me. She was short and to the point. She told me that for every fetus you carry, you risk developmental disorders because you shorten the time they can grow in the womb. With quadruplets, the estimated delivery time is usually 30 weeks gestation. And most mothers who carry quadruplets are on complete bed rest by 21 weeks. She explained to me that for quads, the odds of two or more of them having moderate to severe disabilities was very high. With quadruplets my chances of losing the entire pregnancy was 25 percent. If I were to reduce to twins that rate would plummet to just seven percent.

I knew that I had some control over my destiny. I had a choice. If I did the selective reduction I could almost guarantee that I would have two healthy babies. Or I could do nothing, which would put all of them and me at risk for permanent damage.

That was my first decision as a mother. I decided that I would do the reduction from quadruplets to twins, to ensure their health and my health.

Once Roger and I arrived in Philadelphia for the first of two appointments, the reality of the situation became overwhelming. I was scared to be there, but even more scared to *not* be there. They did chorionic villus testing on the two fetuses that were in an optimal position for testing. We would have to wait seven days to find out the results.

After seven days had gone by, I took a deep breath and telephoned the doctor's office. I was told that the two babies tested were perfect. No chromosomal abnormalities, no Down syndrome. That was a huge relief. We would have to return to Philadelphia in seven days to have the actual selective reduction performed.

That day came quickly. The nurse did an ultrasound first to check all four and to measure exactly where each of them was in my uterus. Then the doctor came in, confirmed the positioning, and talked about what he would need to do. He looked just like to the crazy doctor from the movie *Back to the Future,* but he was a very kind and compassionate man. When he injected the long needle into my belly for the first time, I wanted to jump off the table. I actually envisioned myself doing it. Not because of the physical pain, but because I knew he was injecting the needle in to the fetus' heart to stop it from beating. And when he finished with the first, he made another injection into the second. After waiting 15 minutes, they did an ultrasound to check for heartbeats. And they both were still. No longer did their little hearts beat.

My twins that remained were strong. The pregnancy progressed smoothly until 35 weeks. At that point I suddenly developed severe preeclampsia. My blood pressure was very high and I had extensive swelling. It was time for my babies to come out.

My twins, Adam and Abby, were born at 35 weeks and two days. They were perfect. No N.I.C.U., no special lights, no tubes or wires. There they were, finally, my two little angels I had dreamed of for so very long.

I will always think of Adam and Abby as my lucky charms. I believe it was pure luck that positioned them where they were to be selected for testing. I feel that by making the difficult decision I did in letting the other two babies go, I gave my twins a fighting chance.

Though my marriage did not sustain the stress, I have no regrets about making the decisions I made. My children, whom I fought so long and so hard for, are my future. A future that I once thought had no purpose. Now I know exactly what my purpose in life is—it is to raise those two little people, who melt my heart each and every day, to be fighters and to never give up.

14

Corinne's Story "My Journey of Loss and Endurance"

I am the face of abortion—not a role I would have chosen, but a role I have grown to accept. I am currently a stay-at-home mom, however I worked as a medical professional at a well-respected health institution for the first 10 years of my professional life. I hold a Bachelor of Science degree and a Master of Science degree from a prestigious university. I am a home-room mother. I have high moral standards and values, and am an active member of my church. I am hardly what members of the far right must picture when they think of the word abortion…yet I am the face of abortion—the face most political activists do not even consider when taking their stance.

We have two healthy, beautiful sons who are the light of our lives. In December 2005, we were elated to find out that we were expecting another child—it took us almost a year to conceive and we were over the moon. We had so many dreams and hopes for that baby…the child that would complete our family and make us a family of five. Imagine our excitement when we found out we were having a daughter. I spent hours daydreaming of pastels, hair ribbons, dolls, and teaching my daughter everything she would need to know to be a responsible young woman. And then our dreams were shattered in an instant—and our lives changed forever. Yes, I am the face of abortion.

Our daughter was prenatally diagnosed with trisomy 21, Down syndrome. She was suffering from intrauterine growth restriction—she was over 60 percent behind in growth for her gestational age. We sought the assistance of specialists at a prominent children's hospital in the Midwest—a facility known world-wide for its excellent medical care in pediatrics. They were unable to give us definitive answers, as our baby was too small to see accurately on the ultrasound. They would say that she "most likely had a cardiac defect which would require surgery" and that there "appeared to be problems with her bowel." And there was no doubt that due to her diagnosis, our daughter would be mentally retarded.

The pain and anguish we felt went to the depths of our souls. We cried, we screamed, we researched and cried some more. What should we do? How can we help our daughter in this hopeless situation? Would she be in physical pain? Would she suffer? We considered the best possible outcome—perhaps our daughter would only be mildly mentally retarded. Would she suffer at the hands of her peers, ostracized and hurt because she was different? As her friends turned into young women, and our daughter remained forever stuck in her childhood, would she have any peers at all? Unfortunately, modern medicine does have its limitations. There was absolutely no way to know what our daughter's cognitive functioning would be. And in our case, due to her small size, there was no way to determine her physical impairments before time ran out and we would no longer have a choice, before we would be able to choose what was best for our daughter.

In early April 2006, at 20 weeks gestation, after careful deliberation and much soul-searching, we decided to give our beautiful daughter back to God. We took her off "life support" so that she could be whole and happy in Heaven—something she would never experience on this Earth. We knew that while we loved her with all our hearts, our love alone could not protect her from inevitable pain, whether it was physical or emotional. We chose to suffer so she wouldn't have to. Letting go of our precious daughter was the hardest decision we had ever made.

Labor and delivery was not an option due to my having previous c-sections, so we chose to terminate by dilation and evacuation (D&E). The termination was not without complications, due to a number of factors. My uterus was perforated and repaired and I was hospitalized for several days. Physical recovery was a long road; emotional recovery even longer. I lost track of time that spring and summer, as I spent many days sobbing for my baby girl and all we had lost. My heart literally hurt, broken from the intense grief I was experiencing. I spent many sleepless nights with my mind wandering, pondering the many what-ifs. I spent countless hours on the Internet reaching out for support, as support in real life was fleeting. Due to the area of the country in which we live, we did not feel like we could be completely honest about the circumstances surrounding our loss…people can be very judgmental and unforgiving. The close friends we did confide in tried their best to be helpful, but had difficulty comprehending the magnitude of our loss. My parents supported our decision completely, yet were unable to provide the compassion and understanding that I so desperately needed. I don't think our baby girl ever seemed real to them.

Not a day goes by that I don't think of baby Maddie and wish that she had been healthy…wish that we'd never been faced with a poor prenatal diagnosis, wish that our souls had not been shattered to the core by this experience. Our arms are empty and our hearts are heavy, but we know we made the right choice for our daughter.

After further uterine surgery, a failed attempt at in vitro fertilization, two failed adoptions, and two years on a roller coaster of shattered dreams, I am miraculously expecting a healthy baby boy. I have once again experienced the elation of another pregnancy, the terror that we might receive another poor prenatal diagnosis, and the relief that everything is indeed going to be alright this time. And while my heart is healing with the promise of a new life, I know I will never forget my precious baby girl and the many lessons she has taught me on this journey. I am forever changed by the brief time I shared with her and I know her spirit lives on in my heart.

*In loving memory of Madeline Elizabeth

"Long after a blossom fades, its memory remains forever"

15

Dana's Story **"Wanted"**

*I am not a doctor. I am not a scientist. I am not a therapist.
I am not an expert by any stretch of the imagination. I am a
wife, a mother, a woman. A woman who was faced with an
unimaginable choice. And, I am not alone. There are thousands
of women who have been faced with the exact same choice. As
science advances, more and more women will find themselves
where I did - where we did. Out of love and compassion and
kindness and despair we made a choice. This is my story... This
is all of our stories.*

Pregnancy was the easy part, or so I thought. At the age of thirty-two I had
my first child. After trying to conceive for just over a year, my husband and I
were blessed with a textbook pregnancy that ended in the arrival of a strong
and robust little boy. He was everything. Seventeen months later we sought
to bring another child into our family and marveled that it took only one try.
We did not know then that this tiny baby who took shape so immediately
would leave before we ever had a chance to hold it. We did not know that we
would be the ones to end our child's life, prematurely.

I was just nine weeks pregnant and panicked. The slightest amount of
blood glared back from my underwear. I called my doctor and followed
her instructions: *no heavy lifting, no sex, take it easy.* My husband was home
within minutes. My emotions took over as I imagined our baby's life to be in
danger. I hadn't bled during my first pregnancy and knew it could not be a
good sign. That night I feared our baby had died. I called my doctor the next
morning and she told me to come in.

With much trepidation I entered the exam room. And, to my surprise,
I saw my baby's beating heart up on the screen and burst into tears. I was so

relieved and comforted by the steady heartbeat—simply overjoyed. At that moment I believed the baby was thriving. I thought the problem was me; my body. There was a blood clot behind my placenta and the doctor said she'd monitor me. *Everything would be fine*, she said, if I continued to *take it easy* over the next couple of weeks.

With the arrival of my second trimester, we believed everything would be okay—that we were out of the woods. The blood clot had long since disappeared and I was feeling better, stronger. Checking in weekly with my doctors I had watched the baby grow from no more than a tiny blinking bean into a flailing baby with arms and legs. The baby was active with a strong heartbeat—growing each day nestled safely within me.

When I was thirteen weeks pregnant, I returned to the same hospital where I delivered my son just a year and a half earlier. I was alone. As I walked through the lobby and rode to the fifth floor I found myself wishing I could go back to the day my son was born. I smiled at the thought of delivering our next baby in such a warm and comfortable place. I was feeling thankful for all that I had and would have, as I made my way to the perinatology department. I was there for a routine nuchal translucency screening—a test that measures fluid accumulation behind a baby's neck between the ninth and thirteenth weeks of pregnancy. NT scans, as they are commonly referred to, indicate possible chromosomal abnormalities. I had never heard of this test before my second pregnancy, as it was not offered to me during my first. My doctor explained that it was just like an ultrasound and suggested I make an appointment. They were becoming *more and more common* she said.

When I arrived at the perinatology department the receptionist informed me I had made a mistake. The number written on the referral was that of the radiology department, not perinatology. When I called to schedule the appointment I had inadvertently scheduled a routine ultrasound with radiology. I asked if she could fit me in? I spoke of childcare arrangements and the hour-long drive from the city. After a few phone calls and a little persistence, she was able to squeeze me in—just barely.

Trisomy 18. Trisomy 13. Down syndrome. A pamphlet the receptionist handed to me listed these conditions—glancing at it, I didn't give them much thought. I knew that women over thirty-five ran a greater risk of having a child with Down syndrome, but we had conceived this baby when I was thirty-three. We had no history of birth defects in our families. I had *no reason to worry*. The only thing I felt before the screening was excitement for yet another opportunity to view the baby.

I entered the exam room and prepared myself. As the sonographer guided her wand across my abdomen I fell further in love with the baby up on the screen. It was sucking its thumb and kicking. I commented how strange it was to see the baby moving and not be able to feel it. I remembered that same surprising feeling with my first pregnancy during early ultrasounds. And the baby's heart…watching it, I became lost in its rhythm. Every beat seemed to say… *I am here. I am here. I am really here.* How wonderful it was to see the life inside me.

The sonographer left to get the doctor while I stared at my baby's frozen profile. It was settled, I was in love. There was no longer a question as to whether or not I would love this baby as much as my first—a question that had surfaced since first learning we were pregnant. Having been reassured by every mother I'd consulted on the matter, I now knew they were right. There was plenty of room for this tiny little being in my life. Just as my belly was expanding to accommodate this child, so was my heart.

As I waited in the chilly exam room, the doctor came in and introduced himself. He shook my hand and cautiously stated there were some *concerns* with the baby…

A thick nuchal fold.

Abnormalities with the feet and one of the hands.

I heard the words but I didn't understand them. How could a doctor I had never met before tell me the baby I had just spent the last thirty minutes admiring and falling in love with was NOT okay?

I sat there in a fog as the doctor went on about a test, a test they could do the very next day called CVS. There was a 1/200 chance of miscarriage—I knew I couldn't make that kind of decision without talking to my husband first. How could I risk *our* baby's life?! I told the doctor I was going to my obstetrician's office. He told me he'd call her with his findings before I got there. I was not connecting the dots.

As I left the exam room and made my way down the hall I took out my phone to call my husband. I had trouble dialing, then trouble connecting. When I heard his voice I tried to tell him what the doctor had said—I started to understand what was going on. It was in that hallway when everything came crashing down around me. I crouched in a doorway and attempted to tell my husband something was wrong with our baby. I couldn't get it all out. The pieces just didn't fit. My husband was calm. I was slowly working up to hysteria. He asked questions about what the doctor had told me. I tried to catch my breath and left him hanging on the line. Everything was all jumbled up inside of me.

 The next thing I remember is looking up at a kind face—a stranger was standing in front of me. She took my arm and asked where I had come from. She led me back to the perinatology office where the composed *Me* had left just minutes earlier. The sonographer, the same woman who had performed my screening, brought me back to the exam room—my baby's profile still on the screen. I couldn't look. She said she would call the genetic counselor and ask if she could meet with me. After my unsolicited and tearful apology she kindly acknowledged, *it's a lot right now.* The counselor agreed to meet me in ten minutes. I numbly thanked the sonographer and redialed my husband. This time he talked of trains and schedules. He'd be on the next one. I was an hour away from his office and told him not to come. I would meet with the genetic counselor and then go to my doctor. That was all I could manage to give him as I made my way back to the waiting room—the same room where I sat reading a pamphlet just a half an hour before.

I waited for what felt like forever, trying to make sense of what was happening. As the genetic counselor led me into her office, I was strangely calm. She talked about chromosomes. *Twenty-three and twenty-three make forty-six. When there is only one "X" chromosome and no "Y" chromosome you have something called Turner syndrome. When there is an extra chromosome it is called a trisomy.* I recognized that word from the pamphlet. I tried to take in everything she said; a crash course in genetics. Our baby had a thick nuchal fold. This was not normal. The doctor believed he saw bilateral clubfeet and a problem with the left hand. She then told me about chorionic villus sampling. A needle is inserted through the abdomen to draw cells from the placenta. The chance of miscarriage was 1/100, but really 1/200 she said. They could get me in the next morning, a Wednesday. The test would confirm if there were chromosomal abnormalities. Turner syndrome or a trisomy could be determined as early as Monday. She strongly encouraged me to make the appointment, so I did.

I called my husband as I walked across the street to my obstetrician's office. After telling him what the counselor had said, I asked if he could drive me to the hospital the next morning. He offered to call my mother and ask her to stay for a few days to help out with our son. I held onto my belly, just thirteen weeks pregnant and beginning to show. Heading toward what felt like a safe haven, I held on for dear life.

When my doctor of eight years walked in a hugged me, I knew things were bad. She immediately began talking about her sister-in-law who carried a baby with a cystic hygroma. She was a devout Catholic, as was my doctor, who was counseled by her priest to terminate the pregnancy and refused. The cyst grew bigger and the baby was eventually born still. After almost nine months of carrying her child, of wishing and hoping for a miracle—it died. I couldn't figure out why my doctor was telling me this story? She wrote down the name of the condition—cystic hygroma. I looked at her, my face registering confusion. *This is what the doctor saw on your baby. Oh,* was my only response. She continued to write and handed the note to me. It was the name and number of a doctor who did abortions…*In her office, so you won't have to go to the hospital. Oh*, was all I could mutter and left.

It began to rain as I made my way back to the parking garage. I moved quickly, having trouble catching my breath. Within the safety of the car I let it out. My whole body shook as I screamed. And, I still had to drive home. The parking attendant asked if I needed to pull over and sit for a while. Sobbing, I told him I was okay. I needed to get home to my husband and son.

There was a vacant parking space in front of our building. In New York City that is no small feat especially in the rain. My husband and son came down to meet me. I melted in their presence. Home.

Later that night, I searched for information about the conditions the doctors had mentioned. I read about cystic hygromas, clubfeet, Turner syndrome, and trisomies—learning about fetal hydrops, a fatal indicator in utero. Trisomy 13 and trisomy 18 were incompatible with life, while trisomy 21 (Down syndrome) and Turner syndrome held out hope. Turner syndrome only occurs in girls. I read about a program in New Zealand to raise awareness of Turner syndrome and the kinds of lives these women could and did lead. They were of average intelligence but short of stature and infertile. I read about a movement in America, started by individuals with Down syndrome, to educate people on how productive the lives many of them led were. I read and I read and I read. I doubt I slept for even a second that night.

We showed up at the hospital the next morning and met with the genetic counselor. I wanted my husband to hear about the baby from someone other than myself. I was not a doctor or trained in genetics or indicators or outcomes. He needed to hear what I heard, not just what I was able to relate in my unsteady state. I also wanted to ask the counselor if there were signs of fetal hydrops. She said there were not. My hope was renewed and I started to feel like maybe, just maybe, the baby would be okay.

I walked into the exam room armed with my husband. I whimpered the entire time and couldn't look at the baby up on the screen. All I could do was hold my breath and pray the doctor had a steady hand and careful eye. When the doctor asked if I was *okay*, I told him I was sad. He acknowledged…*I know it's a lot right now*. The procedure was over quickly and I held my expanding belly once more as we left the hospital—again, holding on for dear life.

The two days following the CVS were spent resting and researching. I was convinced our baby had Turner's syndrome and would be okay in the end. My husband and I were preparing ourselves to have a child with challenges. We were ready to change our lives to accommodate our baby. A small baby we loved– who we loved even more as each day passed.

There were no complications from the CVS. It was Friday and we knew we had to get through the weekend before learning the test results. I didn't think

I could be alone when the doctor called, so my husband made arrangements to stay home from work that Monday. It was still Friday afternoon when the phone rang, so I didn't expect my doctor to be on the other end. She told me that our baby had trisomy 21, Down syndrome. I made it through the telephone conversation, and then cried with relief that our baby had a chance at life. But, fear and uncertainty quickly crowded in and it felt like too much. I called my husband and told him the news. It was after that phone call that my research became solely focused. The only thing I could think about was how to get more information about Down syndrome—more information about our baby.

I searched the Internet and read and then searched some more. I walked over to the bookstore in the pouring rain and read all I could find on Down syndrome. I remember reading a book written by the brother of a boy with Down syndrome. It hit me then, what kind of impact would this baby have on my toddler? I saw continuous references to heart defects in the literature; half of all children with Down syndrome have congenital heart defects. Low muscle tone, seizures, compromised immune systems, congenital hypothyroidism, impaired vision, hearing loss, mental impairment, and early onset of Alzheimer's were just some of the medical conditions commonly associated with Down syndrome. The information was too much and too little at the same time. It told me everything about Down syndrome, but virtually nothing about the baby I was carrying.

My husband and I were filled with uncertainty. For the first time we discussed the possibility of ending the pregnancy, an idea that thoroughly depleted us. We didn't want this to be the outcome, we wanted to bring this child into the world and give it the best life we could. But, with only the information we had—a large cystic hygroma, clubfeet, and stunted growth of the left fingers—we needed more.

My husband agreed to call the genetic counselor and ask her new questions we had come up with… *Is there a way to detect the physical or mental severity of Down syndrome in utero? How early can a heart defect be identified? Could she give us a referral for a second opinion? Given the information we already had, what were the chances our baby would make it to term?* And, a question we hadn't really discussed beforehand—*Was our baby a boy or a girl?*

My husband called after speaking with both the genetic counselor and the perinatologist who performed the initial screening and CVS. They referred us to a major teaching hospital for a second opinion. I arranged everything for the next morning…I called the back-up childcare center at my husband's work and begged for a last minute placement. I called my obstetrician and asked her to fax our records to the teaching hospital. I called the woman who coordinated our visit and learned the names of the doctors we would meet with. And, I made one last phone call to an acquaintance of mine—a woman I'd met through my son's swimming class. She worked in a nearby OB/GYN clinic as an anesthesiologist. I knew they performed abortions and I wanted to put things in place, just in case our baby's prognosis was worse than we already understood it to be. I made an appointment for Wednesday morning at her clinic. I had no intention of keeping it.

We were impressed by the warmth and efficiency of the staff at the teaching hospital. Soon, we were in a dark room with a sonographer who was taking pictures and measurements of our son. Yes, son. The son we had hoped for and dreamt of. The son who would inherit our older son's clothing and crib. We both smiled when we learned we were having a boy. An irrational response perhaps, given the circumstances, but a response straight from our hearts. We loved our son. We wanted to find out something (anything!) at this appointment that would help us prepare for his arrival. For his life. My husband watched intently as the baby's image swirled around on the screen. I craned my neck but caught only glimpses. I was excited to see him. For the first time in a week I was hopeful.

After about thirty minutes the doctor entered the room and introduced himself. He had been monitoring the sonogram from another room. As he spoke with the sonographer there was a knock on the door. A resident entered and asked if she could observe the examination. Being a teacher, I have always been an advocate of firsthand learning. Under any other circumstance I would have welcomed this young doctor. But, this was a very private experience. Deep down in my heart I knew it might be the last time we saw our son. I declined.

The doctor and sonographer continued to look at different parts of our baby. I could tell that most of what they saw was good. The kidneys were *normal*, I remembered hearing one of them say. The sonographer thought she saw an abnormality with the left hand. Not surprising, given the findings from the first screening. The feet appeared to be normal, not clubbed. A small token—a little bit of progress.

Soon came the heart and our baby's fate was becoming clearer. I wasn't frightened or tearful or even devastated as I heard the doctor and sonographer discuss our baby's heart. But, I knew things were not normal. Words like artery and ventricle and valve and left chamber were heard as I continued to watch the monitor. I suddenly understood this would be my last viewing. He appeared beautiful on that black and white screen. I can't say for certain what my husband was thinking during those last few minutes, but I can say that it was calm and peaceful in the room. We all felt it. There were no tears.

The exam lasted well over an hour and the doctor met with us in a separate room afterwards. He was kind and competent. The left side of our baby's heart had not formed properly. It was defective. Although it functioned adequately in utero, once our baby was born it could not support him. Our son would need a series of three open-heart surgeries to stay alive—one within days of being born. He had a 50/50 chance of making it to term, the same odds the first doctor had given. The doctor talked about the rest of my pregnancy and what it would look like. He recommended I transfer my care to their department immediately. The small hospital where I had delivered my first son was not equipped to deal with such a birth. The surgeons at the hospital, some of the best in the country, would care for our baby once he was born. I have always considered myself fortunate to live in New York City with access to some of the best medical care in the world. As the doctor spoke, I believed our baby would be in the best hands possible should we decide to continue with the pregnancy. In my heart, I felt we were already in those hands.

My husband and I stepped out of the hospital and into the noonday sun feeling sad but so very thankful. A day earlier we had been told by the genetic counselor that a heart condition could not be diagnosed prior to eighteen weeks. We knew that if we waited an entire month, we would most likely not be able to end the pregnancy. Having carried our first son for a full forty weeks plus, we knew that each day counted. Each day, we believed, our baby became more of a person and the bond would strengthen. Once the baby's movements could be felt in my womb, the decision to end a pregnancy would have been too much to bear. We knew the prognosis of our son's heart defect that day was a gift. A gift from two people, professionals, who took the time to look carefully at our baby. We also knew that babies need affection and warmth and closeness and nourishment during the first year of life. Safety. Our baby would have none of these. He would be taken from our arms, cut open, and sewn back together. His heart would be stopped. His ribs would be broken. His brain would be put on ice. He would most likely sustain brain damage during the surgeries. He would experience all of these things if he were *lucky* enough to be born alive. He would experience them again and again. We were his parents and we could not let this happen to our son. We knew what we had to do, even though it went against every fiber of our being.

That night I called to confirm my appointment at the clinic. I called and arranged for a babysitter the next morning. Then, I tiptoed into my son's room. I listened to him breath—his chest rising and falling. As he slept, my heart swelled. In the comfortable darkness I wept for the little brother he would never meet. I did not make a sound—only tears. The rest of the night I spent in my husband's arms, crying and trying to come to terms with what we were going to do the next morning. I kept thinking…tomorrow at this time my baby would be gone. I did not sleep.

The next morning we took a cab to the clinic. From the moment I entered the building I began to tear and then sob. I could not stop. My husband filled out the paperwork as best he could. With a shaky hand I signed away all of the hopes and dreams we had but a week earlier. I knew there would be an ultrasound to confirm the baby's size and age. As I lay on the table with my eyes closed and my heart throbbing, my husband watched our son moving about on the screen. I so envied his strength. That day was the hardest of my life.

The woman who performed the ultrasound asked for our co-pay after she finished…It cost thirty dollars to end our son's life.

My husband and I clung to each other from that point on. I kept thinking I only had to be strong for a little while longer. When my husband talked of leaving, of letting nature take its course, we both knew that we could not run away. If we did, our son might have to endure more pain in his short life than either of us had in our thirty-four years. We stayed for him.

When the anesthesiologist arrived she reached out and hugged me. I knew of her turbulent history with respect to pregnancy and loss. I knew she understood. She assured me that since I was having general anesthesia the baby would *not feel a thing*. She told me how sorry she was I had to be there. She told me I would have closure soon. She led me to a gurney and stroked my hair as I shook and cried and wailed.

Her face was the last thing I remembered before the blackness.

Waking up facedown I was groggy but quickly aware. A nurse led me to a recliner where I sat for about an hour. My body was numb. My head was strangely quiet. Others joined me, young women who had safely averted unplanned pregnancies, the only kind of abortion I knew—until now. Not only had I terminated a wanted pregnancy, but also I had an abortion. The plain and simple truth—the bitter word so hard to swallow—stuck in my throat as I mourned the loss of my baby.

My husband took me home and I slipped into our bedroom without my son or the sitter seeing me. I crawled under the covers to hide from the world. I kept going over everything again and again in my head. I felt violated and empty and utterly alone. I think I may have slept, fully clothed, for just over an hour. It was the first sleep I remembered having in over a week.

I awoke to my little boy at the side of my bed calling *Mommy*. His father had taken him to lunch and they had brought me back some food. I picked at it as my son cuddled up beside me. I breathed in his warmth and beauty. At that moment he was everything.

Physically I was fine. Empty, but fine. I had little blood loss. No aches. No pains. Emotionally I was a wreck—feeling relieved and sad and guilt-ridden and frightened all at the same time. I missed my baby and wept for my vacant womb. I vacillated between grief and pure exhaustion.

That night my husband called our family and told them what we had done. I asked him not to call my father. He had never known I was pregnant. My father-in-law, who was a Catholic priest for fourteen years before leaving the priesthood to raise a family, offered his love and support unconditionally. The rest of our family did the same. My husband told our parents we were grieving and needed time. We would not be taking phone calls. We would not be reading e-mails.

I did not sleep that night.

The next morning my husband took my son to work with him. I had the whole day to myself. The plan was to catch up on some sleep—to rest. I couldn't. My mind kept going over the previous day's events.... Yesterday at this time my baby was still alive.... Yesterday at this time my baby was being ripped from my womb.... Yesterday at this time my son was gone. I couldn't turn these thoughts off. I ventured into my toddler's bedroom and began to clean. Before long the entire apartment was clean.

When I finally let myself lie back and rest I began bleeding, this time more heavily than the day before. As I climbed into bed that night I was nervous. I eventually fell asleep and awoke to find the bed soaked with blood. I ran to the bathroom. More blood. I was frightened. It was the middle of the night so I called a medical hotline. The woman on the other end asked a number of questions and then advised me to go to the nearest emergency room. I dreaded the thought of leaving my husband and son at 1:30 in the morning to go to the ER, but I was just scared enough to go. I told my husband I'd call him within the hour and left. I caught a cab and was at the hospital within minutes. From that point on I waited. It took time to be admitted and more time to be seen. I was not a priority in the ER that night. I had to relate my story to strangers who made insensitive comments like...I hope you had it done *in a clean place*. I saw the word *ABORTION* scrawled across my chart. The nurse inserted an IV to replenish my fluids and the needle dug into my arm. The doctor inserted a speculum and I throbbed in discomfort. And then I was told everything looked *normal*. A visit to my doctor's office was recommended. I left that cold and sterile ER at 5:30 AM.

The next morning my doctor was at the hospital, so I was to be seen by another doctor I knew from my first pregnancy. The doctor entered the room and performed an ultrasound. My uterus now looked gray and empty—hollow. Just days before it had held my baby. I couldn't cope. I cried. Sobbed. The doctor asked me to meet her in her office as soon as I was dressed.

The doctor was kind. She told me I did the only thing I could have. I shouldn't have any misgivings. She was sympathetic and expressed concern for my wellbeing. She called and spoke with the doctor who performed the abortion to ask if there had been any complications or concerns on his part. He assured her everything went smoothly. I then confided in her that I was not sleeping or eating. She wrote me two prescriptions—one for sleep and one for the bleeding—and then gave me her home phone number. She encouraged me to call if I had any questions. She scheduled a follow-up appointment and I stumbled out of the office to find my husband waiting outside.

The days that followed blended together. I spent them with my son. He kept me busy and gave me reasons to smile each day. When he would go down for a nap or to sleep for the night I would spend time searching for information online. I looked for information about anesthesia and its effect on a fetus, as well as information on fetal pain and development. I couldn't come to terms with how my baby had died and longed for some kind of validation. Some kind of release from the horrible guilt I was experiencing. I began to look for something that would help me get out of the very dark and uncomfortable place I was in.

I called my insurance company for the names of doctors and therapists in my area. Some years ago I was attacked in my home by a stranger—a random act. Beaten. Strangled. Left for dead. I lived. After addressing my physical injuries—surgery for a broken and dislocated jaw, bolsters for pummeled ears, stitches for a cut forehead, and bruises from head to toe—the hospital released me. A colleague reached out and referred me to a trauma therapist, and so began my emotional recovery. Writing, running, and talking about what happened that night helped me to remember, confront, and accept it— a journey that culminated in my running a marathon, and in the prosecution of the man who attacked me a year earlier. Could therapy help me through this trauma? Probably. Ultimately, though, I did not to pursue it. I wasn't prepared to pick a name from a random list of doctors. I also wasn't prepared to call doctors I did know and ask for a referral. The aftermath of losing my baby was terribly isolating. Nobody, it seemed, could understand what I had been through. In addition to feeling misunderstood by people who knew, I also felt judged—as if I had done something wrong. Since I wasn't willing to put myself *out there* any further than I already was, I pushed the idea of therapy out of my mind.

I owe much of my healing to my son—a small, innocent child who knew not what I had done. In the week preceding the termination and those that followed, my son's behavior changed. Physically, he became more intimate. Kisses and hugs were given and received and savored. Each night before bedtime our family would lie down on his bedroom floor, snuggled together.

In my mind I would imagine the four of us there—safe. Our son's routines were interrupted due to last minute appointments and my recovery needs. He took random trips to the back-up childcare center at my husband's work. He missed classes and didn't get as much physical activity as he was used to. I made every effort not to cry in his presence, and did so on only one occasion. Seeking support outside the home would have meant leaving my son with a babysitter. The time I spent with him was my sanest—I didn't want to spare even a second.

I began to search for support groups online. It seemed like a logical place to look. Less than a week after my pregnancy ended I found a web site which published stories of women who had terminated wanted pregnancies. All of a sudden I was not alone.

I read stories written by women who had gone through the same thing I had. Women who had experienced the same love, the same disbelief, the same heartache, and ultimately the same grief. Although the diagnoses differed, each woman acted in what she felt was the best interest of her child and her family. Every baby was loved. Every baby was wanted. And, every baby was eventually let go.

Eight days after making the decision to end our child's life and seven days after ending it—I told my story. At 2:12 PM on a Tuesday afternoon, while my son was sleeping peacefully in the next room, I wrote these words…

My Story

I lost my son last week. We terminated the pregnancy at 14 weeks due to a completely unexpected diagnosis of trisomy 21 and hypoplastic left heart syndrome the week before. The doctors said that if the baby made it to term (50/50 chance) he would require open-heart surgery within days of being born, another one within a year and a transplant by the age of 5. With Down syndrome it was unlikely he would receive a heart. My husband and I faced a decision we never imagined we would…to take our young son's life or watch him die a very slow and painful death—helplessly. I'm still numb from the experience. My 20 month old helps me to smile and even laugh each day, but at night I am very sad, am having violent dreams/flashbacks and have difficulty sleeping. It's almost like I'm straddling two worlds. My husband is back to work fulltime. He's experiencing a very different kind of stress than me. We are supportive of one another though. I really just wanted to get my story out there. I think we made the best decision we could for our family. I'm thankful for wonderful doctors, for second opinions, and options. I do not feel like we were dealt an unfair hand. I do not feel angry, just sad.

I wrote these words for strangers to read—words I could not yet say to my family or friends. I shared my story with these women because they understood. They welcomed me with open arms. No questions. No judgments.

Every day I spent time online reading and writing. I asked questions and shared how I was feeling. When physical or emotional things came up, invariably, someone was able to offer reassurance—we were all on this journey together. There were women who lived in Australia and Italy and Canada and Thailand and South Africa and Germany and England and the United States. There were women who lived in my own neighborhood, whom I eventually met and befriended. I would later learn there were people I'd known for years who silently shared similar experiences. A whole new world was unfolding—one I could have never imagined existed before being thrust into it. A world that is not openly talked about and is rarely written about. A world that is expanding much too quickly. A world in need of a voice.... *Why not mine?*

16

Dawn's Story: "Making the Childfree Choice after a Heartbreaking Choice"

My story begins in my own childhood. I never had any maternal instincts then. I preferred to play with Career Barbie dolls over any baby doll. I had no desire whatsoever to have children and no problem telling that to anyone. Once I became an adult, I made sure any man I dated knew that up front. I was very fortunate to meet and marry a man who loved me for myself without regard to fertility or fecundity. Little did I know how very important that kind of love would become.

I was absolutely shocked when I came down with "baby rabies" in my early 30's after 11 years of marriage. It seemed as if everyone around me had gotten pregnant, so it was time for me to do the same if I were ever going to try. I had some reservations about whether I could physically or mentally handle pregnancy, but I pushed them to the back of my mind and decided to give it a shot. I dedicated myself to the idea of being pregnant in the same way I had pursued my college and career goals, trying to prepare myself as thoroughly as possible. My husband felt ambivalent but was willing to take the chance. In retrospect, this leap of faith was one of the worst decisions we ever made.

I managed to get pregnant within a few months of our trying, but the pregnancy was ectopic. I avoided major surgery only because the fetus was within one centimeter's size of requiring the fallopian tube to be removed. After that, I was really afraid to try again. We waited a year, but then we discovered that it was not going to be so easy the second time around. The fallopian tube was scarred shut from the earlier pregnancy. I was getting very stressed out from trying, so we began to rethink our decision to be parents. We decided to continue trying for no more than three months. We both agreed we didn't want any fertility treatments that involved drugs or surgery; therefore, I chose a reproductive specialist who used noninvasive methods. After my initial consultation and evaluation (no treatment), I was surprised to find out I was pregnant without any professional help.

I had exactly two weeks of normal pregnancy after the home pregnancy test stick turned blue. My husband and I were very happy during that brief time. We began looking at ways to turn our extra bedroom into a nursery, reading baby books, and thinking about how we could set up our schedules that fall for parental leave. We even had fun when we argued about baby names. The very day I went to work and announced we were expecting, I began spotting and ended up in the emergency room with a threatened miscarriage. When the ultrasound technician showed us the first picture of the embryo with the beating heart, my husband and I were both really excited and started to think things might work out. That turned out to be a false hope as things went from bad to worse.

I was on bed rest for what was supposed to be one week. At the end of the week, my husband took me for a drive to pick up some fast food. I became really queasy during the drive and ended up coming home to throw up. At the time we joked about how cute it was that I had my first bout of morning sickness. Within a week, I was hospitalized with hyperemesis gravidarum (HG).

HG is much more than morning sickness; it's like the worst food poisoning anyone has ever had, only much more persistent. A 2005 article from Medical News Today reported that the weight loss, malnutrition, and unceasing nausea and vomiting from HG can cause severe problems for both mothers and fetuses. The Hyperemesis Education & Research Foundation has noted that women may experience dehydration, Wernicke's encephalopathy, electrolyte imbalances, tachycardia, hypoglycemia, severe headaches, esophageal damage, renal failure, and jaundice, in addition to extreme anxiety and depression. Complications for the fetus include an increased risk of miscarriage, low birth weight, and premature labor and delivery.

This condition is so physically, mentally, and financially debilitating that afflicted women often limit the size of their biological families and some choose to terminate a wanted pregnancy due to inadequate treatment. If it is untreated, is treated improperly, or causes serious complications, HG may even result in maternal death. Sadly, many doctors believe that the condition is primarily psychological and treat it as such. I knew none of this when I received my diagnosis, but I was about to become the poster child for poor obstetrical management of HG.

I couldn't hold down any food or water and had a high amount of ketones in my urine from dehydration and starvation. The hospitalization was a very difficult experience. The doctors and nurses could not start an IV because I was so dehydrated, and I have terrible veins anyway; they tried 14 times. No one on duty or on call could put in a PICC line or a central line, so they were going to have to call someone in who was not expecting to work. At that point, it was 3:00 AM on a Sunday, so I refused to allow it. I told them to wait until the morning, retest me, and then have someone from the day shift put it in if necessary. I somehow willed myself to keep down enough water and juice to get my ketones low enough so that I would be allowed to be discharged. The doctors gave me Phenergan, but I was allergic to it. Next they tried Zofran. The Zofran stopped the vomiting but not the nausea. Nevertheless, I was glad to get home. I hoped that would break the cycle and get me back to a normal level of morning sickness.

Unfortunately, things got even worse after that. The gynecologist I had been seeing did not deliver babies, so I had to transfer to a different doctor. The gynecologist wanted me to see her brother; however, since he was in the same office with her, I had seen how rude his staff was and how late he always ran. I was also uncomfortable with the fact that the practice was Fundamentalist Catholic and emphasized that the health of the fetus was always to be put first. I asked for another recommendation. While I waited for a new doctor, I had one more trip to the emergency room with dehydration and anxiety as the diagnosis. The staff could not start an IV on that visit either. Eventually my gynecologist sent me to someone she had worked with before who had since joined a mega-practice on my side of town.

When I called the office, I discovered that he too no longer delivered babies but had an associate with immediate openings. That should have been my first clue that I was about to get an awful doctor. At my first appointment, I explained to him about the HG and how the current medicines did not seem to be working for me. I was not sleeping or eating and needed help. His solution was to send me home with a prescription for Xanax and advice to sniff a lemon, eat crackers, and go back to work. At that point, I could not have made it to the car without puking, much less driven 20 miles to work.

I quickly discovered that the Xanax was making me worse. I felt like an addict as I nearly crawled out of my skin waiting to be able to take the next dose after only a couple of hours. And then it became ineffective altogether. The lemon was equally useless and came to symbolize my choice of doctor more than anything else. I was in and out of his office several times over the next six weeks. I was rapidly losing weight and becoming mentally unbalanced from lack of sleep. I had multiple panic attacks daily. On the rare occasions I did sleep, I had horrible nightmares. And the nausea and vomiting just did not stop. I reached a point where I could keep nothing down. I would get sick standing in the shower; I would get sick in bed; I would get sick getting out of bed for any reason. I was extremely constipated from the Zofran, and as far as I could tell, it was doing nothing else for me. Due to previous experiences, I had discovered I was allergic to all the other standard nausea medications. In short, nothing was working for me.

The doctor's solution was to blame me for the problem. He asked me about the quality of my marriage and intimated that something had to be wrong between my husband and me. He also said that I must have severe psychological problems that caused me to not want the baby and that I should think about what my real feelings were concerning the pregnancy. He seemed to think that whipping out the fetal heart monitor and letting me hear the heartbeat would bring out a maternal instinct in me that would somehow magically make the condition disappear.

In just a few short weeks, my life changed from picking baby names and nursery furniture to trying to keep myself from starving to death. I spent hours on the Internet each day looking for a solution. I ordered every morning sickness remedy available. None of them did a thing for me. I found hyperemesis support groups online and learned that I should be seeing a specialist called a perinatologist, preferably someone who had a lot of experience in treating the condition. When I called and asked for a referral, the doctor refused to provide one. Instead, he sent me to a psychiatrist. She was a patient of his and made it very clear to me that she was working me into her busy schedule as a personal favor to my doctor.

She spent 30 minutes with me, 20 of which she was on her cell phone taking personal calls. Her main concern was the health of the fetus rather than my condition. She diagnosed me as "borderline bipolar" and sent me home with an antidepressant that she said either would help or push me into full-blown mania. Given that I was already on the edge of madness, hearing that did not inspire me to follow her advice.

I cannot even begin to describe the horror my life had become. I couldn't stand the smell of my own bed sheets. The sound of my dog's licking me in attempts to comfort me would make me vomit. I could not tolerate loud noises or sudden movements at all. All I could do was lie in bed, try to keep down water or JELL-O, and vomit periodically. I was averaging less than two hours of sleep per night, none of it restful. And no one would help me. My husband and I felt absolutely powerless over the medical establishment, and I was just too weak to fight any longer. I began to have very serious thoughts of killing myself or doing something to cause a miscarriage regardless of how it would affect me physically; that's when I realized that abortion was truly the only way out of my suffering. My insurance did not allow me to see another doctor without a referral from the obstetrician. I was too sick to do the legwork to find one outside the system on my own and could not have afforded the out-of-pocket expense in any case. My primary care doctor refused to help me, saying that he would not overrule an obstetrician on matters of pregnancy. I was getting very close to 12 weeks' gestation. I went through a period of four days when I neither ate nor slept at all. I was vomiting bile and blood. My throat was raw from the acid burns.

We made one last visit to the obstetrician. My husband and I tried to impress upon him how very sick I was. I had lost 23 pounds in eight weeks and could not even walk on my own because I was so weak. He asked me about the stupid lemon again. I had it in a bag, dutifully carrying it with me to the end (right next to the gallon-size bag half-filled with blood-streaked bile I had thrown up during the car ride there). I told him that I did not want to end the pregnancy, but I felt that I had no choice. I asked him if there were something else, anything else he could do for me, if he would send me to see someone else for a second opinion. He replied that my only options at that point were termination or allowing him to hospitalize me, insert a feeding tube, and "experiment" on me. (Yes, he actually used that word.) He said he could not guarantee any sort of outcome for either me or the baby. He left my husband and me alone so we could discuss the situation.

Neither of us had any confidence in him at that point, so we agreed that abortion was the least bad option. All I could think about was being stuck in a hospital, not being able to leave with that guy as Dr. Frankenstein and my body as his project. My husband was very upset about our being put in that position and said that he would need time to "consider [his] options" and that "all bets [were] off" after the termination was over. I knew this meant he was considering leaving me, something we agreed would never happen to our marriage. I became very angry with him. He knew how much I had suffered over the previous eight weeks and that I hadn't wanted things to turn out the way they had. I felt as if he were blaming me.

When the doctor returned, we told him we had decided together to terminate the pregnancy. He told us he would not do it, so we would have to go to an abortion clinic. He gave us the address and telephone number and said, "You don't need an appointment. Just show up." Even as sick as I was, I knew that was wrong. I believe he was trying to dissuade me from getting the procedure, hoping I would give up if I were turned away. I called the clinic as soon as I got home and made an appointment for two days later.

At first, my husband did not want to take me for the procedure because he didn't think he could go through with it. I arranged for a friend to take me but made it clear to my husband that I thought it was his obligation to see it through with me. Finally, at midnight the night before, he changed his mind but said he would not go into the procedure room with me. It turned out he couldn't have anyway, but I was very upset by his decision. Again, I felt as if my lack of strength and willpower caused this.

When the day of the abortion came, we had to drive through protesters and weave through sidewalk counselors. I said nothing but felt like puking on every single one of them. Those people have no idea what brings any woman to such a decision; I felt as if they were judging me. I was a nervous wreck the whole time I was at the clinic. My husband sat next to me and held my hand, but he would not look at me or say even one word, making me even more jittery as I contemplated the state of my marriage. Even the ultrasound was a cause for anxiety as it revealed the fetus was already two weeks smaller than it should have been due to my malnutrition. The women around me were a microcosm of society: husbands with wives, boyfriends with girlfriends, parents with daughters, friends with friends, in all ages from teens to 40s and all races. It was the day before Mother's Day. The television in the waiting area blared commercials and news programs commemorating that fact. And all of us, the soon-to-be-unpregnant and our loved ones, sat there watching and listening silently.

I asked a lot of questions and was very concerned about possible negative outcomes. At first, the clinic staff seemed to welcome this. Then, when they found out I was not employed in the medical field, they became annoyed. The procedure itself did not go as easily as it should have because the nurse could not start an IV. When I tried to explain why and tell her where she would have a better chance of inserting the catheter, she rudely told me she did not want to hear it and that she knew what she was doing. She called in another nurse, but neither they nor the doctor was able to start the IV. My abortion was done with only a little nitrous oxide gas and no anesthesia other than a local to the cervix.

The ride home from the clinic was one of the longest of my life. My husband and I barely spoke. All I could think about was my anger over the loss of the baby and possible loss of my marriage. Adding insult to injury, once I was home I continued to vomit for a few days after the termination. I remember *kneeling* over the toilet crying, "It's not fair. I thought this was supposed to stop!" I was still so weak from not eating or sleeping that it took me a couple of weeks to be out of bed on a regular basis.

Although my husband was doing his best to be supportive, he was in a lot of pain too. During the first few months, it was almost like having a roommate instead of a spouse. He took care of me, but he withdrew deeply into himself and spent a lot of time on the computer. I was terribly afraid and anxious because I thought he didn't love me anymore and still blamed me for what happened. I began to feel a lot of anger toward him because I felt we had done the best we could under the circumstances and I hated feeling as if he held me responsible for something I could not have controlled.

Above all, he did not want to talk about any of it (though he was willing to listen to me once in awhile). So I did the only thing I could. I found support from my friends, family, and rabbi. A friend found me a new psychiatrist, one who actually cared about me and worked with me to find a good combination of medication and talk therapy. It turned out I was not bipolar, just extremely anxious. (Who wouldn't be after all that?) The medications made me able to function well enough to get back to work. My colleagues were very supportive and helped me get back into my daily routine. But the one thing I needed to make me feel better, the reassurance of my husband that all was going to be okay, was still missing.

It took nearly six months before he was able to open up to me about how deeply the experience hurt him. He said that he didn't blame me; he blamed himself for not being able to help me. He said that he wanted to take care of me and felt as if he had failed at his job as a husband. Most importantly, he said that he'd never stopped loving me. We agreed to commit ourselves fully to the marriage and work things out. We made it through that difficult time and came out stronger and closer than ever.

At that time, we also had a heartfelt talk about our parenting future. Given that hyperemesis is not only likely to recur but also to be worse in subsequent pregnancies, we'd already decided that another pregnancy was not an option. But we also decided that we didn't want to pursue any other form of having children. My husband is an amazing man with a good heart. I thank God every day for sending him to me. He agreed to have a vasectomy so I would not have to fear getting pregnant again or undergo another surgical procedure myself. Realizing that I had a choice and never had to subject myself to this kind of horror again was an enormous relief.

At that point I felt as if several huge burdens had been taken from me, but the one issue that still lingered was my crippling anxiety. Even after I began to feel better about the termination, the anxiety did not abate and I didn't feel like myself. The doctors told me it was all psychological in nature and related to the termination; however, my periods were extremely erratic. No one wanted to pursue testing on me after I made it clear that I did not want a future pregnancy. Women who don't want to make babies don't merit treatment for reproductive organ issues in many doctors' eyes.

Finally, after a year of no periods, a year of period cycles between 11 and 61 days, and another six months of no periods, I found a doctor who was willing to run hormone tests. It turned out I was in premature ovarian failure, a type of early menopause that needs treatment in order to prevent osteoporosis and heart disease. It's amazing how much hormone imbalance affects anxiety levels! With proper hormone replacement, I am much better now. As a result, I no longer take daily psychiatric medications and need rescue medications only occasionally.

The aftermath of this experience is something that I'll never get over, mainly because of the extremely poor medical treatment I received. I made the best choice that I could at a time when there were no good choices for me. I will never be ashamed of or regretful for doing what I had to do. I realize things might have turned out differently had I received better care; however, there is no way to know for certain what the outcome would have been. I am grateful that this choice to terminate was available to me; it relieved my suffering at a time when nothing else would have given the conditions. I am blessed to have a wonderful marriage, a successful career, and a great network of family and friends who, for the most part, stood by me throughout all of this. Despite all the bad that came from my situation, those people helped me realize the strength within myself to get through it.

Overall I am content with my situation and happy with the childfree life I have built with my husband. It is a bit odd, however, to be in a kind of no woman's land. Some people who never wanted kids or don't like children consider me not to be "really" childfree because we tried to become parents. Some who've suffered hyperemesis or pregnancy loss consider my ordeal to be not as bad as theirs, either because I made the choice to end my pregnancy myself or because I decided not to try again and am happy with that decision. I choose not to let those people define my identity or my experience. I still have problems with anxiety from time to time (as I did before this), but I am much better than I was five years ago when this journey began for me. I finally have the optimal combination of good medical help I can trust and a strong personal support system (both online and in "real" life).

For any woman who finds herself in the situation of facing a termination, whether it is as a result of her own health or that of her baby, I want this story to be a message of hope. Things will not always be as horrible as they seem at the time of this experience. It will take time and work, but healing can and will happen. I will always be thankful to everyone who helped me along the way, and I hope this story and the others in this book provide some comfort. You are stronger than you think you are, and you are not alone!

17

Ellen's Story "Bittersweet Blessings"

As I write this story, it has been one year since I said goodbye to my first child, Kylie Ann. My husband and I had been married four years when we decided to start a family. I was 28 years old and he was 31 years old. We stopped birth control in November of 2004. I was surprised that it took 13 months to conceive. It happened when we were visiting his family in Australia. I was absolutely elated when, a month after returning home, I took a home pregnancy test and it was positive. I immediately started taking prenatal vitamins and extra folic acid. I couldn't hold the news in and told everyone I knew within two weeks of finding out. I worked in the healthcare industry and told all of my patients and co-workers. They were all thrilled for me. Morning sickness started pretty quickly and tended to last all day. I was very tired throughout the months of January and February, but so happy to be expecting. Our due date was set for September 24, 2006. Overall, I had a very easy first trimester.

Every doctor visit was very easy and smooth, and we were given little ultrasound pictures of our peanut, which we showed to everyone. My husband was over the moon with joy and started calling the baby "Ricey," because we read that she was the size of a grain of rice on one of my weekly Internet baby updates. I started to show a little bit in March, but could still wear my regular clothes. We hoped for a boy, but agreed that we would be very happy with either gender.

As I started the second trimester, I began to feel a lot more energetic. We were remodeling our bathroom, as we were only five months away from having a baby to take care of. It was very stressful since we were doing all of the remodeling work ourselves. My only symptom of pregnancy at that point was the dizziness I would feel when I worked hard in the hot garden. I wore my bikini with pride, showing off my little belly!

Our big doctor's appointment was during my 18th week of pregnancy, on April 26th. We were literally unable to sleep the night before, wondering about whether we were having a boy or a girl. It never dawned on us that we would also be having tests to determine if the baby was healthy. All we cared about was that it was alive and what colors we would choose for the baby's bedroom. I was very eager to clean out our guest bedroom in preparation for the baby, but jokingly said I would wait until I found out that everything was viable since I hadn't yet felt any movement.

We had the standard abdominal ultrasound and were told that we were having a girl! I laughed and told my husband that I was sorry. But we were so thrilled. We already had a name—Kylie Ann. The ultrasound technician told us that the doctor had gone out on a delivery and would be back soon, and we were to wait in the lobby. So that was what we did, and in the meantime we called our parents and friends to tell them we were having a daughter! Everyone was thrilled and my mother stopped by the office to look at the ultrasound photos. Kylie had the most beautiful profile I could imagine.

It took the doctor about an hour and a half to get back to the office. When she came into the exam room, she apologized profusely for being so late. We told her we didn't care; we were on top of the world. She said, "Well wait a minute, we saw something on the scan that we need to talk about." She then explained that Kylie had a significant-sized myelomeningocele, or spina bifida, affecting her spine from at least the lumbar level down. My husband and I both worked in rehabilitation and we knew that meant definite paralysis. Later on, my husband told me that he noticed that it looked like Kylie had two spines on the ultrasound, but that he thought it might have been just a blurry image. It turned out that her vertebrae were separated like an open zipper. My husband's face turned absolutely white when we heard the diagnosis. I cried like a baby. The doctor said to stay calm, that she would refer us to a perinatologist as soon as possible, and then she wrote the diagnosis on a piece of paper for us to research. She also mentioned that the baby had hydrocephalus, or fluid on the brain. That was at 18 weeks and four days, and the baby already had a "lemon-shaped" head from the excess fluid. My heart absolutely stopped. They sent us out the back door of the office and said that we would hear from the perinatologist soon.

When I got into my car, there were pink flowers on the dashboard. My husband had gone out while we were waiting and put them in my car before we received the bad news. I felt so bad for him. On the way home, I had to call my friends and family back and tell them that all was not well and that we just had to wait to find out more. My mother was devastated and my friends were shocked, but we all agreed that we would try to stay calm.

I went home and started scouring the Internet to find out everything I could about the diagnosis. It was everything I remembered from therapy school—the best case scenario being a person who has a shunt in his or her brain and no control of the bowel and bladder. The worst case is retardation, severe paralysis, deformity of the legs, and death in childhood. It appeared from the scan that Kylie was affected from the L4–L5 level down, which meant that she could possibly stand with braces. I went to bed and prayed for a miracle. Unfortunately, I knew in my heart that it would be bad, no matter what. I have worked with these children. They always had some cognitive delays, had to learn to live with wearing a diaper their whole life, and had to undergo multiple surgeries.

I went to work the next day and had to tell everyone that the baby was very sick and that we were waiting to hear more. I lived in a conservative area of the southern United States and I could see the look on people's faces when I talked about it. They knew that I was considering termination. It was very uncomfortable. I called the perinatologist's office about 9:00 AM and begged to be seen that day. They asked me to come in about noon.

I met my husband and mother there. They both looked like death. The doctor was very nice, very thorough and very gentle. As he performed the ultrasound we could see a big bubble in the back of Kylie's spine. He told us that it started at the T11 level. That was much higher than we originally thought. It meant that she would never sit up alone, much less stand. I was hysterical. My mother didn't understand what he was saying, but she knew it was bad because I kept looking at my husband and saying, "What are we going to do?" The doctor gave me the impression that he was very pro-life. He told us that we had a beautiful baby and we should go home and relax before we made any decisions. He then performed an amniocentesis to rule out any genetic syndromes. I actually hoped in a way that there would be more things wrong to make the decision easier.

We all went into a conference room with a genetic counselor, who gave us information on many different options. One option was to be a part of a study, being done in the Carolinas, to have in utero surgery to close the hole in the baby's spine and possibly stop the hydrocephalus; another option was do nothing and have a cesarean section when the baby was full term; and yet another option was to terminate the pregnancy. We talked for a very long time; I cried incessantly. The in utero surgery was still considered experimental and came with no guarantees. If I chose that option, I would need to have the surgery at around 25 weeks, and then live in the Carolinas on bed rest afterwards. I would have to quit work and my husband would have to come home alone. Once I reached full-term I would deliver by scheduled c-section. The in utero surgery would not change anything about the baby's paralysis, and carried significant risks to us both. Also, only half of the people who apply for the surgery actually meet the criteria to be in the study group. So even if I were to apply that day, I might find out a week later that I wasn't selected.

I decided to call another number, which was to a women's clinic in Atlanta that performed abortions. The woman who answered the phone told me that they were only performed on Fridays and Saturdays and that if I waited another week I would have to have a labor and delivery (L&D) termination. However, if I went ahead now it would be a dilation and evacuation (D&E) termination under anesthesia. I asked her if there were any openings for the following day, as it was a Thursday afternoon. There were, so I booked a space for the next morning and went home. It was all a very strange and quick decision, but one that I knew was right in my heart and had known was right since the previous day.

There we were, standing in the parking lot of the hospital; me on my phone speaking with an abortion clinic, and my husband on his phone speaking with his crying mother. But as soon as the decision was made, there was a certain weight lifted off of our shoulders. We both knew exactly what our child would require to survive, and it was more than we could bear. My mother had offered to quit her job and take care of Kylie full-time, but I knew that it would be too hard on her. How could my mother lift a paralyzed child when she grew to more that 30 or 40 pounds? How could any of us? In my work I had not only seen what the condition can do to the patient, but also to the caregivers. They become very isolated and sad people. That was not what we wanted for our lives or for Kylie's life.

At 4:00 the next morning, we started the six hour drive to Atlanta. I was fortunate enough to have a very good friend there who was a neonatal nurse. She was totally supportive of our decision and we stayed with her and her husband. But first we had to go to the clinic. After waiting in a heavily guarded waiting room for about 30 minutes, we were taken to a private waiting room with a very comfortable couch (which had a big teddy bear sitting on it) and soft lighting. We spent the morning undergoing counseling, filling out paperwork, and waiting. We also had to have one last ultrasound. It absolutely killed me to look at Kylie for what I knew would be the last time. My husband and I both had to turn away from the monitor.

Finally, at about 11:00 AM I was given a Xanax. It completely knocked me out for about an hour. My poor husband was stuck there holding me while I slept. They then took me into a room to insert the laminaria. The doctor who performed the insertion was very gentle and I felt nothing. We left shortly thereafter and spent the rest of the day and night relaxing at my friend's house. She had a baby girl of her own at the time, but it didn't bother me. She was such a sweet baby. It made me very hopeful for the future. I was so thankful that I was able to stay there instead of some hotel.

Early the next morning we went back to the clinic and I was taken to the operating room. At that point, I really broke down. It was a terrifying-looking room with another patient in the corner. I started sobbing and telling the nurse and doctor how I wanted my baby but that she was sick. The anesthesiologist was an older lady who said, "Now you have to stop crying, or you'll choke, okay? C'mon…," so I calmed down. Then two young female doctors from Emory University came in and told me they would perform the D&E. I thanked them and fell asleep.

When I awoke I immediately started crying and asked if they saw my baby. The nurse said, "No, honey." It was at that point I realized that maybe labor would have been better, as I would have been able to see Kylie. To this day I don't know what would have been the best option for me. I opted not to get Kylie's ashes, and now I second guess that decision too.

I was quickly ushered into the bathroom to clean up. I bled everywhere but didn't care because I was so dazed from the medication. I got myself dressed and was sent out the back door where my husband was waiting in the car. He was apparently treated pretty coldly by the staff and was very worried about me. But I actually felt fine physically. We drove back to my friend's house in somewhat decent spirits.

That night was spent on my friend's couch, taking many phone calls from friends and family. Most were totally supportive, but one person called and asked if I knew what I was doing. I told her, "Of course!" In my opinion, she was just very naïve. We passed the time watching television and eating junk food. It was very calming.

We went home on Sunday, and my mom offered to bring a casserole over. That was when my world started to break down. My mom brought my brother with her, and my husband and I ended up serving them dinner. It was awful. The next day, which was a Monday, my husband went back to work. I almost did too, but was convinced by a co-worker to take one more day off. So I spent the day working on the bathroom remodeling. I couldn't stop crying.

I went back to work on Tuesday. Over the course of the next two months, life got very difficult. I started counseling with my husband, which helped tremendously, as I became convinced that I was going to burn in hell for my selfish ways. I was able to work through those thoughts with counseling. I came to the conclusion that I would make the same decision if I had to do it over again, right or wrong. But it was so hard to face all the people who knew I was pregnant and to decide how much I would tell them. I refused to pretend that it was some kind of miscarriage. I was totally honest with everyone.

On top of that, I became very angry at my husband anytime he was not willing to try to conceive. One weekend, two months after our loss, I became so enraged at him and so anxious that I left the house and checked into a motel. In the motel room I slept for about 16 hours, which was good for me, I guess, but really cruel to him. My poor husband spent the weekend calling friends and family looking for me. He really thought I was going to hurt myself. In fact, on Mother's Day that May I put our loaded .45 in my mouth in front of him. That gun has been hidden from me ever since.

I was very fortunate that somehow, in the midst of all of that horror and chaos, I successfully conceived again. I don't really know how things would have turned out if I hadn't. I know I would have come out of this in one piece regardless. I have become a much more compassionate yet more cynical person. I still get angry at people who conceive quickly and skate through their pregnancy with their only worry being not knowing if they are having a boy or a girl. That was us once, but never again. I still count the blessings in my life as much as I can, and one of those blessings is the fact that I was allowed to make this choice for myself, my husband, and my sweet, precious little daughter. I am also blessed by the love I feel for her which grows every day.

18

Emme Bea's Story "Christopher's Gift"

In the Spring of 2005 I was 36 years old and found myself at a crossroads. The company for whom I worked for over 13 years was closing and offered me a large severance package. I found myself without a job for the first time in 20 years. I planned to enjoy the summer, maybe do some traveling, and take my time in looking for another job.

My husband G and I had been very casually trying to get pregnant for two years. I had polycystic ovarian syndrome (PCOS) and had gone off birth control pills with the hope that we could conceive naturally. Though I knew that my particular condition made it difficult to get pregnant, I didn't want to allow trying for a baby to become a stressor. I didn't want to chart, to pee on any sticks, to count days, to take drugs, to have "calendar sex," or to become "crazy fertility lady." I had watched my sister go through that in her efforts to have a family and I wanted no part of it. I had been with my husband for 16 years, married for 11, and knew that being childfree was something I could live with. What I thought I couldn't live with was turning our lives into a medical pressure cooker in an effort to build a family when we were already so happy with our family of two. I wanted a baby to add to our love, not to cause it undue pressure. (That, ladies and gentlemen, is called "foreshadowing" in the biz. Take note, and feel free to laugh at me all you want.)

One week after my last day of work, I conceived our baby. When my period didn't start on time, I bought a pregnancy test, almost on a lark. I didn't think I could be pregnant, but I was planning a birthday party for G and wanted to make sure I could have a few drinks. Hot damn and stop the presses! Right there in the little electronic display window was the word "pregnant." I was pregnant! My body worked! And we did it naturally and without intervention and at a time in my life that really made sense. With me being out of a job, we decided that I would stay home the first couple years of the baby's life and just enjoy him or her. Wasn't that what the universe was telling us? Lost job, big severance package, and a new baby? Of course it was! Oh happy day, it was a joyful time.

At my first prenatal appointment, I skipped in and out of the office rubbing my belly. My OB, (let's call him Dr. Idaho because he later moved there) had blood drawn and I signed a bunch of papers authorizing different tests. We discussed what to expect in the first trimester, and scheduled my first ultrasound. Overall, it was a very uneventful visit. Based on my last menstrual cycle, Dr. Idaho estimated that I was six weeks pregnant and said, "See you next month!" You could almost read the thought bubble over my head that read "Tra la la, not a care in the world, life is good, tra la la!" I can still feel that happy, ignorant, naïve hope that was propelling me through the early days of that pregnancy. On Mother's Day, I sent out an e-mail to all my friends and family and it was entitled, "Happy Mother's Day… to ME?" It was meaningful to me to make that announcement on Mother's Day as it was the second Mother's Day without my own mother who had passed the previous year from lung cancer. I felt she was looking down on us and smiling.

Fast forward to my second prenatal visit, and if this were a movie, you'd hear the big scratch of the needle on the vinyl record of my happy tra la la music. SCREEEECH went my happy song as Dr. Idaho went over my chart and said, "Oh, by the way, your blood work came back positive for being a carrier for cystic fibrosis." He said it so casually, so nonchalantly and with absolutely no concern. Apparently one of the papers I signed at my first prenatal appointment authorized a blood test to screen for the cystic fibrosis (CF) gene. I didn't realize this as I was too busy skipping and singing and picking out nursery colors and baby names to be concerned with what papers I had signed. Not that I wouldn't have signed them, but I wasn't focusing on what those papers meant. Dr. Idaho went on to allay my fears and lay out what being a carrier of CF meant. The fact that I alone was a carrier meant nothing really. But we would need to have my husband G tested for carrier status. Then we *might* have to worry. Dr. Idaho mentioned that in the five years he had been testing for CF, he never had a patient's partner also test positive, so we shouldn't worry. Easier said than done. I left his office on lead feet and went home to confer with Dr. Google.

What I learned online was that we were about to enter a game of chance and the odds were in our favor. First, one out of every 20 Caucasian Americans of eastern European descent carry the recessive gene that causes

CF. The chance of two carriers hooking up and procreating is one in 800. I liked those odds. I focused on those odds. I didn't want to think that G's chances were one in 20; I wanted to focus on the lower odds of the *both* of us being positive. If your partner also is a carrier, then the odds get a little scarier. Any baby conceived by two carriers of CF has a 50 percent chance of being a carrier, a 25 percent chance of not even having the CF gene, and a 25 percent chance of having both recessive genes and being affected with cystic fibrosis.

G went and had blood drawn for the test and I settled in to learn as much about CF as I possibly could. I was 10 weeks pregnant and the happy, skippy days of my pregnancy were officially over. Treatment for cystic fibrosis has come a long way in the last 20 years. Life expectancy has almost tripled and many patients can live into their twenties and thirties. However, it remains 100 percent fatal, there is no cure for it, and there is no way to predict how severely the disease may manifest itself. Cystic fibrosis affects the exocrine (mucus) glands of the lungs, liver, pancreas, and intestines, causing progressive disability due to multisystem failure. Thick mucus production, as well as a compromised immune system, results in frequent lung infections, including repeated cases of pneumonia. Children with CF go through daily physical therapy treatments to clear their lungs, are often hospitalized due to the constant threat of lung infections, may have to have bowel surgery right after birth, are often home schooled to reduce the threat of illness, and are unnaturally aware of their own mortality. CF is painful, incurable, and cruel. And my baby might have had it.

A week went by and we still didn't have the results of G's blood test. After some frustrating telephone calls, we learned that the lab had lost his sample and they would need to pull another sample to be tested. I was now 11 weeks pregnant and waiting for the news that my husband wasn't a carrier. Tick tock went the clock. The calendar pages slowly tore away and I entered week 12. G's results finally came back…he was also a carrier of CF.

Dr. Idaho had me make an appointment with a perinatologist to schedule an amniocentesis. I was so ignorant about prenatal testing that I didn't even know what a perinatologist was. In making the appointment, I was told I needed to meet with a genetic counselor prior to the amniocentesis. I was 13 weeks pregnant when we sat down and spoke to the genetic counselor to discuss our testing options. We discussed cystic fibrosis, the different mutations, and our results. I quickly learned that I knew more about CF than the well-meaning and sweet genetic counselor. What I didn't know then, but she told me, was that I had just missed the gestational window of opportunity to have a prenatal test called chorionic villus sampling (CVS) that could test for CF weeks before an amniocentesis is even possible. A CVS is similar to an amniocentesis in that a needle is inserted into the uterus to retrieve genetic material to test. However, in a CVS, placental material is removed, not amniotic fluid. A CVS is typically scheduled between 10 to 12 weeks gestation. If you miss that window of testing, you must wait for an amniocentesis, which is generally scheduled no earlier than 16 weeks gestation. Though slightly riskier, a CVS will give you earlier results. When testing for cystic fibrosis, CVS results can be back as soon as 10 days after the test, but for an amniocentesis it usually takes four to five weeks for results. The time it takes to get cystic fibrosis results back is much longer than if testing for either aneuploidies or sex chromosome abnormalities. If testing for aneuploidies (an abnormal number of chromosomes) such as Down syndrome, a simple count of the chromosomes is all that is done and results can often take as little as three days. With cystic fibrosis however, there is no speeding up of the process as they must grow the culture in a lab until the sample is large enough to test the seventh chromosome to determine the genetic makeup. CVS results can come back much sooner than amniocentesis results because the genetic material retrieved from the placenta in a CVS is more concentrated than the genetic material present in the amniotic fluid retrieved from an amniocentesis; therefore, you don't have to grow it as long before testing. Due to the lab's snafu in losing G's blood sample, we just missed our opportunity to know as early as 13 weeks whether or not our baby had a fatal disease and would now have to wait for almost two more months to know the status.

At 16 weeks I had my amniocentesis. The ultrasound technician that did the preceding scan was, I believe, clearly aware of our situation and clearly biased against terminating. She wasn't exactly subtle in letting us know this. Before the scan, I had to sign a paper stating that I was counseled about my options to terminate the pregnancy (I was not). I asked the technician about this clause and she said, "Twenty-four weeks, now you've been counseled." I said, "Twenty-four weeks? For what?" She said, "You can legally abort your baby in this state up to 24 weeks. That's what I'm supposed to tell you." That was the only counseling I received on termination. G and I knew it was an option. G was sure that he didn't want to put a child through a life of illness but I wasn't sure of anything. I knew I didn't want my child to suffer, but I was not ready to make any real decision before I had to. During the ultrasound, we learned our baby was a boy. It was so bittersweet seeing that perfectly forming little baby mugging for the camera and knowing that he may be fatally ill. The technician kept saying things like, "What a cutie. What a blessing. What a gorgeous child." On the two ultrasound pictures she printed out, they both have the phrase, "What a cutie!" printed over the image. The only photos I have of my son are printed with her propaganda.

I get sick thinking about it. As I lay on that table watching those images, tears silently rolled down my eyes and into my ears. I had puddles of tears in my ears and a heart that was growing for this child even as it was breaking with the possibilities of what might lie ahead. The amniocentesis itself was uneventful, relatively pain free and quick. We left the office and went home to await our fate.

How was I going to get through this time? How would I survive? I wanted so badly to enjoy the pregnancy. I was in love with my baby already. I had seen him move on the ultrasound. I watched my belly grow. Despite wanting to distance ourselves, we found it impossible not to begin making plans, even as we knew we had a 25 percent chance that those plans would be ruined. I wouldn't buy maternity clothes or anything for the baby, but I couldn't stop myself from hoping.

I was hiding all this from my family and most of my friends. I could see their curious looks when I couldn't muster up the enthusiasm they thought I should have in the glow of my second trimester. My mother had passed away the previous year and I didn't want to put my father through further worry, he was still so very fragile after her death. I was being strong for me, for my family, for my husband and for my baby. I kept going over and over the odds in my head. My baby had a 75 percent chance of being healthy. Still, it was hard not to focus on the one in four chance that he might be sick.

Because the percentages were still in our favor, I had convinced myself that even if he were sick, we would continue with the pregnancy. I had to tell myself that in order to keep going. We picked out a name; Christopher, and against our better judgment, began to say things like, "After we find out he's okay we'll set up the nursery, pick a registry, etc." I would rub my belly and talk to Christopher and beg him to be healthy. The weeks between that first glimmer of something possibly being wrong to the call from my genetic counselor dragged by in a slow, excruciating haze. On a Friday morning, four and a half weeks after my amniocentesis, the phone rang. G had just gone in to take a shower so I was alone when I listened to the genetic counselor on the other end saying "I'm so sorry but…." After the obligatory discussions on the chances of the test being wrong (no chance), I curled up in a fetal position and began to cry, holding my belly, holding my baby, my son. I knew that second that I couldn't put this child I loved so much through a life of pain, sickness, hospitalizations, surgeries, procedures, and isolation. I knew I would let him go. G came out of the shower, saw me crying and just knew. He lay down next to me, spooning me and joining in mourning for our son that was still with us.

I made a call to my OB, but he was out of the office. I left a message for him to call me back. I made a series of other phone calls while I waited to hear from him. I called a friend of mine that had lost a baby girl due to a heart condition after fighting for almost a year. I told her of my situation and asked her what it was like to have a terminally ill child and watch it die. She told me unequivocally that if she had the chance to end her daughter's suffering prenatally she would have done so. I called a former coworker with whom I had kept in sporadic contact with since we last worked together. I knew he had lost a son to cystic fibrosis and I wanted to speak to him. His son was three years old when he died. He understood why I would consider termination and he offered me support without judgment regardless of what we chose to do. I then called my mother-in-law. She was the one family member we told while we were waiting for results and she gave me the strength I needed during that long summer. She felt very strongly that the best thing to do for our child and our marriage was to let our son go. She was an anchor my husband and I held onto during those stormy days.

I then called Planned Parenthood, who recommended a local clinic that would support a late second trimester termination. I called them and made an appointment for the following Tuesday. I would be almost 21 weeks pregnant by then. They told me that at that gestational age, they only performed labor and delivery (L&D) terminations. I did not want an L&D, but felt I had no choice. I couldn't imagine laboring for hours to deliver a baby that was not meant for this world. I was heartbroken and unable to further research my options regarding location and type of termination. In the next five days I settled into a fog of sadness and tears. I was feeling my baby move and each kick was a literal stab in my gut. I threw out my prenatal vitamins and the two maternity shirts I had bought. I hid my *What to Expect When You're Expecting* book. It was no help to me now. I needed a "What to Expect When You're Going to Terminate a Pregnancy You Wanted So Badly" book. I spoke with my dad and my friends, and sent an e-mail to my siblings explaining what we were going through and asking them to not call me for awhile. I didn't want to talk to anyone except my dad and my mother-in-law. I made them my spokespersons and made everyone talk to them if they wanted to find out about me or pass me a message.

Tuesday morning rolled around. I now feel like I have total recall of every moment of that day. We went to the clinic and it was *not* what I was expecting. It had a large waiting area that was literally packed to overflowing. Each chair was occupied and I was given a clipboard with paperwork to fill out. I stood while I filled out the paperwork and looked around. The waiting room was populated with people that didn't seem to be waiting to abort their babies. There were obviously-young girls there with their friends or family, and there was a strange air of disconnect—like we were all waiting to get our teeth cleaned. There was a large television on in the waiting room and it was blaring an old episode of "Family Feud." After each un-guessed answer was revealed, the people in the room would repeat it like little cult members. "Name a food that would make you gain weight if you eat too much of it." As the answers would show on the screen, the people in the waiting room would echo "haaammmburrrggggerrrr" or "iiiccce crrreeeeaaammm." The floor was scratched linoleum, the chairs were mismatched plastic. The vertical blinds were broken or missing and none of us were allowed to bring purses or bags for fear of protesters bringing in contraband or worse. So there we all were, with our IDs in our pockets and our eyes glued to "Family Feud." It was at that moment when I heard a voice in my head, as clearly as I heard the people on television. It said, "Your son deserves better than this." I turned to my husband and said, "I need to get out of here." Without another word G and I put the unfinished paperwork on the counter and walked out.

I went home and called my OB and he gave me the name of a doctor that performs late-term terminations for medical reasons in the quiet solace of his office. I called that doctor's office and told them my situation. They told me to come in immediately. While I was on the way, they had my OB fax over my paperwork. When I arrived I found a regular OB/GYN practice with two clean, open waiting areas. One area was for the happily pregnant clients of the doctor, and the other room had a separate entrance and was for those women, like me, that had chosen to end their pregnancies.

I went in to see the doctor, who I'll call Dr. B. He had a technician perform an ultrasound on me to determine the age of the fetus and then had me wait my "turn." This place was quiet and I could tell that the doctor and his staff believed very strongly that the women who came to them deserved respect and compassion. The doctor was so kind and gentle and understanding. Also, he only did dilation and evacuation (D&E) terminations, saving me my fear of labor and delivery. He explained the procedure to me and asked if I had any questions. I broke down when I asked if my baby would feel anything. No, I would be under twilight sedation and the baby would be immediately sedated even before I felt the effects of the anesthesia. It would be a two-day procedure: laminaria to open the cervix on the first day and the actual procedure on the second day. After the exam and discussion, I was sent to wait in the waiting room until it was time for the laminaria insertion.

As I waited, I noticed a television was on in the waiting room. It was showing an old episode of "Yes, Dear" where the main fictional character was pregnant and was being filmed for the show "A Baby Story." Are you *kidding me*? *Seriously*? G had someone change the channel, but not before I had to see happy grandparents and happy parents and a happy birth. Yeah, thanks, that was nice.

Next, as we continued what seemed like a decade of waiting, G read over the lab results we brought with us and noticed something that made him question the accuracy of the test. It listed my DNA sample in two places and assigned that sample a number. He noticed the number was different in two places. He thought, "Oh my god, what if they tested the wrong sample? What if our baby *isn't* affected?" Get on your roller coaster, we're going for another ride. We had Dr. B call Dr. Idaho who in turn called the lab that did the testing. After 45 minutes which felt like a lifetime, the answer came back; the sample numbers we saw were blind numbers used to ensure that the tests were accurate and they tested two samples to ensure that the results were the same each time. So yes, indeed, the results were not only accurate, they were double tested and checked. I can't even begin to explain what it was like to sit and wait to hear those words. I'm very glad that every avenue was checked and I would not have been able to continue if I wasn't sure, but my heart was literally ground into a pulp to think that there may have been a reprieve and then learn that there was indeed no hope.

After that, there was no more waiting. While the laminaria was inserted I cried and cried. I heard one nurse whisper to another, "cystic fibrosis." Then that nurse came and held my hand and stroked my shoulder and hair while they continued with the insertion. They had to stop periodically as my uncontrollable sobs were making my muscles tense up very badly. Finally it was over. I got dressed and walked like a zombie out to the waiting room and into the arms of my husband. As G and I were going down in the elevator I let out a primal scream. I screamed for my son that was going to be gone the next day and for the life he should have had if he were healthy. I cried all the way home. Truthfully, what I refer to as "Laminaria Day" was worse than the actual procedure the following day. Not because of the pain, but because I had begun something that I couldn't stop. I couldn't fool myself that I would change my mind at the last minute. Even so, I knew that what I was doing was the right thing for my son. I was giving him a life of love and comfort and not allowing him a single moment of pain and suffering. It was the hardest thing I had ever done, but it was also the surest thing I had ever done. No one goes into that room undecided and if they say they are, they are kidding themselves. I don't believe that anyone ends a pregnancy if they are not 110 percent sure that what they are doing is right and good. However, knowing that and doing so with a light heart are two different things. My heart was heavy, my soul was bruised, and my spirit was broken. But my son would never know pain or fear and that is why we did it.

The following day we returned for the actual termination and, as I mentioned, it was not as bad as the previous day. When I awoke from the sedation, the nurse that had assisted in the laminaria insertion was sitting with me, holding my arm. She administered to me and, after some time, I was ready to go home. Home to heal, home to lick my wounds, and home to try to figure out how to go on.

The next week I never left my home. I would take long showers two and three times a day so I could cry unfettered without worrying if I would upset G. It felt like I was in the middle of some kind of weird grief hangover. I dreamed I was still pregnant and could feel my son moving. I have vivid memories of this time. Little vignettes that continue, even now, to play through my mind. I remember seeing G cutting our front yard through the window and stopping to speak to our next-door neighbor. I watched the pantomime of the neighbor smiling and asking how I was doing and then seeing her face fall as he told her we "lost" the baby. I remember answering the doorbell and finding another pair of neighbors smiling and holding a bouquet of flowers. They had just heard I was pregnant and were bringing me a congratulatory card and flowers. I was momentarily confused. I didn't know how to be gracious and informative at the same time. "Thanks, but I 'lost' the baby." They gave me the flowers and the card anyway. My belly was empty but I had a congratulations card celebrating a new life.

I remember preparing for Hurricane Katrina. We live in south Florida and she was heading our way less than two weeks after the termination. G was working and I had to summon up the strength to leave the house to get hurricane supplies. It was the first time I ventured out. I remember being in Home Depot, with my breasts leaking milk for a baby that was gone, and crying on the cell phone to my dad, sobbing, "But I can't find the damn thing!" Whatever it was I was looking for was either not where it should have been or not where my clouded eyes could find it. I don't know why I thought my dad, who lived five hours away, could help.

I remember going to dinner on my birthday and drinking wine. I hadn't had wine in five months. I didn't want wine, I wanted a healthy baby. I was measuring my life in terms of before the termination and after, of when I was pregnant and when I was not. I wanted to be normal. I wanted to not grieve. I wanted the pain and hurt to stop. I wanted to be whole again and I didn't know how to make that happen.

I searched for relief on my computer. (When all else fails, Google to the rescue!) I found an online support group for women like me that was like a light at the end of the tunnel. I had thought I was alone, but I was not. There were women out there just like me that were going through this journey. Those women offered me hope and friendship and understanding in a way my family and friends could not. I will be forever grateful for those women and the strength they were able to help me find in myself. For a short while, I truly thought I would go insane from the grief, but I did not. Each day I got a bit better, a bit stronger. I found I could still laugh. I could still smile. I could still hope.

During the summer, while I was getting my degree in genetics from the University of Google, I learned of a way to have a baby that would practically ensure a healthy CF-free outcome. I learned of a procedure called pre-implantation genetic diagnosis (PGD), which is done hand in hand with in vitro fertilization. I filed this information away in the back of my head and discarded it as being too expensive and too risky. I wasn't prepared emotionally or physically to even think about it. But one night after our termination, while lying with my husband in bed, he whispered to me, "You know, I've read about this thing called PGD…." Prior to that, I had no idea that he even knew about it or even cared to research it. I was wrong. He was hurting as much as I was and was pained to see me so devastated. He wanted a way to make me happy, to offer me hope, to fix in his own way what was broken. That one little sentence showed me how much he loved me, and how far he was willing to go to bring joy back to his wife.

I began to look into PGD in earnest. Basically, a woman goes through a regular IVF cycle, but before the embryos are transferred into her uterus, a single cell is removed from each one and is tested to ensure it isn't affected with the disease you're testing for; in my case we would test for cystic fibrosis. After the tests are done, only healthy embryos are transferred and if you're very lucky, one (or more) implants and you have a normal pregnancy after that point.

Shortly after my son's diagnosis I had pretty much decided we would be childfree. I knew that I could not go through another termination and I couldn't bear the thought of conceiving naturally now that I had the knowledge of what was at stake. After learning about PGD I began thinking about trying for a baby again, and it felt strange. I found a reproductive endocrinologist with PGD experience and met him for a consult. I was actually hoping he would talk me out of it. But I left there thinking that it was something we could do. Hey, I still had that fat severance package just itching to be blown on something, why not use it trying for hope? I did a lot of soul-searching and ultimately decided that I needed to honor my son's memory by taking the chance to have a healthy baby. We went through too much to give up. Here's where that foreshadowing comes in. Remember when I said I didn't want to be *that* woman who went crazy with the fertility treatments? Well, in order to ensure a healthy baby, that's what I became. With IVF, you jump in with both feet and go hog wild with syringes and drugs and calendars and hope. I went from a casual "let's just see what happens" kind of conception ideology to a crazy syringe-wielding, self-injecting IVF veteran.

I found myself back in a world of fighting percentages. There was a less than 40 percent chance of becoming pregnant, but even before you get to the point where healthy embryos are transferred, you have to pay your money and take your chances. Who knew I'd become a gambler? I had already lost so much counting on even better odds than that, why was I trying? Because I had to. I had to give my body the chance to carry a healthy baby. So what gave me the strength to go on and how did I know it would lead me first through despair and then to a happy ending? I didn't know, and I don't know where I got the courage to try. I gathered strength from my family, from my friends, and a great deal from the women I came to know in my online support group. But the truth is I think I needed to try. I needed to feel like I was actively participating in my own healing. I needed to fight for my happiness and fight to control my own destiny. I wanted to be able to say "I *made* this good thing happen" instead of "this bad thing happened to me." I wanted to be more than the sum of my grief and sadness. I wanted to be happy again and I wanted to believe that I deserved a happy ending.

This story does have a happy ending. We went for it, and after our first IVF cycle we learned we were indeed pregnant with a healthy baby boy. Our healthy son was born in November 2006. I often think of him as a gift that was given to us by the brother that came before him, for if it weren't for our first son, Christopher, we would not have the unbridled joy of being Justin's parents today. There's not a day that passes that I don't think of the son I let go, even as I hold and love the one I fought so hard to make. I would never ever want to go back to relive those dark days of the summer of 2005 again, but I will be forever grateful for the destination to which that rocky road brought me.

19

Jen's Story "My Greatest Gift"

One year ago today, I embarked on a journey that would change my life in ways I could never have possibly expected or imagined. One year ago today, I said goodbye to our baby girl, Emily Grace. Although I never got the chance to see her, to hold her, or to gaze at her tiny face, mysteriously, she has somehow managed to be responsible for shaping the person I am today. Her spirit lives within me, and with each day that passes, I am in awe at how she continues to bless me, to guide me, and to nourish my spirit with all that she illuminates for me. She is a gift, and I am honored that I was given the privilege of being touched by her love and by her short, yet profoundly significant life.

If you would have asked me one year ago where I thought I might find myself today, I am afraid that my answer would have painted a picture of a place in time containing little other than hopelessness, disbelief, and despair. It is hard to believe that an entire year has already passed since what I would easily consider the worst chapter of my life. After our heartbreaking choice, I was convinced that I was irreparably broken, and that I would never recover. No one could have told me otherwise. I had little faith that I would ever be happy again. What I did not realize back then, was that I was never quite as happy as I thought I was to begin with, and that I would learn so much in the short year to come.

When I reflect upon my experience, it seems strange to me that my faith in God did not waver. Each day, however, I certainly did endlessly question why it had happened to me. Each day I puzzled over what I could have possibly done in my life or another to deserve such pain. I cringed every time someone spoke the words "Everything happens for a reason," or "Don't worry, you can have another one," or "It just wasn't meant to be." On many days, I felt like I was just teetering on the edge of sanity, trying desperately to process what had happened. There could be no reason for it. There could not just be "another" Emily. If it was not meant to be, then why was she given to us only to be taken away? Was it arrogant of me to think that I was somehow supposed to be exempt from bad things happening to me? Maybe it was because until then, nothing "bad" had ever happened to me.

Each day I searched for solace, and was left empty when none came. I felt like it was on many levels, my failure, because I had let so many people down. From the beginning, I never completely bonded with the pregnancy. It was different somehow than when I was pregnant with my first daughter, Hannah. With this pregnancy I did not realize why I felt somewhat detached. When I now reflect back to that time, I think that maybe some part of me must have known all along that something was not right.

I felt as though I had let Steve, my husband, down. He so wanted the baby. I could almost physically feel his heart sink with a nearly audible thud upon his hearing the news that I would need to have another ultrasound, because "there was a problem." I can still see him sitting there in the chair in the corner of the ultrasound room with his knees apart, holding his head in his hands. Even worse, I felt as though I had let my daughter down. I had failed miserably, in a way that could not be fixed or taken back. I felt Hannah's heart break when we told her only days before her sixth birthday that the baby might have to go to Heaven to be with God. She so wanted a baby sister. I felt a pain like no other when she wrapped her arms around my waist, buried her face into my big pregnant belly, and sobbed as only one quiet word came out…"Baby…" I could not fix this.

As if coming to the dark realization that the child you are carrying in what you thought to be the safety and protection of your womb has something fatally wrong with her is not devastating enough, learning of what would have to happen to end her suffering was far harder to digest. We were told that I should not carry to term, that doing so posed serious risks to my health. Emily's condition was "100 percent fatal," and there was "0 percent survivability," meaning there was zero hope. We knew we would have to terminate the pregnancy. I was sure that it would be taken care of in a hospital, but that was not the case.

At nearly 22 weeks gestation, the procedure I was to have was considered a "late-term abortion." I would just make the cutoff to be able to still opt to have a dilation and evacuation (D&E) procedure. "No one does these here," we were told, as if no doctor in our entire metropolis wished to be associated with people like us, who were about to do what we planned on doing. I began to feel like I was the only one in the world that it had ever happened to, that it was somehow my fault, and that we were about to do something unspeakably wrong. "There's a doctor in another city that does these procedures, and we send everyone to him," we were matter-of-factly informed. "We've never heard any complaints about him. And by the way, your insurance won't cover this," added salt to the already painful wound, and "but you should appeal the bill from the clinic," offered no comfort whatsoever. I was numb with disbelief that it was even happening. We were given the clinic's information, and escorted out the back door of the perinatologist's office into the parking lot. I had never felt as alone as I did at that moment.

In the days leading up to our trip to the clinic, I felt as if I were almost mechanical, and that all of the non-crucial parts of me were switched off—like components of a circuit breaker or fuse box. I walked around as if my mind and body were relying on their auto-pilot functions, trying to appear as if life was perfectly normal in the surreal situation. I did housework, shopped for groceries, shopped for a blanket small enough for a nearly 22 week-old fetus, and made burial arrangements by phone for our baby. It was just like any other day after you find out that your baby is going to die. I look back to what seemed like an eternity, wondering how I was able to function. I still was not entirely convinced that it was truly happening. I remained unable to wrap my brain around it, and remained in a robotic state for as long as I could.

Steve and I arrived at the clinic. I had read stories of protesters, and was relieved when there were none outside. We were told beforehand that we could park behind the building if that was a concern.

I was dumbfounded by what was happening to me. How could it possibly be that a week before I was expecting a perfectly healthy baby to complete our perfectly normal, happy, uneventful life, and that day, I found myself sitting in the lobby of an abortion clinic waiting for my number to come up, as if I were at a counter in the Twilight Zone Deli? It was all so very wrong. Somewhere, somehow, the whole story had taken a very wrong turn. I looked at least seven months pregnant. I wanted to disappear.

I just wanted it to be over with. I prayed that God would just make her die inside of me, before I was forced to make the decision for her. It was not supposed to be up to me. Then the guilt swept over me. Over with? I just wanted to go home and be with my six-year-old little girl. I missed her. I reached into my pocket and felt the little purple crystal she had given me earlier that morning. It was attached to a necklace that was a thin black satin rope. It was the special one—one of her favorites. Before we left for the clinic, she had placed it in my hand, and then gently closed mine around it with hers before she kissed me goodbye. "Mommy, I want you to take this with you so you can remember me when you're at the doctor's." As if I could forget that sweet angel face of hers. She is so special and loves me like no one else can.

The night before, she had climbed up into my bed. I was feeling especially sorry for myself, and was trying to prepare myself for what was to come the next day. "Mommy, can I sleep in your bed?" she asked. "No, honey, Mommy is tired and needs to rest. You need to sleep in your own bed tonight," I told her gently. I was too tired to argue. Her big brown eyes welled up just enough to wet the bases of her thick, black, wing-like lower lashes. Her little pink lips formed the most perfect tiny rosebud, just like they had since the day she was born. I had instantaneously fallen in love with that little face. My thoughts then shifted to Emily. Would I ever see her face? "But Mommy," she said with an ever so slightly furrowed brow, her voice cracking just a tiny bit, "I was just thinking that if I laid here with you, I could hold your hand until you fall asleep. That way, it will make you be not so sad about the baby for a little while." "Okay, just for a little while," I said. How do you say no to that? There is no one like her. I am so blessed.

When it was my turn to go back, we were given several prescriptions to fill—one to help me relax, one to help me sleep, one for pain, and two antibiotics. We could leave and check into the hotel we were to stay at for the night. After we filled the prescriptions, we were to come back, after I had taken the one to help me relax. Then, we would fill out the paperwork, and they would start what was to be the first of the two-day procedure. On the first day, they would insert the laminaria, which were sticks made from seaweed, the nurse explained, into my cervix, to force dilation. Thankfully, I would be put out for it. At that time, they would insert a needle into my belly, and then into the baby's heart, and the medication would stop her heartbeat. Emily would not feel anything, because she would be asleep, just as I would be. The administrator asked how we would be paying for it. I gave her my debit card and signed the receipt. There was a receipt for it? When I came to, I was crying. We went back to the hotel to wait until the next day, when they would take her out.

That night was excruciating, both emotionally and physically. I became aware that my belly was still for the first time in weeks. I knew she was gone. I no longer felt her little kicks. There was no movement at all. The cramping began early that evening. I could not keep any pain medication down. I had a fever and chills, and could not stay warm. I was trembling from the pain, or maybe it was the fever. I could not sleep or get comfortable. When morning came, the cramping got worse. I got into the shower, wanting to just rinse the sweat off of me, thinking we could head to the clinic, and that they might agree to take me early. I vomited again in the shower, but nothing came out. When I looked down, there was clotted blood in the tub. I figured then that I might be in labor, and prayed that I would not deliver in the hotel room. I got dressed and waited on my knees with my body bent over the bed for

Steve to get back from taking our bags down to the car. I was definitely having contractions now. When he returned, he helped me down the hallway, where we were greeted by the stares of a few of the housekeeping crew, then down the stairs, and into the car. I could tell he was scared, but we did not talk about it on the car ride over to the clinic.

When we arrived at the clinic, they took me back right away. I said one last prayer…"God, please don't let me die…" When it was over, I asked to see her. The nurse told me that because I had spiked a high fever and became combative during the procedure, they had to work quickly. I had not dilated enough. She told me I kept thrashing and kicking, pulling my IVs out several times. "We weren't able to keep her intact," she said. Groggy from the sedation, I said that I still wanted to see her. I cried and asked her why they could not just cover up the bad parts and let me see her.

The nurse then told me, very gently, yet very bluntly, that all of the parts were bad, and that she would be unrecognizable as a baby. Although she advised strongly against it, she reluctantly offered to bring her parts out to me on the tray they had her on if I still needed to see her. A tray? My baby was in parts on a tray? Again, I shrank away from reality. Steve pleaded with me to stop pursuing it, and I did. The doctor left for a moment, then came back from around the corner, holding his cell phone. He had taken pictures of her, with only her feet showing on the screen. In his own way, he was trying to console us, I think. We looked at the pictures. Her feet were small and red. One was bigger than the other, and the smaller foot was not fully formed. He said that it was one of the more severe cases of skeletal dysplasia he had seen. It was textbook, in fact. The nurse later offered to personally drive Emily's remains to the funeral home. It did not really matter.

The day of the funeral, my milk decided to come in. One last sick joke nature had to squeeze in, as if I could take anymore. I stood in the shower and wept. My soul had never felt as empty as it did at that moment. Did I even still have a soul? I was not certain. It just would not stop, would it? Each time during the experience, when I thought I had reached my lowest point, somehow, something managed to drag me down deeper, to a depth that I never knew existed.

I got out of the shower and tried to get dressed. What the heck was I supposed to wear? I stood in the closet, looking down at my once pregnant belly, which still looked deceptively pregnant, while milk dripped onto the carpet. I stared at the tiny red puncture mark where the needle had been inserted in my belly just days before to stop Emily's heart. Why didn't I think about buying something to wear earlier that week? I felt dizzy and weak as I rifled impatiently through my closet. Everything was either obviously maternity, or too small. I pulled out a dress from the back rack. I had splurged and bought it about a month earlier at the Motherhood shop to wear at Emily's baby shower, which was to be given by my childhood friend for me in just a few weeks. It was a black sundress, with little white dots. Just underneath the bust line was a thin pink satin ribbon, tied neatly in a bow. It was perfect. How perfectly ironic it was that I was putting on a dress that I was supposed to wear to my child's baby shower, to instead wear to her funeral. Again, I reassured myself that it could not possibly be really happening, so what did it matter?

After I was dressed, I looked at myself in the bathroom mirror. I looked like a corpse. My eyes were dull, my face pale and gray as stone. I felt brittle and as fragile as an old empty eggshell. I began to have thoughts of what was to transpire at the funeral. If anyone picked up on my mental state, or saw me break down, they would surely think that I was an unfit mother, and would try to take Hannah from me. I could not let that happen. To prevent such a breakdown, I went to the medicine cabinet and took what I recall to be at least one of every prescription I was given from the clinic. That would do the job nicely. That would surely numb me to the point that I could not feel, and if I could not feel, then I could remain composed. My only concern would be to get through the service without vomiting, falling, or passing out. I could do that. I was a good mother.

At the service I felt as if I were in a thick fog. As we sat in the front of the chapel, I stared at her tiny casket, which was draped with a spray of beautiful tiny pink roses that my mother had insisted on getting for her. It was incomprehensibly tiny. I heard a baby cry in the background. I thought I was beginning to lose my grip. How could I be sure that she was really in there? Should I ask them to check one last time? Did they wrap her in the quilt I had given them? Did they swaddle her remains neatly like how I would have done? If she was in pieces, did they arrange them the right way? Did they put all of her in there? What would the right way even be? Did they place something around her body to keep it from rolling about when they put it in the car to drive her to the cemetery? Please God, do not let her be in a baggie. Did any of it really matter at this point? I went to a place in my mind, where no one should ever go. I avoided eye contact with anyone for the most part. A part of me felt strangely ashamed. I was not sure why. I could barely focus. I still felt feverish and clammy. Hannah was cold. They had the air conditioner set too low in the chapel. I wrapped Hannah up in my sweater and hugged her tight against my side. I had to be strong for her, yet she was my anchor that was keeping me from drifting out of reality. She looked so pretty that day.

We proceeded to the cemetery, where the rabbi struggled as he searched for a few more words of consolation and wisdom. There was nothing more to say. Then we left. I could not bear to stay to see her being lowered into the ground. I could not watch the dirt go on top of her. It looked like it was going to rain. I had a vision of her grave being filled with mud. I was at my threshold. I needed to leave. The funeral director picked one of the small pink roses from her casket and handed it to me. "I thought you might want to keep one of these," she said. Some people came back to the house, had something to eat and drink, and left. My medication was starting to wear off by then. So that was it? It was over? Now what?

The hours, the days, the weeks, and the months following have been an epic adventure to say the very least. It has been a spiritual journey for me, as well as a spiritual awakening. I never would have dreamed that the one thing I would gain from the experience would be gratitude. But that is exactly the gift I have been given by all of it. While it has been the single most painful event in my life, as well as my single greatest loss, on the other side of that same coin is that it has also been my single greatest gift.

I feel Emily's spirit in me. She is with me always and in all ways. She is a part of my past, my present, and my future. She is part of the very different person that I was just one year ago. She is a part of the person I am today, and she will be a part of the person I hope to become. Sometimes, on a quiet day, I can feel her brush my cheek when the wind blows. Other times, when a butterfly crosses my path, and then lingers for longer than usual, I am convinced that it is her.

The life lessons that have emerged from the ashes of my pain are immeasurable. I want to share just a few of them with you. Life is not fair. Things do not happen for a reason. No one is immune from suffering. When something terrible like that happens, something that knocks the wind out of you, making you certain you have reached your threshold for pain, asking why won't change it. Knowing why won't change it. However, you can change, and you can choose to find the message in all of it. Otherwise, this awful thing has had no meaning. Emily's life would have had no meaning. I refuse to accept that.

I have learned to be more compassionate. I now try my best to refrain from judging others. I have realized that I do not know what I would do in someone's situation until I am faced with her situation. I may have an idea of what I would do, but I know now that I cannot truly know. I have learned to be a better friend. When I see that someone needs help, I reach out and make my greatest effort to be there for her in whatever way I can. By helping others, I have realized that I can heal myself. I have learned to love myself unconditionally. I have realized that by loving myself, there is more of myself to give. The more I give of myself, the more I find that I receive in return. That is the only way I know how to make any sense of all of it.

It has all come full circle, starting with a passage I read one year, as I felt helpless and hopeless. I printed these words off my computer, and I keep them with me at all times. They are like sacred scripture to me:

"Many people voice the thought, 'I will never be the same person again' as if that is so terrible. Let me offer a reframe for that comment. No, you will never be the same again...You must believe that there is now a greater purpose in your life... your baby's spirit is with you always. Honor that spirit by living well. Seek to grow in compassion and understanding for others. Renew your faith in your Creator. Reach out and give back. The love you felt for your baby will always be with you, and you can turn that love around and with it, be there for others in this sometimes heartless world. Find the message. I guarantee it is there waiting for you."

I like to think that I have found the message, or at least a small portion of it. I have faith that I will continue to receive the remainder of the message as time continues to heal my heart. I am willing to listen. I am happy to say that I am living well. And for the first time in my life, I believe I have found what it truly means to be happy. It cannot go without mentioning that there are still days when I struggle. I have accepted that there will always be days that are difficult, and that happiness and contentment take hard work, as does everything that is worth having in this life. It has taken a lot of work and looking inward to get to the point where I have been able to see that out of my deepest sorrow was born my greatest inner peace. I can say today with confidence that I know who I am, and I know the kind of person I want to be. All I can hope is that I continue to evolve as an eternal student of life and to give of myself. I am a work in progress.

And to think that all of this is because of one perfect tiny soul who left her beautiful, indelible footprint on my heart. Emily Grace. I love you. You will always be my butterfly. Today I let you go, with the peace of knowing that I need not say goodbye. Be free.

20

Jennifer's Story "Expecting"

Wednesday after work I got my blood drawn. The doctor had explained—
something about birth defects—but I wasn't concerned with the details.
I expected that my first baby would be healthy. My biggest worry on the
way home from my last appointment was that we decided not to find out
the baby's gender, yet we had a nursery to decorate! Yellow for the walls?
White and pale green for the nursery bedding? I had made it into the second
trimester. Four months of morning sickness were starting to give way to the
thrill of anticipation with late-night Internet forays into the world of crib
bedding and baby registries.

When I got home from work Friday evening, my doctor had left me a
voice mail. The sound of his voice made me feel dizzy. What was that test for?
I called the answering service. To my surprise, the doctor called me back even
though it was after 6:00 PM. He told me that my test came back with odds
of one in 10 for Down syndrome. A level II ultrasound and amniocentesis
were scheduled for Tuesday. He tried to be reassuring. I sat on the kitchen
floor and felt my heart sinking beneath me into the hardwood floor, through
the concrete and into the earth. My husband counted out nine dish towels
and then a 10th to show me what 'nine out of ten' looks like—a 90 percent
chance all is well! He scolded me for not having a more positive outlook. I
stayed on the kitchen floor and stared at the legs of the kitchen table, trying
without success to pull my heart back up from below.

Saturday we went to the hardware store and out to lunch, trying to keep
busy.

Sunday I went to the library. As I paced through the aisles trying to
distract myself from the knot of worry in my chest, I thought about giving
my baby a bath. Even if there's something wrong, I could still give the baby
a bath. I thought of my husband and his dishtowels and forced a smile to

myself. Shaking off the dread for a moment, I started making a list of baby bath things I would need: baby towels, washcloths, shampoo, baby wash, a rubber ducky and of course a little plastic tub.

Monday I called in sick and stayed in my pink fleece maternity pajamas on the floor in the nursery, listening to the Christmas lullabies that my friend had recently sent for the baby. It was only September but I thought the Christmas spirit could help.

Tuesday we woke up in darkness. The baby was hungry—my stomach growled urgently so I ate cereal, the kind I had specially picked out to make sure the baby would get plenty of nutrients. We drove to the doctor's office and waited. When it was finally our turn, the ultrasound technician was quiet as she poked my belly so she could get a better view. "The baby's all bunched up," she explained. Muddled shapes flashed on the screen as she pointed out the heart, fingers, brain, leg, spine, and the fingers again. But the technician wouldn't look at us. I asked if everything looked okay and she said she wasn't trained to interpret the results. My heart was frozen still; I held my breath.

The doctor came in and looked me in the eye through his black-rimmed round glasses. I searched his expression, trying to prepare myself for what was about to come out of his mouth: "There are complications." The medical terms that followed seemed to be slurred into a shapeless mix of syllables. I asked him to repeat the words: cystic hygroma and signs of a chromosomal problem, and the baby will pass in a matter of days or weeks.

My husband squeezed my hand hard. His question sounded like an accusation: "What do you mean by 'pass'?" I responded flatly without meeting his eyes, "He means the baby is going to die." I looked up at the doctor, "Definitely die?" He nodded and said, "The fluid is filling her lungs and her stomach, see there? See that right there? Fluid filling her lungs. It's consistent with Down syndrome or Turner syndrome."

I looked at my husband but still couldn't meet his eyes. I bought cereal for this baby and I didn't drink caffeine and I walked and I ate salad. And still I couldn't make her right. I started to shake with grief and rage.

The doctor said, "These situations always have happy endings, I swear they do, you'll see, you'll have a healthy baby, you will." The rest of his words started to pile on top of each other: here are your options for now, you should really have the amnio, you'll regret it if you don't and we can't tell if it's a boy or girl because it's so bunched up in there, I'm telling you these stories have happy endings. Eventually they took us out the back entrance; I guess so people wouldn't hear me. I sat down on the elevator floor, shaking harder with each floor we passed on the way down until we reached the bottom and my husband had to lift me with both arms so I could stand.

I talked to several doctors that day in order to get multiple opinions. They were extremely supportive of me. I felt that my baby was suffering since she was essentially suffocating and starving to death and stood no chance of survival. So my mind was made up. It was killing me to think of her suffering and I wanted to proceed quickly.

Hours later, a different doctor studied my face for a brief moment before beginning his work. He explained the procedure and then went about the business of starting to dilate my cervix.

Wednesday we woke up in darkness and went to the hospital. I couldn't stop crying even to say my name to the nurse. It was raining and I wore a white maternity shirt and maternity jeans. When I woke up from surgery I asked if the baby's heart had already stopped beating and I heard hushed voices saying in unison, "It was very slow, very slow." A nurse leaned in close to my head and said, "Honey this happened to me, and a year to the day later, I had a healthy baby." This was the first moment that it had yet occurred to me that I wasn't the only one on earth to endure this kind of loss.

When we got home, I stared out the window at the leaves on the neighbors' trees turning red. I didn't leave the house for two weeks and the leaves were brown by then. All I remember of those weeks is that I didn't like the night because it meant that morning would come and I would have to wake up. I hated waking up because I had to endure that split second of not remembering, then remembering. The remembering would come from my gut—not from my womb, but from my stomach, which was no longer hungry. Daily I curled up on the nursery floor and cried, shaking for hours at a time.

A few months later, I woke up hungry again. I bought healthy cereal again, and I didn't drink caffeine and I walked and I ate salad. This time I did not expect that everything would turn out fine, and yet it did. On the first anniversary of our angel's death, we celebrated our healthy newborn daughter's five-week "birthday."

Slowly my heart has ascended from the earth beneath the kitchen floor, up through the concrete and back into life, pulled up from above. With each passing year, I have expected that my grief will diminish, time will heal, and new babies will erase my first daughter's memory. But this has not been the case. My angel lives with me, in me, around me, in my daughters, in the paint on the nursery wall, in the blankets and the books that we had bought her. I feel her near me always, and I know that she knows that we let her go so she would be free from the pain she was enduring. While I no longer expect that everything will turn out right just because I expect that it will, our angel taught us to believe that out of darkness light will come eventually.

21

Jenny's Story "It is Not the Length of Life, But the Depth of Life"

I first learned of my pregnancy in February 2007. I came home from the grocery store one day, promptly ate an entire tub of potato salad, and then passed out asleep without even putting the rest of the groceries away. That was my "Aha!" moment, and soon after I bought a home pregnancy test, although I didn't really think I could be pregnant. The line turned blue very quickly, and I ran to the bedroom to wake up my husband. We were both so happy. He couldn't stop smiling and I, although worried about becoming a first-time parent, was so happy that my time to be somebody's mom was coming.

I was told by my OB/GYN that everything was going "perfectly," and we soon told family and friends about the pregnancy. Everyone was very happy for us. My husband and I decided to go on one last vacation to Palm Springs before we had children. The entire weekend was filled with conversations of our future, what our child would be like, and if it were a boy or girl. I suspected it was a boy, but my husband, Jeff, suspected twin girls. My hCG levels, which tell the body to prepare for a pregnancy, were very high and my OB/GYN told us that could indicate a multiple pregnancy. Hearing that, of course, both terrified and excited me.

The happiest day of my pregnancy was during my first ultrasound. The ultrasound technician had the screen turned away from me, but my husband could still see it. I almost did not mind that I couldn't see the screen because I was able to watch my husband's face. He was engrossed in that screen, and probably didn't notice me watching his unfettered happiness. After a few moments, he turned away long enough to mouth the word "one" and raise up his index finger. I was so happy; we had our own family.

The gifts and well wishes began. We received many wonderful and thoughtful gifts from family and friends. Our happiness and excitement grew, and I very much looked forward to the second trimester when I wouldn't feel so exhausted and sick. I was ready to put on my maternity clothes, and I bought a small stuffed monkey for my little baby that was to be coming in October.

As a librarian I read voraciously, although sometimes I felt like too much information would worry me needlessly. I happened upon a pregnancy book which I liked very much because of the color pictures. Jeff and I looked at the book every week to see how our baby had changed. In the book, they mentioned something that seemed to be a standard test called a nuchal translucency (NT). As Jeff and I were leaving after a routine appointment with my OB/GYN, I casually asked the doctor in the hall, "So next time we do the nuchal translucency?" He said, "We don't do them here but will schedule you for one. They aren't really *routine* but we can get you an appointment. It has to been done in a certain time window so we need to get you in right away."

I approached the date of the NT test with much apprehension, and even wrote in my online journal about the "feeling of dread" I got when I thought about it. I received the normal, "Oh you'll be fine, you're just worried" type of responses from people. I almost cancelled the NT test three or four times, but I didn't.

The day of our NT, Jeff and I were looking forward to learning our baby's sex and didn't worry about anything being wrong. The ultrasound began; our baby was very still and had to be thumped a bit to get a good reading of the nuchal translucency. The technician informed us that our baby had a high reading and that we would have to wait to discuss it with the perinatologist. At that point, we did not feel a sense of urgency so we waited patiently. The doctor came in and informed us that our baby appeared very swollen and sick. He told us that the high nuchal translucency reading could have been indicative of Turner syndrome or some other genetic defect.

Both my husband and I were in shock. At one point I said, "This is heartbreaking." The doctor said there were three choices; to do nothing, to terminate the pregnancy, or to do further testing. We opted for further testing and requested a chorionic villus sampling (CVS) test. The doctor left. My guttural sobs and screams must have terrified the other expectant mothers in the waiting room. Those screams were the sound of my heart breaking. The days after were very much a blur.

In the days before and after the CVS, my husband and I took walks, did as much research as we could, and talked about our future. During one of our walks, I placed my hand on my belly and said, "Goodbye Peanut." Jeff and I both broke down in tears and mourned for the first time, knowing we were saying goodbye to our dream of a healthy baby.

During that emotionally charged time there were enumerable pressures, like our next visit to the perinatologist for the CVS. The CVS was equally emotionally and physically painful.

Physically, it was difficult for the doctor to get a sample. He tried to get a transcervical sample but could not. Unfortunately, I had a very sensitive cervix. The feeling of a slight "pinch," as it is described in medical literature, was inaccurate in my experience.

After many very painful attempts transcervically, the doctor opted for the transabdominal method. It was not very painful at all. The ultrasound screen was turned off at my request; I felt I could not face the sight of my sick baby. The doctor was very patient and, upon leaving, his nurse gave us an informational handout which included the Internet address for the *A Heartbreaking Choice* support web site.

Waiting for the CVS results was a terrifying and horrible time. The genetic counselor called me at work to give me the results. My baby had trisomy 18.

Trisomy 18 involves an extra copy of chromosome number 18, which can severely affect all organ systems of the body. Many times there are severe cardiac and/or renal malformations. Only five to 10 percent of babies with trisomy 18 survive to their first birthday.

There isn't a way to fully or accurately describe our tragedy. Jeff and I spent many days and nights crying inconsolably and searching for answers that weren't there. "Why did this happen to us? What is best for our baby? How on earth can we let our baby go? How can we let him live? Why can't we fix this?"

We both felt compelled to let our baby go before he felt any pain from his disabling disease. Peanut died on April 1st, 2007 at 13 weeks and three days gestation.

I think it is important for parents to know there really is no right way to get through a tragedy such as ours. I live with regret, but I believe I would regret it immeasurably more had I borne my son and watched him exist in pain. I feel that parents who lose a child by termination for medical reasons are not truly ever given a chance to grieve publicly, mainly I believe, due to the stigma placed on termination. At 13 weeks and three days, I wasn't given an opportunity for labor and delivery, but had a dilation and extraction (D&E) procedure. I was less fearful of that choice. I had to fight very hard to get a hospital termination with full sedation and to have my insurance company cover it. I had to deal with a genetic counselor who wanted to tell me the grave news and then farm me off to a clinic to be someone else's problem. I had to listen to the genetic counselor talk on the phone with an abortion clinic in a casual and cheerful way, all the while ignoring the pleas of my husband and myself to have a D&E under full sedation, something the clinic did not offer. At the worst time in a parent's life they are often forced to be their own advocate, when their strength is at its weakest.

My family helped in any way they could. My sisters called with advice and sent food and cards. My father sent us a beautiful note telling us how "helpless" he felt, and donated a substantial amount of money to help us with the ever-increasing medical bills. My mother visited and listened to me cry. They dealt with my eccentric and uncontrollable grief in the best way they could. During my journey of grief I found support in some unexpected and wonderful places, and found zero support in other places where I had expected it.

I realize I was fortunate to have found out about Peanut's problem so early in my pregnancy, when a hospital termination was still possible. I was fortunate to figure out some creative insurance coding so I didn't have a medical bill of $10,000 during the worst time of my life.

There were so many issues that came up so quickly for us, and there was no way to know how to do everything right. When termination is chosen, there is so much pressure to do it all as soon as possible. My main regret is not having Peanut's remains. I have learned that it's possible he was so small that he simply evaporated during cremation, so that is what I choose to believe.

The Saturday before I went to the hospital for my D&E, I had to take a pill called Cytotec. I held in my hand the pill that would start the process of severing my baby physically from my body. At the insistence of mothers who I met on the *BabyCenter Termination for Medical Reasons* message board, I fought my natural reaction to distance myself from him. It was the best advice I had ever gotten. I held the pill and cried and talked to my Peanut. I asked for Peanut's permission to let him go now and the answer was yes. I had been bleeding for almost a week prior to that and I felt he was already trying to leave me.

The day I lost Peanut, I was blessed to have a nurse that shared her own personal story of losing a baby at five months. She took wonderful care of me. She was a good, caring and understanding person. I believe there is a special connection between mothers of deceased babies. When you have the strength to speak of your own story, you find that many other mothers have broken hearts too. That is the silent grief of mothers.

It has not yet been a year since Peanut left us. The only proof I have of his existence is an ultrasound picture and our memories. The world is not kind to grieving people and even less kind to parents who were forced to make hard decisions in this not so black-and-white realm.

Peanut's existence has changed our lives considerably. After living through a tragic event, I learned there is a whole other world filled with people who suffer. I think about my son every day.

My husband and I planted a tree in the local park where we previously strolled, dreaming of Peanut's life. He is honored with a plaque with his name and my favorite quote, "It is not the length of life, but the depth." by Ralph Waldo Emerson. Jeff and I now go to the same park and mourn Peanut.

22

Jess' Story "I Miss Them Both"

My husband and I decided after much pondering that we were finally at a place in our lives where a child would make it complete. I was 31 years old and he was 34 years old, we had just bought a house, and it just seemed right all of a sudden. After only two months of trying I became pregnant. I will never forget that first pregnancy test.

We were going out with friends the next evening and I decided to take a pregnancy test because I didn't want to drink any alcohol if I could be pregnant. Not giving it much thought I took the first test, left the bathroom, and forgot it. Fifteen minutes later I went in and saw two lines. My heart was in my throat! I figured it must have been positive because it sat for too long. Two tests later with positive results and I was out of my mind. I couldn't believe it had happened so soon and I wanted to tell the world. My husband was at work and I was very hesitant to tell him over the phone so I called my doctor. I worked as a nurse and I was pretty close to the girls in the office and to my doctor. They were all excited for us. Since I had already taken three home pregnancy tests they told me I didn't need to come in. They made my first appointment for a few weeks from then to do the blood work. After about two hours I couldn't hold it in anymore and I called my husband. He was in shock. Too cute! So that he could see the words "pregnant" on the test stick I went out and bought a digital pregnancy test.

That whole night we just looked at each other saying we couldn't believe it. We wasted no time and called our parents. My stepmother was not so nice, telling me (in a very unkind way) that I shouldn't be telling people I was pregnant so soon because something bad would happen (little did she know how right she'd be.) I stopped talking to her at that point. There were many other reasons but that was the icing on the cake. The next night at dinner we announced to our friends our good news. They were shocked because no one thought we planned to have kids, but they were all very supportive.

So the months passed and we were happy. I was nervous a lot. For some reason I felt the need to pray that the baby would be okay all of the time. I also had really bad shortness of breath and, even though my doctor said it was normal, I was in fear for my life over it. I knew most of those emotions were normal in pregnancy. At what would turn out to be our final prenatal visit, my doctor asked when we wanted to go for our first ultrasound. I wanted to go right then. All I wanted to know was if it was a boy or a girl. I could have sworn it was a boy (I ended up being wrong). We couldn't go that day, Wednesday, but there was an opening on Friday. We grabbed it. If I had known then what I know now, I would have gone for the ultrasound on the following Monday.

So off we were for our first ultrasound at 18 weeks. We went in and saw our little baby on the screen moving around like a wild one. The technician was quiet and seemed to take forever. I saw things on the screen that looked strange to me, like extra digits on the hands (polydactyly), but hoped I just didn't know what I was looking at. Then the technician left the room, came back, and said she needed more pictures. I knew right then something was very wrong. She took the pictures, printed our ultrasound photos, and said we needed to speak to our doctor. So we arrived at his office, he looked morbid and said "Please have a seat." I hate those words. They never mean anything good. They were the first words I heard after my mother died when I was 17 years old.

He went on to tell us about all of the anomalies that were seen on the ultrasound which likely pointed to a diagnosis of trisomy 13: holoprosencephaly, no forebrain, calcified kidneys, no stomach, polydactyly, severe heart defects, and cleft lip and palate. The only words I really remembered hearing at that point were "not compatible with life." My husband and I cried so loudly in his office and so did my doctor (he had lost his own child just a few months prior.) Before I even learned anything else about the diagnosis, I knew in my heart what we must do. My doctor arranged an appointment for a level II ultrasound at the prenatal diagnostic center. It was Friday and they couldn't see us until the following Wednesday. The waiting was pure torture. I prayed harder than I ever had; I bargained with God…you name it. It didn't work.

We went in for the level II ultrasound and the likely diagnosis was confirmed. It looked like trisomy 13. We spoke to a genetic counselor and made our decision right there in her office. We chose to do a dilation and evacuation (D&E) termination. Neither of us could bear to go through labor and delivery and see our very broken daughter. I pray she forgives us for that. I almost feel like I was weak by not being able to see her, but I knew I would not recover well from that. We had a picture of her in our minds we wanted to keep. Also, I never wanted to associate labor and delivery with death.

Our parents had come with us to the ultrasound appointment and my dad drove us home. My husband and I couldn't see straight. Our world became a very realistic version of hell. We never knew something like this could happen; no one ever talked of such things. Even being a student nurse, this was never covered in my obstetrics course.

After the level II ultrasound we had to wait another week for the D&E. During that time we chose to have an amniocentesis done because we wanted to make sure that our genes didn't cause the problem and because we wanted to know the gender of our baby. The gender was the only thing they couldn't see on the ultrasound. The amniocentesis results revealed that our child did have trisomy 13.

My local hospital was a Catholic one, which I had not previously known, and they refused to help us with making our heartbreaking choice. My doctor to this day is fighting them tooth and nail regarding their refusal, and I wrote a letter to the president of the hospital expressing in great detail my anger and disappointment.

We had to go to a clinic. The doctor at the clinic was highly recommended and regarded, so at least I had that to comfort me.

It took three days to complete the D&E termination. Because of my age and not having any prior children, my cervix was very tight. My doctor had to insert laminaria sticks twice. I found it to be very painful and scary. I was put on a table with my legs strapped down in a freezing cold room. The table was raised way up and tilted back. The girl (all of about 21 years old) who was supposed to be counseling me held my hand. I wasn't even allowed to have my husband with me. Then the doctor stuck a needle into my cervix and put the laminaria in. It happened just like that—both days. Those two nights were filled with pain, sadness, and fear. My husband kept his hand on my stomach the entire ride to the clinic on the last day, saying goodbye to our baby.

On that last day we encountered protestors saying "You have options." Yes, and we were exercising one of those options. We walked past them into the waiting room full of teens. I got called into the back, was put under anesthesia and woke up with a bunch of other women in the recovery room. I felt like I was in a factory. They gave me medication to clamp my cervix down, took my vitals and then told me to get up to put my clothes on.

When I stood up blood gushed everywhere. I left a trail of blood to the bathroom, my socks were soaked with it; the nurse just said "Don't worry, it happens all the time." I was dizzy and felt mortified as I tried to clean the blood off of me and the floor. I threw my socks into the trash. I was handed written instructions and sent out the door. I was high from the anesthesia most of the day, but when it wore off the grief was overwhelming. I wasn't pregnant anymore and I felt so unbelievably empty.

We had our memorial service a week after our heartbreaking choice. It was beautiful and healing and both my husband and I felt like we had closure.

We have a place to go to feel close to Hailey, which was what we named our daughter. It's been a few months now and each day gets better. I tend to move through grief quickly, having been through it many times in my life.

It will always hurt, just not as frequently, and some days are worse than others. Not a day goes by where I don't think about my daughter and what should have been. I should be fat and happy right now. I should have my little girl. While I think of these things I also realize the reality being what it is. She is gone and I will meet her again one day. Until then, she is with her grandma. I am crying right now. God, I miss them both.

23

Jessica's Story "Our Brief But Bright Light"

It has been almost seven weeks since I terminated my pregnancy with my son Conner, at 22 weeks. There are some things that have already gotten easier to handle. There are other feelings that I am dealing with which I never fathomed when we made the decision to end the pregnancy.

I think I always knew something was wrong with the pregnancy. I felt it, but I wasn't at all prepared for it. I had a healthy two-year-old daughter, and the two pregnancies couldn't have been any more different. With my daughter, I knew exactly when I became pregnant. With Conner, I was nearly eight weeks along before I had to go to the doctor's office to figure out how far along I was. I had lost my father to lung cancer two days after we had conceived Conner. I was so distraught about my loss that I wasn't paying attention to my body and missed all the pregnancy signs. We had just started trying to get pregnant prior to losing my father, but hadn't thought it would happen so quickly. Another difference between the two pregnancies was that with my daughter, I felt sick the entire nine months. With Conner, I never felt sick. When I went in for my check-ups, the doctor would ask me if I had any complaints. I always told her my only complaint was that I didn't 'feel' pregnant and that it worried me.

It was a high risk pregnancy because I have Type 1 (insulin dependent) diabetes. I spent six months before each pregnancy working on my blood sugar levels and getting the okay from my doctors before we started trying to get pregnant. Diabetics' babies have a higher heart defect rate, among other possible complications. I believe I would have been more prepared had that been Conner's diagnosis, but that was not the case. During our level II ultrasound at 19 weeks, the technician left the room to summon the doctor.

I understood that it was standard procedure for the doctor to be the one to review the results with the parents, but we were left alone in the exam room for a very long time. I commented to my husband that something must have been wrong and even during the small talk once the doctor arrived, I was dreading the worst. We were told the baby's long bones, those in the arms and legs, were measuring at five weeks behind. We were told that it was most likely a condition called skeletal dysplasia, but we were given no more information at that point.

My husband and I had met at the hospital after work for the ultrasound and therefore had two separate cars. The ride home for me was long and lonely after getting the news of our baby's issues. At that point I was thinking we would have a special needs child and my thoughts centered on what affect that would have on my two-year-old daughter's life. I also spent time pondering whether God had played a role in our recent move to a new colonial-style home that had one bedroom on the main floor. Maybe we had sold our previous home and found this one for a reason?

Once I arrived home, however, with the help of the Internet, my husband and I discovered that skeletal dysplasia was not what we had been imagining. The prognosis ranged from a healthy, but disproportionately short-statured person to fatal. The more we read, the more dire our outlook became. It was at that point that we read one web site which recommended that medical termination of pregnancy should be offered to all parents in this situation. I was so naïve before then that I hadn't even realized parents had the option to terminate a pregnancy due to a poor prenatal diagnosis. And I had absolutely no idea it could be done so late in pregnancy.

It was impossible to sleep that night for both my husband and I. I had irrational fears that God would somehow punish me for even considering termination. I worried that something would happen to my husband and daughter. I hoped and prayed the original diagnosis was wrong, even though I myself could tell the long bones didn't look quite right on the ultrasound.

It took about a week before we could get in for additional testing—the longest week of my life. Testing included a fetal MRI and many more ultrasounds, including 3D. The size of the baby's chest is the determining factor in whether or not skeletal dysplasia is fatal. Our baby's chest size continued to measure borderline. We were told that there are hundreds of types of skeletal dysplasia and that they would be unable to give us a definite diagnosis until after the baby was delivered. Not knowing was incredibly stressful on us. We wanted answers and all we could be given was speculation.

The hospital had us participate in a Multidisciplinary Conference. It was me, my husband, a genetic counselor, my Maternal Fetal Specialist doctor, a Fetal Imaging expert, a Pediatric Genetics doctor and two social workers. We also asked my mother-in-law and father-in-law to attend with us. Before the conference, my husband and I had discussed termination as an option. One moment I would be leaning toward it and he would be leaning away. The very next moment we both would have switched sides. We were so unsure at that point that we wanted more opinions and we knew my in-laws would have only our best interests at heart. We were positive they would support our decision either way. We were grateful to have them there because my father-in-law was able to get the doctors to admit that they were confident the baby would not survive. We had been hoping for that honest admission because many of our questions about the prognosis had been met with vague answers due to the complexities of distinguishing the differences between the different types of skeletal dysplasia.

The day at the hospital for the conference was bittersweet. We were in a conference room getting the worst news of our lives and, at the same time, my sister-in-law was upstairs in labor and delivery. My in-laws, no doubt, were on a roller coaster of emotion that day. My sister-in-law was sympathetic to our situation and was nice enough to assure us that she understood if we did not make it to the hospital to meet the new baby. We still went to visit the next day though, and it was surprisingly easy for me. I couldn't have been happier to have an adorable, healthy new nephew. And I certainly couldn't let pregnant ladies or babies upset me. In addition to my newborn nephew, I had two acquaintances due the day after my due date, two close friends due two weeks after me, and my very best friend was due a month after me. I don't resent those ladies at all. If anything, I fear that my situation may have made them worry about their own babies. All women deserve to have a blissful, worry-free pregnancy. No one should face the possibility that their baby could die.

My husband and I had about two weeks to decide whether to terminate or not. People had started commenting that I was looking pregnant and I would politely grin. People were asking me how the ultrasound went and I would ignore them. I would shut my office door for hours and just cry. I would cry my whole commute home from work daily. I would cry every time my daughter cried. Sometimes I could hide it, other times I could not.

We wavered back and forth on our decision, but once we confirmed that no organs from our baby could be donated, we decided to terminate. There was almost a sense of relief when the decision had been made. There were so many unknowns over the last three weeks that it was good to know what was going to happen. We were in control of our lives after weeks of spinning wildly. However, the feeling of being in control by no means took away the hurt.

When my father died, I had thought I would never feel a greater sadness. I was wrong. I had tremendous grief again and I didn't have my dad there to help me through it. My dad would have made my decision seem easy. He would have been able to take the emotions out of the situation and tell me that we shouldn't bring a terminally sick baby into the world. And he would have told me that I shouldn't worry about things I have no control over. It may come off to others as callous, but instead, my dad's words always managed to have a calming effect on me. And that would be it. Kind of a, "You made your choice, it is the right choice, end of discussion" thing. It would have made me more confident in our decision.

My best friend was able to help fill the void left from my dad. She had been the first person I called when my dad died and she was also the only person I told about my ultrasound results. After 20 years of friendship I could count on her for sound advice, understanding, and sympathy. She was a listening ear but never judged and admitted she would have no idea what she would do in my situation. She checked in on me almost daily. She was a dedicated friend and the only non-family member to know we were terminating. I was lucky to have her and can't imagine the situation without her e-mails and telephone calls. While the ultimate decision came down to me and my husband, we were lucky to have such a strong support system surrounding us.

We chose labor and delivery over a dilation and extraction (D&E). The choice was easy for us because we were told that with skeletal dysplasia a D&E would make the official diagnosis after birth much more difficult. We had an absolute desire to know exactly what had gone wrong. We needed confirmation that it was a mutation and not something in our genes. I had extreme fear that it was something we may have passed down to our two-year-old daughter and that somewhere down the road, she would be faced with the same decision.

I was numb the entire stay in the hospital. The doctors and nursing staff were incredible. They handled everything with professionalism and understanding. We were kept at a distance from the happy deliveries on the labor and delivery floor and our room door was marked with a picture of a flower with teardrops on it so everyone that entered would know what we were facing. It was not as horrendous as I had imagined. There were brief moments of laughter between my husband and me as we tried to use humor to break through the stress. However, there were more moments of pure grief. My husband, despite his own intense pain, was my rock and never wavered to ensure I was as comfortable as possible.

Though somewhat painful physically, the delivery itself was quite uneventful and the doctors were happy with how things had progressed. We had chosen not to find out the sex of the baby until he was born, but somehow we both knew it would be a boy, and we were right. He was absolutely tiny. We gave him the name we had picked out for our daughter had she been a boy. It was devastating, yet still somehow peaceful to hold him. He had never been given a chance and for that I was angry. But it wasn't his fault and he deserves all of the love we have for him.

We spent several hours with Conner. It was exhausting to have delivered a baby and then deal with the rush of emotions that followed. Without a doubt, he had his sister's nose and I will cherish that for the rest of my life. It was heartbreaking to give him back to the nurse. I felt guilty for wanting to get home to my daughter. The doctors kept us the night after delivery and it was upsetting to wake up the following morning knowing it was all over. It was even more devastating to walk out of the hospital without a baby. That was my lowest point. I will never forget that moment and I will look back on it every time I think times in my life are bad. I pray nothing will ever compare to the devastation I felt at that moment.

We informed our closest friends only that we had lost the baby, not about the details or the difficult decision we had faced. We were flooded with messages of condolence and thoughtful gifts. I felt somewhat guilty for getting people's sympathy, knowing that some might not agree with our decision to end the pregnancy. I was able to get past that guilt by realizing that they do not know what it is like to walk in our shoes. Before this, I was someone who had said I would not terminate a pregnancy. My mind changed quickly when faced with four months of carrying a baby who had no chance of survival. I like to think that after what we went through, we do indeed deserve sympathy. I spent hours reading the thoughtful responses we received from our friends. It was nice to feel so much love, even if it was in sorrow.

Not many people asked questions and though I was in some ways grateful for that, I also had a strong need to talk about Conner. My husband's friend's wife stepped up upon hearing our news. I had always liked her, but for whatever reason, I only spent time with her occasionally. Her outpouring of sympathy was of tremendous comfort to me. She actually asked what I needed and made sure to deliver. Most people tried to avoid any conversation about Conner in an effort to prevent me from getting upset. But this friend was an outlet for all my anxiety and heartbreak and I continue to talk to her about Conner more than any other person. I know that Conner has a very special place in her heart and for that I am incredibly thankful.

Other friends surprised us by telling us of things they had gone through that we had not known about. Though the stories were very different, it was nice to know that we were not alone. We did struggle with people comparing our loss to a miscarriage. We would have much rather lost the baby naturally than have to make the decision ourselves. I have to remind myself, though, that their miscarriages were devastating to them and my story simply reminds them of themselves and their own loss of a baby they loved. Looking back, I should have been more sympathetic when they miscarried. I am hoping to be the person that steps up when devastation hits my friends' lives in the future. And I regret not having been there for them in the past.

Another issue we struggled with was the constant remarks of "God's will" and "it is all his plan." As my husband so eloquently put it, "God has a shitty plan." I don't believe this is the work of God. I see it as more of a scientific glitch. Our faith has definitely been tested and this is one arena in which I have not yet found closure. I was raised Catholic and have begun to look into converting to another religion. I still believe in God, but feel like a hypocrite practicing a religion that does not believe in termination for medical reasons. I have no intention of going to confession to be forgiven for a sin that I should never have had to face.

Both my sister and a close co-worker are very religious women. Before my husband and I made the decision to terminate, they both knew of the decision we were facing. I felt like they did their best to bite their tongues to ensure their religious beliefs did not overshadow my own decision making. Though I appreciated the respect they had over the decision I was faced with, I almost wanted them to lay it on the table for me. I felt ready for a fight over the whole religious question. I wanted them to explain to me how I could have faith in a God who I couldn't see or touch, when I already had faith in my doctors whom I had built strong relationships with over the years. I wanted them to tell me how I could expect miracles from God, when I started to blame him for all the devastating stories I had been reading about innocent babies. If he was responsible for miracles, than how was I supposed to not hold him accountable for the bad things too? In the end, it is best that neither side brought it up. I respect their beliefs and they respect my decision. It all turned out for the best and we still have strong relationships.

Though this time of my life is filled with incredible sadness, I am overcoming the grief slowly. I unwittingly gave my son the name of a street I pass every day on my way home from work. For weeks, I would cry every time I passed the street sign. Then finally last week I caught myself smiling when I passed it.

I don't regret our decision. My only real regret, in fact, is that I did not invite our family to the hospital to hold Conner. It did not cross my mind at the time. I feel Conner deserved every bit of love available. I feel I may have cheated him by only having me and husband at the hospital. I have an enormous amount of love for my son, yet I don't necessarily feel that our parents feel they have a grandson or that our siblings feel they have a nephew.

I feel sad for Conner for that and I feel responsible for not making him a bigger part of their lives. I am working on a memorial for my son and will include our family so we can remember the brief but bright light that will forever be a part of our lives.

This event in my life has led me to be grateful for many things. I am thankful that we easily got pregnant and don't have fertility issues like some parents face. I am grateful to have doctors whom I have strong relationships with and for whom I was able to put my trust into. I am lucky to have a strong support system of family and friends to help us through the sorrow. I am thankful to have such a loving and supportive husband with whom I have a wonderful relationship. I am thankful that I have a daughter who is the light of my life. I will never take either of them for granted and will thank God every day that they are a part of my life. I guess that is the positive in all this—that I am more appreciative of life and those that I love.

I wish that my son had been healthy. I wish that our first car ride with Conner wasn't home from the cemetery with his remains in a small box. I wish that we had never been faced with the decision to end the life of a small child we loved so much. I hope that science brings cures for the devastating prenatal diseases that innocent babies face. I hope that I continue to think of Conner every day and that it comes with less heartache. I hope that my family and friends think of him occasionally and with great love, for he deserves it. But mostly I hope that Conner and my dad are having a good ole' time in Heaven together.

24

Karen's Story "My Journey to Parenthood"

I will never forget the day that my husband and I decided to try to conceive our first child. It all started in February 2004. Ten months earlier, my mother-in-law had been diagnosed with stage four cancer of the intestines. She asked my husband, Steven, if we were ready to start a family. We had been married for 18 months and Steven was back in school, so that was a tough decision. She already had two grandchildren from her other son, but she really wanted to "know" Steven's first child. Steven and I talked about it over the next couple of days and we decided that we wanted to do this. We were going to have a baby.

I stopped birth control only to find that my menses eluded me. My OB/GYN prescribed Prometrium to bring it on every two months and I was told to try Vitex, an herbal remedy, because many women have had success in regulating their cycles that way. It was also recommended that I buy the Clear Blue Easy fertility monitor (CBEFM) because I would better be able to see what was going on with my cycles. But you can only start using the CBEFM once you get your period, so it was only during the months that I menstruated from the medications that I was able to use it. Trying to conceive was much more stressful than I had expected. I always had this picture in my mind that all that was needed was one time in the bedroom (must have gotten that idea from a high school sex education class).

In June 2004, my mother-in-law sadly lost her battle to cancer. My husband took it very hard, as he was extremely close with her. It all happened so fast. It seemed like one day she was doing her favorite pastime, which was shopping, and then next day she was in hospice on IV fluids clinging to life. Steven and his family made the final decision to let her go when the fluids were the only thing sustaining her. That was a hard decision, but they felt it was the right thing to do. Trying to conceive took a back seat to my husband's depression. He tried to hide from it, but it was there, mainly in the form of "performance anxiety." This was a blow to the system because there was no way of getting pregnant that way! Luckily, that cleared up in a few months and we were actively trying to conceive again.

In the spring of 2005, my midwife recommended that I see a reproductive endocrinologist (RE) to help determine if anything was wrong. I was diagnosed as having polycystic ovarian syndrome (PCOS). The RE was not convinced that I had full-blown PCOS, but rather that it was most likely caused by gaining some weight too quickly. It was also discovered that Steven had a nasty, symptomless urinary tract infection that was causing his sperm count to be extremely low. He was put on a regimen of antibiotics, vitamin K, and vitamin E to help with his problem.

I was to start taking Metformin and Clomid to help induce ovulation, along with timed intercourse. In July, I started the Metformin and in August we began our Clomid cycle. Success on the first try! We were the talk of the fertility clinic! Everything was going wonderfully. I was given ultrasounds every week for the first four weeks and I was released to my OB/GYN at nine weeks. I went to my OB every four weeks and she would check my urine, weight, blood pressure, and listen to the baby's heartbeat. I held my breath at every appointment thinking that "This is the time we won't hear the heartbeat." It was very strange because I really didn't have any reason to suspect that anything was wrong, but yet, a suspicion was there nonetheless.

We were sent to a perinatologist for a level II ultrasound at 18 weeks because the birth defect cleft lip and palate runs in my family. Unbeknownst to us, we thought that would be the worst of our problems. We got quite a shock that day! We were warned that the ultrasound technician and doctor did not talk during the scans, so we should not be nervous if the technician and doctor did not speak to us until afterward. And there was silence. Steven and I watched everything on the screen, and tried to figure out what they were looking at.

After the ultrasound was complete, we were told to wait in the doctor's office to speak to him. He told us that the baby had echogenic bowels consistent with cystic fibrosis—of which Steven was NOT a carrier, but I was. In most cases of cystic fibrosis both parents need to be a carrier for the child to be affected. Then the doctor went on to tell us that the amniotic fluid was extremely low. I remember sitting there in complete shock. No expressions, no emotions, just frozen. We were told to go to the diner to get something to eat in an attempt to stimulate the baby. The doctor was not able to see both hands of the baby open, and he felt that was an important thing to see.

We walked out to Steven's truck. I looked at my husband and said, "There's something wrong with our baby!" and I bawled. I could not catch my breath. I didn't know which way was up. How could this be happening to me? This wasn't supposed to happen! We sat there, outside the office, in the truck, for some time. Steven held me as I sobbed uncontrollably. How could I possibly eat after that? After a while, we reluctantly headed to the diner. I managed to consume a small amount of food and some juice. I remember sitting there at the table in stunned silence.

We headed back to the perinatologist's office so that they could finish the scan. They were able to see both hands open. The doctor stayed in the room and talked with us for a little while. Steven asked what the chances of the baby actually being born healthy were and we were told there was a 20 percent chance. We were instructed to come back on Monday for an amniocentesis.

We went back to my parents' house, which was where we lived at the time. My mom was anxiously awaiting details from our appointment and most of all…the sex of the baby. She took one look at me and knew that something was terribly wrong. I blurted out "There's something wrong with the baby!" and fell into her arms. We stood there sobbing for some time. The weekend was hell.

When we went back to the perinatologist's office on Monday we were hoping for a miracle of some kind; that the amniotic fluid level would be normal and that what the doctor saw in the bowels was just a shadow or something. He performed the amniocentesis, and also did some more ultrasound scanning. After the scan, he mentioned that the baby did not have any lungs and with the amniotic fluid level being so low, the lungs would not grow. He also brought up the subject of termination. We were so confused! We were told that the amniocentesis was mainly done to find out what happened since ours was such an unusual case, being that Steven was not found to be a cystic fibrosis carrier. But the reality was that the baby had no chance of survival without lungs. We were devastated!

We rushed over to my OB's office for her opinion and she agreed that termination was a realistic option unless we wanted to carry to term and lose the baby then. We decided to let our angel go. We then spoke about options. I decided that I didn't think labor and delivery was the right option for me. I couldn't bear to deliver my son stillborn. I didn't want my first experience of delivery to be filled with so much sorrow. We decided to go ahead with a dilation and evacuation (D&E).

My OB told us that she would not be able to perform the termination. She had no experience with doing them and wasn't willing to risk doing any damage to me. There was only one doctor she trusted enough to refer me to, but he had likely already retired. She told us she would do some research and find a suitable location for me. I got the call later Monday afternoon that the best place she could find was actually an abortion clinic not too far from where I lived. She felt that because they did them so frequently, the chance of anything going wrong was slim. I don't remember questioning anything more. I wrote the telephone number down and made the call right away. I was able to schedule the D&E for later that week. Being that I was already 19 weeks along, it was to be a two-day D&E procedure. Now, I just needed to make it through the rest of the week.

On Friday morning, my husband and I drove to the clinic. We met first with someone from the financial department to settle the finances and pay our co-pay. I remember sitting in the waiting room listening to people talk around us. I didn't hear the specifics of any conversations, but was aware of the different tones. Some people were talking non-stop, some were laughing with their friends, and some were very quiet and reserved. There were quite a few people there. I was surprised. I don't think that I'll ever forget that waiting room.

I was finally called into the office. We had to meet with the social worker to go over the specifics of the procedure and to be screened for competency. We explained the situation to her about our difficulties conceiving, and how having to give up this baby was heart-wrenching for us. We were in the office for quite a while. She was in disbelief. She was so accustomed to seeing women giving up babies that they did not want, so to have someone giving up their baby that they desperately wanted was hard for her, too. She cried with me. She then reminded us about the protesters who were always there on Saturdays, something we weren't aware of. She apologized that we were not warned about that before.

As we stood up to return to the waiting room, the social worker directed us to a different area to wait so that we didn't have to go back into the general waiting room. I would have to wait for the doctor to insert the laminaria which would begin the dilation process. At the clinic, there was a policy that no one but the patient was allowed to be in the exam room during the laminaria insertion, but the social worker made an exception in my case. My husband held me during the procedure. I could see the pain in his eyes as he watched me go through that agonizing experience. It was so terribly painful and uncomfortable. The cramping started immediately after the doctor was done. It was hard walking down the stairs to leave. On my way down, I ran into the social worker who was on her way back in. She stopped me, gave me the biggest hug, and wished me peace. She will never know how much that meant to me. To this day, I am reminded of her kindness on such a dark day in my life.

That night, at home, was pretty terrible. The cramping was unbelievable. I was not given a narcotic pain medication, but was told to keep a heating pad on myself. That was the first time I remember crying myself to sleep. My mother decided that she really wanted to be there with us for support. I was taken aback by my parents' complete support of our decision to terminate. They were devout Catholics and I didn't know how they were going to react to it. Their support meant everything to me. I knew that we were doing the right thing, but to know my parents were behind me made it a little more bearable.

I didn't sleep much on Friday night and was up much earlier on Saturday morning than I needed to be. So we headed to the clinic early on Saturday. That turned out to be one of the best things we did because we had arrived at the clinic before the protesters showed up. One less thing I had to endure. As we sat in the waiting room for our turn to be called, we found out that under no circumstances would Steven be allowed with me in the procedure room or recovery area. I would have to go alone. Several women were called at a time to go back. We had to change into hospital gowns and wait to be called again to be placed in a bed. Then we were all given Cytotec to further dilate our cervixes. It was very painful. I was all alone, cold, and in pain. I remember hearing girls moaning and screaming from the cramping associated with the Cytotec. I suffered in silence.

An hour later, I was wheeled into the procedure room. The anesthesiologist was very nice. She got me situated on the table and put me under anesthesia very quickly. The next thing I remember was waking up crying and yelling that I wanted my baby. I could not get control of myself. I was completely hysterical. The nurse came over and told me that I had to stop, but I couldn't. After a short while I fell asleep, and then woke up again crying. It was the most alone I had ever felt. I just wished that someone who loved me was there with me, but they weren't.

After the procedure all of the patients had to be able to walk to the bathroom and change their own maxi pad before being released. It just felt so wrong; a line of zombie-like women walking to the bathroom. I was recovering fine so I was given medications and was cleared to leave. Steven and my mom helped me to the car. As I was leaving I saw the last of the protesters packing up. I was just so glad that I didn't have to experience them shouting at me; I had enough of my own guilt, I certainly didn't need any more.

It was a tough road to recovery after that. I had a very hard time. I confined myself inside my bedroom and didn't talk to anyone. I cried more than I had ever cried in my life. My eyes were so swollen from crying that, at one point, I couldn't even open them. I spent my days either crying or sleeping.

Unfortunately, Steven was in the middle of finals at school and needed to focus on studying. He would study in a different room, but brought his cell phone up with him so that I could call him if I needed him. He would take breaks from studying to check on me. One time I called him just to say that I needed a hug, and he came downstairs immediately to lay with me. That meant the world to me.

Two weeks later, I was in my OB's office with an empty womb for my follow-up visit. She checked me over and told us that it was her opinion that there was no need to wait to try to conceive again. She even felt that if I got pregnant again quickly, it could actually help me to heal. Before I left, she gave me a big hug and said how sorry she was. This was extremely poignant because we did not have a close relationship, and it made me feel like she really did care about me.

Shortly after that, I received a telephone call from the perinatologist stating that our baby did indeed have cystic fibrosis and that they needed to do karyotyping to check our chromosomes to see what happened. Ultimately, we were told that it was maternal uniparental disomy 7; which meant that our baby got two copies of my chromosome 7 and nothing from my husband. Unfortunately, the extra copy of chromosome 7 that our baby got was positive for cystic fibrosis. The baby, who we named "Ephraim," was also deemed to have Silver-Russell syndrome, which is most commonly linked with failure to thrive and very short stature. It was also found that I had a homozygous C677T mutation in the MTHFR gene. In short, this means that I lack an enzyme needed to metabolize my homocysteine level; putting me at risk for blood clots and low folate levels; which is linked to neural tube defects. The doctor wasn't completely sure about the reason for the lack of amniotic fluid or the underdevelopment of the baby's lungs. We were told that what happened was a complete fluke and that the chances of it happening again were close to zero.

I decided that I wanted something to commemorate Ephraim's existence. I thought it would be nice to have an original piece of jewelry created in his honor. So I began looking for a jeweler to do the job and to give me a price estimate. I couldn't believe how expensive it was! For one reason or another, it didn't pan out. So I pushed aside the thoughts of the original jewelry and started contemplating a unique tattoo. I was undecided.

Unfortunately, I slipped into a depression. Steven asked me to consider getting some professional help. I did consider it, but I was in no shape to do the research needed to find a therapist, so it didn't happen. Steven and I became very distant. It was difficult for him to handle my depression since he was in pain, too. In the past, when he was in a rough patch, he would turn to his mother or me. Unfortunately, his mom had passed away and I was in no condition to be able to help him. Our pain wasn't something that he could easily "fix," so he didn't know what to do.

He tried to escape. He started to live a different life where there was no stress. He started to push away all aspects of his previous life, including me. I was a reminder of the pain that he was desperately trying to get away from. Unfortunately, this ultimately led to him trying to ease his pain in someone else's arms. I recognized that something was very wrong pretty quickly and we separated. It was then that I sought out a therapist to help me through everything. I quickly dropped all thoughts of commemorating our Ephraim because I assumed that Steven and I were headed for divorce. At that point, I did not want any connection with Steven at all.

Six weeks after our separation, as we were discussing the separation of our assets, Steven admitted that he made a huge mistake and said that he wanted to work things out with me. Sadly, he had done quite a bit of damage to our marriage in that short time and we would have a lot of painful feelings to work through. His life was in a downward spiral, and he asked me for help, which I offered to him without hesitation. I promised to help him get back on track, but I could not promise that we would work things out. He started individual therapy, and eventually we went into couple's therapy. We started dating again and things started moving in the right direction.

In July of 2006, we were doing well and about to move back in together. My desire to have a child was stronger than ever! Knowing that Steven and I were headed back together, I started monitoring my menstrual cycle. After the termination, my cycle had regulated on its own, so I had started using the CBEFM again. When the monitor showed that I was ovulating, I made my move.

It worked—I was pregnant again! Unfortunately, at five weeks I started spotting. I had planned to go to Germany to visit my sister for a couple of weeks, so I panicked and requested that my OB see me right away. She did an ultrasound on her not-so-great ultrasound machine and couldn't really make out what she was seeing. She thought it might have possibly been a twin loss because she saw one perfect sac and a bunch of "shmutz" (as she called it). She sent me to a radiologist. He saw the perfect sac but was confused by all of the clotting that he saw.

Because of the irregularity of the pregnancy, my OB and the radiologist were concerned that it might be a complete molar pregnancy. In a complete molar pregnancy there's no embryo, amniotic sac, or any normal placental tissue. Instead, the placenta forms a mass of cysts that look like a cluster of grapes. It was recommended that I have a D&C before leaving for Germany so that they could do the necessary testing to make sure that it wasn't gestational trophoblastic disease. If that was the case, I might need to have chemotherapy with one or more anti-cancer drugs and have further testing, such as a CAT scan or an MRI, to be sure that the disease hadn't spread beyond the uterus.

The day before my flight to Germany I was wheeled into the operating room for my D&C. I was petrified. The only thoughts going through my head were my experiences at the clinic and waking up hysterically crying. Luckily, this time they made sure that Steven would be right next to me as I woke up. I remember waking up and feeling so thankful for all of the wonderful support from the hospital staff. It was a completely different experience than my D&E.

The pathology report wouldn't be available until I was already in Germany, so I was told to call one week into my vacation for the results. If it was molar, I'd have to start treatment while in Germany. I received the results, and thankfully, it was not molar. It was a blighted ovum, which surprised the doctor because usually with a blighted ovum the sac is not perfectly round as it was in my case. No medications were necessary, and the trip gave me a good distraction.

After we came home, we were told not to wait to try to conceive. However, my menses was a little elusive, again. Steven and I moved back in together in November. I ordered a necklace from a web site which specialized in pregnancy and infant loss jewelry to commemorate my two angels for Ephraim's angel day on December 17th. I also started to design a tattoo that I was thinking about getting.

My menses was regulated by December and we decided to try to conceive again. In February I learned that was pregnant again. I was ecstatic! The third time had to be my charm. But we were not so fortunate. I went directly to the perinatologist for my first ultrasound at six weeks and he saw nothing in my uterus. The mention of an ectopic pregnancy came up, so I was sent for blood work. My hCG level never got above 360, so there was no hope. It was diagnosed as a chemical pregnancy. I miscarried the following weekend. I couldn't believe it.

I decided it was time to get the tattoo that I had been wanting, before I became pregnant again and wouldn't be able to get it. I knew that it had to be done in the first two weeks of my cycle to be sure that I was not pregnant. I set up an appointment with a tattoo artist to draw an original piece of art to put on my back. I gave him a rough idea of what I was looking for and had him work on it. It took several appointments for it to be exactly what I wanted. I was originally going to put my angel Ephraim's name on it, but decided that the tattoo would be for all of my angels.

In order to optimize my chances of conceiving and sustaining a pregnancy, I was advised to use progesterone after ovulating each cycle. It was determined that I had progesterone insufficiency along with the MTHFR mutation. I decided that I wanted complete medical intervention this time, so we went back to the RE. They performed some tests again and sent me for a hysterosalpingogram to make sure there was no uterine scarring from the D&E or the D&C and that my fallopian tubes were clear.

Everything was perfect and the RE did not even find the PCOS! We decided to pursue intrauterine insemination (IUI). Because the PCOS wasn't an issue, I didn't need the Metformin, but it was decided I should still use the Clomid because I had reacted so well to it the first time. Steven's symptomless urinary tract infection was back and that had to be treated with antibiotics. I had one too, which meant we were both on antibiotics.

In May 2007 we went ahead with our first IUI and it was successful! We were beyond happy! At Steven's sperm analysis the month before his numbers were abysmal, but that particular morning they were astounding. We were followed closely by the RE, getting ultrasounds every week and taking progesterone to keep the lil' bugger in there. At six weeks, we saw the glorious heartbeat. At eight weeks, we were back with my OB and the perinatologist. The 12-week nuchal translucency scan was great and there was no need for chorionic villus sampling or amniocentesis.

The level II ultrasound went wonderful! I decided not to find out the sex of the baby. I was just glad that I was finally getting to have my dream baby, no matter what gender it was.

I'm happy to say that on February 17, 2008, we welcomed our second son, Ethan Ephraim, into this world. A happy and healthy seven pound, two ounce bundle of joy!

I have learned quite a bit from my experiences. First and foremost, I learned that you have to speak up for yourself. No one knows what's in your head better than you. I also learned that you have to ask for what you need in terms of support. No one expects you to be able to handle it all. You do not need to be a martyr. Get the help you need when you need it, or feel free to ask for space if that's what you desire. There were many people who wanted to give support, but didn't know how. By telling them exactly what I needed, they were able to help me. Some people will unknowingly say the wrong things, hoping to be supportive. They just don't know any better. I started telling people that just saying "I'm sorry" or "Life isn't fair" was all they needed to say. My mom once told me that she really didn't know how to help me because she had never been in my situation. Knowing that she cared enough to want to try was all the support I needed.

Lastly, this experience taught me how to be a better person. Things in life are not always what they seem. Everyone has their troubles and challenges, and we all need to help each other out. And above all, don't give up!

25

Karen H.'s Story "Gambling With the Odds"

I had lived a charmed life. Usually things fell into place for me quite easily. When I thought about having kids I figured I would just get pregnant and have a baby. I had never been more wrong in my life.

My husband had two brothers with muscular dystrophy. When we decided to have children we went to a genetic counselor to see if we carried the genes for that disease and if we could put our children at risk for inheriting it. While there, the counselor suggested we also test for cystic fibrosis (CF). We said sure, no problem. February 14th, 2002 the counselor called with good and bad news. We were not carriers for the muscular dystrophy genes but we were carriers for the cystic fibrosis genes. We had a 75 percent chance of having a baby that was fine but a 25 percent chance that our baby would have CF. That was just the beginning.

We didn't know what to do. But the more we thought about it we decided to take the gamble. I thought, "Hey, if you were in Vegas with those odds you would go for it." and that is what we did.

I was so naïve about getting pregnant. All I knew was that there was about a week or so in a woman's cycle when she ovulates and that is when she should have intercourse. When it came time for that week we had sex. That was it. There were no kits or medications or taking temperatures. It was just simple. While waiting for my period I went to a tarot card reader. I worked at a university and she was hired to entertain our students during a break. The first thing she said when I sat was "Are you pregnant?" That was just creepy.

In the week or so that I waited to get my period I didn't think much about getting pregnant. I wasn't in a rush. I just figured it would happen when the time was right. One Saturday morning I woke up thinking I was either pregnant or going to get my period that day. I didn't see any signs of my period so I used a home pregnancy test and it came back positive right away. I remember feeling like I had accomplished something so great that it only took one try, but I also knew instinctively that the baby would be sick.

Two weeks later I had my first prenatal appointment. I was given a mountain of paperwork, told about the schedule, and had the usual exam. I felt fine with the exception of a little nausea. When I was 10 weeks pregnant I heard my baby's heartbeat. I just couldn't believe it. It was so loud and strong it filled the room. Afterwards I drove to work in a haze of tears because I just knew I would never meet him. I knew in my heart I was going to end my pregnancy. I just knew it and I was right. Three weeks later I found out through a chorionic villus sampling (CVS) test that I was carrying a baby boy with CF. I was crushed.

That day I once again drove home from work through a haze of tears. It was a Thursday and I had pre-scheduled an appointment for an abortion for the following day. That night I did not sleep. I lay on my couch curled up in a ball just talking to my unborn child, telling him how sorry I was and how much I loved him. I cried so much and so hard that I couldn't move.

The next morning my husband took me to the abortion clinic. I didn't know anything about ending my pregnancy in a hospital. I assumed it had to be done at a clinic. When we arrived we were escorted into a waiting room. I was there with several young girls who were talking and laughing. One girl even talked about wanting to get back to work and then to go out for drinks after her shift.

I was called to meet with a counselor. She wasn't used to meeting with women like me. She didn't normally see women who wanted to keep their babies. I don't think she knew what to say or do with me. I just sat in her office and cried. I couldn't believe I still had tears left.

After that meeting I was escorted upstairs and given a gown and a valium. I changed into the gown and began to feel a little more relaxed as the drug took effect. I was escorted into the surgical room and put into "the position." My husband was on one side of me and a very nice counselor was holding my hand on the other.

The doctor dilated my cervix and began the procedure. I will never forget the sound for the rest of my life. The machine made this horrible suction noise that got loud then quiet then loud again. I couldn't stand the noise as I imagined why it was getting loud. I put a pillow over my head. My husband couldn't handle it so he left. It was over within a few minutes. Just like that I was no longer pregnant.

What followed was a slow recovery. I healed physically within a few weeks. We took a vacation to Aruba. We had a wonderful trip but there was a hint of sadness that would not go away. Mentally I felt horrible. I missed my baby.

About six months later I found the *BabyCenter* web site. While browsing through the message boards I found the *Termination for Medical Reasons* board. I felt like God had handed me a gift. I found so much support from those women. I met so many women just like me whereas before I thought I was the only one. Those women were phenomenal and I was so relieved to find people who really understood what my experience was like, even more so than my own husband.

It has been over four years since I ended my pregnancy. I lost two more pregnancies before I finally had my dear daughter. Neither of those pregnancies was ended by termination and, while I think of them every day, there is a different feel to those losses than my first. My angels are always in my heart and I will never forget them.

26

Kathryn's Story "What Are the Odds?"

The decision to try to have a second child was one not taken lightly by my husband and me. Our first-born son was born with many medical problems and was later diagnosed with a very rare and fatal genetic disorder called Peroxisome biogenesis disorder, Zellweger syndrome spectrum (PBD, ZSS). PBD, ZSS is a genetic disorder which manifests itself after birth in impaired vision, impaired hearing, developmental delays, low muscle tone, an inability to feed, liver dysfunction, and neonatal seizures. Most patients with PBD, ZSS don't survive the first year of life. What made our decision to try to have another baby especially difficult was that both my husband and I were identified as carriers for this autosomal recessive disorder; therefore we had a 25 percent chance of reoccurrence with every future pregnancy.

Unlike some who find out during pregnancy the devastating news that an abnormality has been found, we knew ahead of time of our increased chance of this disorder happening again. We had already decided that we didn't want to bring another child with this disorder into the world, for we knew how they would suffer. We also knew that we could not continue to give the care our living son needed if we were to bring another child into our home that would need the same, if not more, care as him. We knew the demands and the physical, emotional, and financial exhaustion that came with raising a child with disabilities. However, I struggled horribly with the question of whether I could end a life because of the same disorder that my living son had. How could I love my son so much, yet be willing to end another child's life due to the same condition? Spiritually I was torn. I wasn't sure how it would be perceived by God if I went into a pregnancy knowing that I would terminate if the PBD, ZSS recurred. Did I have the right to even do that? Would I be forgiven? Would I still be reunited with my baby someday?

My husband and I debated for years whether we would pursue adoption, just not have any more children, or try to conceive again. At some point I realized that there were no guarantees for any of those options. But I strongly felt that I deserved a healthy baby. I learned that, should I become pregnant again, I could find out ahead of time whether the baby had PBD, ZSS through prenatal testing. That would allow me to spare a child the pain and struggles that my son had to endure. I finally began to see that if I were faced with that situation and ended the pregnancy, it would have nothing to do with the love that I had for my son. It would instead have everything to do with how much love I would have for that new baby. I would love that baby and not want him or her to suffer and would want him or her to have the quality of life that my son didn't have.

We decided to try to become pregnant again and go through prenatal testing via chorionic villus sampling (CVS), agreeing that if we were in the 25 percent again, we would end the pregnancy.

After becoming pregnant only a few months after we began trying, we were devastated when I miscarried. I came to peace with that loss very quickly as I accepted that God had chosen to take our baby's life so that we did not have to face the decision ourselves. We immediately began trying again.

As soon as I began to get discouraged that it wasn't happening, I found out that we were expecting once again. We chose to tell only close family and friends about the pregnancy since we knew the possibility of what we could be faced with. We made it through the first trimester, after many scares with bleeding on and off the entire time, and had finally arrived at the time to get the CVS test done. We were so excited to have made it that far and we were very eager to get the testing done. Our excitement and enthusiasm was brief as our appointment for the CVS test had to be rescheduled a week later due to the coordination of how the specimens would need to be sent to an outside university three states away. We were so disappointed and our anxiety level about the pregnancy only climbed higher. A week later we finally went for the CVS.

Within minutes of seeing our baby girl on the screen we knew something was wrong as another technician, the doctor, and the genetic counselor entered the room. They all stood with concerned and puzzled looks on their faces as they talked about the position of the placenta and if they could reach it. The placenta had attached at the very top backside of my uterus, causing the CVS via the cervix to be very complicated. After two hours and many, many failed attempts they finally said that they could not reach the placenta to collect the specimens.

The genetic counselor made some phone calls and advised us that no one in our state was capable of doing a transabdominal CVS. We were told that we could travel a week later to a hospital five hours away for a transabdominal CVS or we could wait even longer and have an amniocentesis done. We couldn't bear the thought of waiting any longer so they made the arrangements for us to travel the next week to the hospital five hours away.

When we arrived at the hospital for the transabdominal CVS I was taken into a room and prepped for the procedure. The doctor walked in and told us that I could not have the transabdominal CVS after all. He explained that, due to the rare and complex disorder we were testing for, the quantity of the specimen required was much larger than usual and that amount could not be obtained via the abdomen. After viewing the ultrasound, the doctor requested that I allow him to make an attempt to reach the placenta transcervically. Still physically hurting from all of the attempts the week prior, I felt I had no other option if I wanted the testing done. So out of desperation, I permitted him to try. And he did it—it was finally successful!

We reveled in the numerous ultrasound photos of our baby we were able to collect from each appointment. Our celebration was short-lived as we were now on our way home to begin the most dreaded two to four week wait for the results.

Approximately two weeks later I received a call from the genetic counselor. I remember it all too well. I don't think I will ever forget that day. It was a warm, sunny afternoon and I was sitting outside at work having lunch with a few co-workers when my cell phone rang. The genetic counselor immediately asked me if it was an okay time to talk. I told her that it was, but asked if I could call her right back so that I could go to a more private area to talk in case I had any questions. She agreed to that, then added the words that I can still hear her saying so clearly to this day, "Yes, because you will." I don't even recall saying goodbye. I just simply hung up the phone. I immediately knew from the tone in her voice and the words she had said that something was wrong. I left my lunch sitting there and began walking inside the building to the second floor conference room where I knew I would have privacy. As I made my way up the back stairwell I felt empty—like I had just swallowed a ton of air. I was suddenly very aware of my heart pounding and had a sinking feeling in the pit of my stomach. By the time I reached the conference room my eyes were welled up with tears and it felt very hard to breathe.

I very anxiously dialed the phone and the genetic counselor answered on the first ring. She told me that the results we were waiting on were not back yet, but the chromosomal studies that we had agreed to be done in addition to the PBD, ZSS testing had come back with an "incidental finding." That was the same testing that I so naively and ignorantly signed off on. I remember thinking at the time that since they would already have the specimen for the PBD, ZSS testing and insurance would cover the additional testing, why not? The genetic counselor continued to tell me that the direct reading showed a chromosomal make-up of 46xx. I assumed that meant that we were having a healthy baby girl. The genetic counselor then told me that when 30 of the cultured cells were looked at more closely, they all revealed a missing sex chromosome. I remember feeling very anxious, like she couldn't explain it to me fast enough. I responded, "What does this mean?" She told me that it meant we were having a girl with Turner syndrome. I couldn't believe what I was hearing. How could that be? That wasn't what we were the most concerned about. That wasn't what we were primarily testing for. She went on to explain that most people are diagnosed with that syndrome after an abnormal sonogram, yet my sonogram had showed no signs of anything being abnormal. She continued to tell me all of the things that could affect our little girl—from one end of the spectrum to the other. Girls with Turner syndrome tend to be short in stature, infertile, are at risk for heart defects, high blood pressure, kidney problems, diabetes, cataracts, osteoporosis, and thyroid problems. I would also learn that only two percent of fetuses diagnosed with Turner syndrome make it to term. Through the tears I tried to write down notes of what the genetic counselor was telling me. Lastly, she told me not to make any decisions yet because the results for the testing we originally went for were not ready yet. A decision, what decision? How do I make a decision? Turner syndrome wasn't what I knew about. It wasn't what I had researched and experienced first-hand. I had a plan for a baby with PBD, ZSS, but not Turner syndrome. I asked the genetic counselor if people terminated for Turner syndrome, and she said that some do and some don't. I wanted so badly for her to tell me what to do. I knew she couldn't, but I didn't want to decide and I didn't know how to. I knew that we couldn't decide, at that time anyway, since she had advised us to wait for the other test results. If those results came back normal we could have additional testing to try to learn more about the severity of the Turner syndrome.

During that time a very close friend walked into the room. She knew from the way I left lunch that something was very wrong. I hung up the phone and couldn't even look at her. I remember feeling very weak and sitting down in a chair that was beside me. As I sat down I leaned over with my elbows on the table, hands over my face, and stared down at the table as I tried to absorb and make sense of the words that I had just heard. They were echoing over and over again in my head. I couldn't even say them aloud and when I tried, I began sobbing uncontrollably. The only words that came out were, "I can't do this. I just can't do this. This can't be happening."

Somehow, I managed to tell my friend the news I had just received. Then it suddenly hit me that I had to call my husband and tell him. How? The news would just crush him! I tried to figure out in my head what I would say to him, but the thought of uttering those words overwhelmed me and I became sick. I finally gathered myself and dialed the phone. I remember the conversation very clearly. I didn't cry one tear and tried to down play it as much as I could, for his sake. Looking back, I guess I was trying to protect him. I was holding on to the fact that maybe it wouldn't be severe or maybe it would all be a mistake. We ended the conversation, both agreeing and acknowledging that we couldn't make any decisions until the other test results came back.

If the other testing came back okay, I had no idea what we would do. At least with the PBD, ZSS testing we knew what we would do if the baby was affected. We had a road map and we had a plan that took years to decide, and all of a sudden someone threw a fork in the road and we had no idea which direction to go. We were lost. I can honestly say that I was in such a fog that I could not see one foot in front of the other. I prayed and prayed and pleaded with God for the baby to be okay. I did endless reading and researching. I accessed every medical resource I had available to me from co-workers in the medical field, friends, medical professionals, the Internet and even borrowed a friend's biology books. My husband did the same.

My husband felt that we could continue to term. I was not feeling the same, but I didn't know how to tell him. He was so full of hope and I was losing mine. I found myself feeling so guilty when I uttered the words, in a silent desperate prayer, that I just wanted my baby to have the PBD, ZSS. At least then I would know what I was facing. I felt consumed by the guilt for even thinking that. I was also consumed by the fear of not knowing what to do. How was I supposed to make that decision? I didn't want her to suffer and there was no way to know if she would or not. I didn't really want her to have PBD, ZSS, but at least then I would know that I would be making a decision that would be best for her. I felt like I had no strength left. The fear and guilt was consuming me. I pleaded with God to let her have PBD, ZSS so that I would know what to do, or to please just take her at that time. As the hours passed, the reality of the facts began to hit me. There was no turning back and I knew that, no matter what happened, from that point forward a decision would have to be made as to whether or not I would end the pregnancy. That was when my pleading to God turned into desperate cries to take the baby at that time and not be faced with the decision to terminate.

Only 48 hours after the first set of results came back I received the call that our daughter had received both of our mutated genes and was fully affected with PBD, ZSS as well as the Turner syndrome. I felt relieved. I knew without a doubt that our daughter would suffer and what decision had to be made. I wouldn't choose a life of suffering for anyone and that was why I knew that I had to let her go. I didn't want to let her go but I knew I had to. I felt horrible and guilty for feeling so relieved. How could I feel relief when I knew that I had just made the decision to end our daughter's life? The genetic counselor told me to not feel guilty or horrible and said that what I was experiencing was "the comfort of a decision." She was right. But a part of me was furious and devastated at what was happening to us and to our baby. I called my husband and told him the results and that I was ending the pregnancy.

I was able to talk to my doctor the next day to try to set everything up. It was Friday afternoon and I was told that I would have to wait until the following Wednesday to have a dilation and evacuation (D&E) termination. I couldn't have the procedure done locally. My OB was capable and willing to do it, but the hospitals in the area would not allow it. I had to travel two hours away to a hospital that was willing to accommodate me. I was fortunate enough to have insurance that was willing to pay for the procedure if it was done in a hospital setting. I was very grateful for the coverage as I have since learned that many women, unfortunately, have to travel a great distance to a clinic where they receive no sympathy and are treated disrespectfully. To add insult to injury, they often have to pay out of their own pocket for that kind of experience.

The days leading up to the procedure were horrible. They reminded me of the saying, "The calm before the storm." My husband chose to bottle it all up and remain as busy as he could. He busied himself by working in the yard, building a two-level flowerbed and even installing a new irrigation system. I, on the other hand, spent my time reading the book *A Time to Decide, A Time to Heal* which the genetic counselor had sent to me via overnight mail, along with a sympathy card. When I wasn't reading, I was trying to figure out in my mind a way to say goodbye to my daughter. At one point during the days before the D&E I went to the bathroom and found blood. I froze and thought immediately "This is okay." I thought, "Now I won't have to do this." I prayed right then and there that it was a sign that I would miscarry and I begged that she be taken peacefully so that we wouldn't have to follow through with the termination. I never saw another drop of blood.

The day before I was scheduled to go in for the D&E I remember waking up and having a complete feeling of anxiety rush over me as I realized that day would be the last day I would be pregnant. That night I lay in bed and held my belly as if I were holding her. I told her how sorry I was, how I didn't want to do it, how much I would miss her and I begged for her forgiveness. It was in those moments that I decided on her name—Kayla Marie. It was also the first moment I realized that I could feel her life moving from within me.

The next morning as I stood in the shower and washed my belly, I stopped and rubbed it knowing that the next time I stood in the shower there wouldn't be a cute little bump where my baby girl was. As we began our trip to the hospital I had to take some Cytotec pills to start the process which would end with my baby girl's death. I was supposed to have already taken them, but I found myself in the passenger seat of the car staring at the pills in my hand. As I placed them in my mouth I knew that was it. It was really happening; my baby of only 16 weeks would die that day. When we arrived at the hospital, I could feel the effects of the Cytotec as I tried to walk across the parking garage. The contractions made it very difficult to walk. Once inside, we found our way to Labor & Delivery. We arrived at the double doors, pressed the button, and a nurse responded by asking, "May I help you?" My husband just looked at me blankly for a moment as if we didn't know how to say what we were there for. He simply said my name and they buzzed us through the doors. The nurse handed me three papers to complete and sign. The last page, about halfway down, had a section to be filled out regarding care of the newborn baby. I skipped that section and signed below. The nurse handed the page back to me, commenting that I had skipped a section. Holding back the tears I asked her "What do you want me to write?" She then realized quickly what the section was asking for and simply apologized and as she pulled the papers back to her side of the counter. She directed me to go into the room directly behind me.

I walked in the room that was filled with nurses ready to take care of me. I wanted to tell all of them how much I loved my baby, how much I wanted her, how it was not supposed to happen like it did, how I did everything I was supposed to, and how it was not supposed to end like it was going to. But I didn't say anything as my eyes quickly moved around the room and I saw the hospital bed, my hospital gown, and, over in the corner, the infant warmer that normally would hold a healthy newborn baby. The nurses had thrown a towel over the infant warmer in an attempt to prevent me from seeing it. The reality of it all hit me hard at that moment.

We were there for hours, but it didn't seem like that long to me as I was kept distracted by the nurses and doctors. I was given some medicine to calm me down and the doctors and nurses were wonderful and sympathetic to us. After all of the preparations were done, it was time. I gave my husband a hug and kiss and told him I loved him as the nurse wheeled me to a room just outside the operating room. After a few minutes the nurse said they were ready and, as I stood up, I felt like everything was moving in slow motion. I stood there for a moment before I hesitantly walked into the operating room and sat on the operating table. I was told to lean over into the nurse while I received a spinal block. The nurse walked up and placed a warm blanket over my legs. With one glimpse she told me with her eyes how sorry she was. As I leaned my head on her shoulder she held both my hands in my lap and told me it was going to be okay. I sat there thinking to myself, "No, this isn't okay." and wondering how it ever could be.

As I sat frozen still with my head rested on the nurse's shoulder I remembered doing something similar years earlier when giving birth to my son. Only this time I would have no baby to see, no baby to hold, and no baby to take home. I looked through my tears, which were now a steady stream down my face, at the instruments that surrounded me, the people moving about, and finally my doctor coming through the operating room doors. It almost looked like a scene out of a movie. But it wasn't a movie—it was my life. I wanted to scream, I wanted to run out of there, and I wanted someone to wake me up from the horrible nightmare. But they couldn't. It wasn't a nightmare. It was really happening. I didn't speak a word as I would soon be numb physically; I was already numb emotionally. I wanted to pray, but couldn't. I didn't know what to say.

I continued, in my mind, to tell my baby girl how sorry I was and how much I loved her and didn't want her to go. For a moment, I was scared for myself and my own life. I instantly felt guilty and selfish for even thinking about myself. How could I think about myself when my baby girl's life was about to end at any moment? I was hoping that she was already asleep, but I knew that once they finished administering the drugs to me that she would be asleep. I wanted her to be taken peacefully and was overwhelmed by thoughts that she might not be. I was devastated and terrified at the same time. They placed a sheet in front of me to obscure my view. As I lay there I felt them lifting my legs into what felt like slings instead of stirrups. Once it was determined that I was numb enough, they commented that I was ready. I had a moment of panic as I feared them starting the procedure with me still being awake. I very quickly and clearly exclaimed that I was aware of everything that was going on. The anesthesiologist told me not to worry as she finished administering medication into my IV. I don't remember anything else from the operating room after that point.

The next thing I remember, I was back in my hospital room and was hysterical. The reality of what had just happened hit me like a freight train. I couldn't breathe and I felt like I was suffocating. I screamed as loud as I could while I cried from a place so deep down inside me I didn't even know it existed. I was devastated. I had nothing left in that moment. I wasn't pregnant anymore, my baby was gone, and I had nothing to show from the pregnancy with her. I had nothing to show that she was real and that she existed not just in my heart, my mind and my body. She was a real person and I had nothing to remember her by. Even though I knew beforehand that I did not want to go through a labor and delivery termination, I was mad that I had the D&E because I didn't have footprints from my daughter. Who would have thought that would have meant so much to me? I would have never guessed that I would have reacted that way. I was mad that I didn't have any recent sonogram pictures of her since I hadn't had a sonogram in weeks. I remember clearly opening my eyes to a room full of medical staff as I was having a container shoved in front of me because I told them I needed to throw up. I found out later that no one heard my screams and few people understood the moans and mumbles that were coming out of me. I was in a state of grief that no one could ever prepare for. Apparently, they knew that from my body movements, shaking, and crying which made it obvious. Although my screams were clear in my mind, the people in my room only caught bits and pieces of my mumbles.

After a few hours we were able to go home. That was the hardest thing I had ever done in my life up until that point.

I made a decision that no mother should ever have to make. Even though I knew it was always a possibility that we would be faced with it, I could have never fully prepared myself for it. Making the hypothetical decision to end your child's life and actually ending it are completely different. I unfortunately know that now.

The following weeks were dark. There were days when I looked in the mirror and couldn't recognize the person staring back at me. I did everything I could to disconnect and keep all of the pain, anger and guilt pushed under the surface, but I couldn't.

I wanted the pain to stop, even if only for a day. The thoughts and feelings that I was experiencing were of magnitudes that I wish I hadn't known existed. I began pulling way from others around me as I had a hard time communicating and relating with them. I either couldn't find the words to use or was too afraid to utter the words for fear that they wouldn't begin to understand. I also felt a little ashamed about it all. I continued to isolate myself, believing that others could not possibly understand what I was going through. People that truly cared for me and supported me surrounded me, yet I felt so alone.

As the days turned into weeks and the weeks into months the darkness slowly began to lift. The time had finally arrived that my desire to try to conceive again overcame my sadness and fears. I found out I was pregnant again only four months after letting our little girl go. But my dreams were quickly shattered once again when we lost that baby to miscarriage. During that miscarriage all of the pain, anger and guilt that I had managed to keep pushed down finally surfaced. I couldn't stop thinking about my little girl that I had lost and all of a sudden I found myself in a dark place full of rage.

I came to the conclusion that the reason I couldn't recognize myself anymore was because a piece of me was gone. A piece of me must have died with my daughter. At one point, a part of me wished I had just died with her. I not only began to not recognize myself but I didn't like who I was becoming. I was angry. I hated the fact that some days I didn't know how to be me anymore. I hated the fact that some days I felt like I couldn't cope. I hated the fact that some days I was consumed by it all. I hated the fact that I didn't feel like a good mom or wife anymore. I hated the fact that I couldn't relate to others around me anymore. I hated that I felt sorry for myself sometimes, that I was unhappy a lot of times, that I wondered if my own husband regretted being with me, and that I was hating everything so much. I knew that hating was such a useless, wasteful emotion that takes so much of your energy that could be put into something positive, and yet there I was. I was alone and hating everything that surrounded me, including myself. That was when I realized that I needed to somehow find a way to pull myself out of the deep, dark, lonely pit that I felt trapped in. I needed to do it not just for my family that needed me, but for myself too. Though my dreams kept shattering, my hope somehow still remained.

We immediately tried to conceive again as soon as I was physically able to. The first month we tried to conceive I became pregnant. I was terrified yet excited and hopeful at the same time. I took progesterone everyday in hopes that it would help me hold onto the pregnancy and every other week I anxiously waited to see the heartbeat on the sonogram screen. When I was around 10 weeks pregnant I told my husband that we were having a boy. I just knew it was a boy that time. At 11 weeks we went and had the CVS testing done. Everything went so smoothly. Everyone, including us, was so excited and so full of hope. We were hopeful for the baby we had been dreaming of and waiting so long for. We went home so full of hope as we waited the two to four weeks for the CVS results.

A little over a week later, while my husband and I were out to dinner with friends, we received the phone call. The baby was a boy and he was fully affected with PBD, ZSS. We had hit the 25 percent chance again. I couldn't believe it. At first I was in denial. It had to be a mistake. The results were not even supposed to be ready yet. It wasn't a mistake. I was so angry that God could allow us to be faced with that again. Why? I became numb emotionally to it all. The next few days were a blur. They called me on Monday to let me know that I was on the schedule for Wednesday to end the pregnancy.

Wednesday morning arrived and there I sat, barely one month away from the one year anniversary since we chose to give our little girl back to

God. The situation was the same—with the Cytotec pills in my hand as I sat in the passenger seat of the car on our trip to the same hospital. We arrived at the hospital and found our way to Labor & Delivery again. We went through those same double doors and I completed and signed those same papers, again skipping the section about care for the newborn baby. This time I knew what to expect and requested that I be sedated earlier on than before. As soon as I received my spinal block they granted my request and the next thing I remember was being moved off of the operating room table. It was in that moment that it all hit me. My baby boy that I had only just begun to know was gone. As I write this, it has only been three days since we let our baby boy go.

In the flowerbed that my husband made the week we gave our little girl back to God sits a statue of a little girl angel in remembrance of our little girl. At some point I will likely get a little boy statue, in remembrance of our baby boy, to sit beside her. I realize that I don't need these tangible reminders of my angels in order to heal. But having something to look after and nurture brings me a tiny bit of peace during the sad times. Having something tangible, like a statue or a memory book, affirms to myself and to others that my babies did exist, that they weren't a figment of my imagination, and that I can still honor their importance in my life. I know that my babies are not lost, they are in Heaven together, happy, healthy, and playing as their bodies would have never permitted them to do here with us. Until the day comes that we meet again, I will carry them in my heart forever.

I don't know what the future holds for us. I do hope that I will one day be able to feel hopeful again as I have before. I know there are others that have the same odds as we do and have gone on to have beautiful, healthy babies placed in their arms. Those are the stories that give me hope. My husband and I still have that dream of holding a healthy baby in our arms, but we don't know if that dream will ever become a reality for us. We don't know why this happened to us. Part of me feels that I will never truly know that answer. I no longer feel the need to ask for forgiveness. I believe that God knows what is in my heart. I don't struggle with the guilt of it all as I did before. I felt his love and knew that he was with me when the guilt and fear consumed me. I believe he knows my pain and that God was with me and helped me through the horrible decisions. I was once told that sometimes the miracle isn't the healing we prayed for or the healthy baby we so desperately wanted but that we are able to make it through such an experience. Whatever the future does hold for us I do still hope that the day will come when I can lay our healthy baby down to sleep and ask his or her four angel brothers and sisters to look after him or her.

Along with my hopes and dreams of having a healthy baby to hold one day, I also hope that the day will come when other women who face this unfortunate and devastating situation will not have to suffer in silence. It saddens me that, due to the many moral, ethical, religious and political issues that surround these choices, so many women, including myself, have been forced to keep this secret from people they encounter everyday and even from their own families. Some women are denied these services entirely and are not able to obtain the level of care that they need and deserve during such a tragedy. I am grateful for the care that I received throughout all of my experiences. I don't think I would be where I am today if it were not for the wonderful support and care that I had received.

Through these heartbreaking choices that I have had to make I have learned just how many of us there really are and wonder how many more are out there suffering silently. We share a bond that no mothers should ever have to share. However, we do. We have all had to make that heartbreaking, gut wrenching decision to put our babies first and set them free of any pain and suffering. Unfortunately for now, we all share this bond behind closed doors, hidden from the judgment of others that, fortunately for them, have never walked in our shoes and hopefully never will have to.

Raising a child with disabilities caused by a fatal disorder and making a heart breaking choice twice has shown me the horrible, dark side of this world and yet it has also shown me the compassion and love in this world as well. It has changed my views in every aspect of my life and I feel as though I see the world through a different set of eyes now. I have come to realize that my world did not crumble and fall apart, although it can still feel that way at times. It has only been twisted and turned in new directions that I never expected, and while I continue on this journey it will continue to do so. I don't know what awaits us around the next turn. I know that I will keep moving forward, one step at a time. If I fall again or the road seems too steep, I can only hope that my family and friends, who may not know what it is like to walk in my shoes, will be there to at least walk beside me and hold my hand along the way.

27

Kendall's Story **"My Son, My Teacher"**

My long awaited journey into motherhood began the day I found out I was pregnant with my son. He was my lifeline the day my brother died and I thought the world was ending. He was the glimmer of hope that was offered to family members that horrible week when we had four family members die. He was my everything; and then he was gone.

My husband and I found out we were expecting a baby at the end of September 2005. We were so excited! Finally, we were starting a family. The following week my brother and cousin were killed in a car wreck, then my aunt died from cancer, and my husband's uncle died in his sleep. In the midst of our overwhelming sadness we still had hope because our baby was coming.

On December 12, 2005 I had my triple screen blood test. One week later, during a regular appointment with my OB, he informed me that my AFP level on the triple screen test came back elevated. The normal AFP level is less than 2.5 ng/mL and mine measured at 2.54 ng/mL. He assured me that I shouldn't worry. We both felt confident that it would come back a "false positive," but I was scheduled for a level II ultrasound later that week anyway.

On December 22nd (my daddy's birthday) my husband, mom, and I met with the genetic counselor who informed us of what the elevated AFP levels could indicate. According to the statistics we had a less than one-half of one percent chance that anything was wrong with the baby. We were so excited about the ultrasound and started debating whether or not to find out the sex.

Thirty minutes later our world crashed around us. The doctor and sonographer began the level II ultrasound by taking measurements and showing us all the baby's major parts, but they slowed down when they got to the spine. My son had his back up against the placenta and they couldn't get a very good view, but what they could see was not good. The baby had spina bifida. There was definitely an opening in the lumbar region of the spine from L1–L3 but they couldn't tell us any more than that. Then they proceeded to scan the baby's heart, which showed an echogenic focus that could have been indicative of Down syndrome. The only good news was that the baby's brain appeared normal and, at that point, there was no clubbing of the feet.

We then met with the genetic counselor who tried to give us all the possible outcomes of the diagnosis and tried to answer my family's questions while I sat quietly crying, completely numb. Unfortunately, I had a medical background and knew that things were serious. I was devastated. We decided to have the amniocentesis and then go home and try to process everything.

We decided at that point to continue the pregnancy because we had so many unanswered questions and were unwilling to end the pregnancy when the worst-case scenario appeared to be only that the baby wouldn't be able to walk. We scheduled another level II ultrasound and anxiously awaited our amniocentesis results. We were cautiously excited when the amniocentesis came back normal but unfortunately the worst was still to come.

A couple of days before the level II ultrasound I noticed a change in the baby's movement patterns. He began to move for shorter periods of time and not as often. I tried to convince myself that it was because I was stressed, but I couldn't shake the feeling of impending doom. I realize that may sound overly dramatic to some, but it is honestly how I felt. We went to our next doctor's appointment and discussed with the doctor what the possible outcomes were for our child. My husband really wanted to know exactly what the outcome would be and found it frustrating that there were no concrete answers.

We discussed the possibility of hydrocephalus (water in the brain) and what that could mean for our son. At that point the baby had not shown any signs of hydrocephalus but my husband had been reading up on how babies with spina bifida often develop this condition in utero. Our doctor reassured us that the baby's brain looked fine and that we would monitor for hydrocephalus, but that there was little to be done at that point.

The doctor then began our level II ultrasound. Little did we know that we were about to be dealt another blow. We found that the baby's spina bifida lesion was larger than they had originally thought. It appeared to be located from L1–L5. The most horrible part was that the baby had developed ventriculomegaly—enlarged ventricles of the brain caused by excess cerebrospinal fluid. At that point, it had yet to affect the size of the baby's head. I lay on the table crying and knowing in my heart that my son was not going to make it.

When we got home my husband wanted to discuss termination but I was absolutely against it. I was in complete denial about the baby's condition and the eventual outcome. I tried really hard to start arguments with my husband so that I wouldn't have to face reality. Luckily, I had a wonderful husband who let me vent while softly continuing to encourage me to face what was happening.

We returned to the doctor 10 days later at 22 weeks and five days, and found that the baby's brain measurements were the same. That made the situation even more difficult. His fetal movements had continued to decrease and I was beginning to return to reality. We asked our doctor about options for termination and he explained that, unfortunately, we had passed the deadline in our state, so our only remaining option was to go to a clinic in Wichita, Kansas. My husband and I decided to take the weekend and really focus on each other and the decision that was ahead of us.

We sat down on Friday night and read the book *A Time to Decide, a Time to Heal.* We completely unloaded to one another about how we felt, what were afraid of, and what we thought our future looked like. I confessed that I felt enormous amounts of guilt; he was my son, it was my job to protect him, and I was failing miserably. My husband confessed that he was scared to bring a child in the world who may never have an understanding of himself or his place in this world. That weekend broke our spirits, but we were still able to come together. We decided that we had to make the toughest decision of our lives and end our pregnancy.

I contacted the doctor's office and made my appointment at the Wichita clinic for the following Monday. I was warned that there would be protestors outside of the clinic and that I would have to pass through a metal detector to enter the clinic. The woman on the phone was very nice and almost started crying herself when I broke down.

I was petrified when we left home on that Superbowl Sunday. I was so afraid that I would wake up the next day and not recognize myself. I was afraid I would emerge from the clinic broken and unable to be fixed. I thought I would lose my son, my marriage, and myself. I was also angry. I was angry with God that he allowed this to happen. I was angry with my husband that he couldn't fix it. Mostly I was angry with myself because I hadn't been able to save my son.

That Monday I arrived at the clinic and met with other couples who were there for similar reasons. As a group, we watched a video about the procedure and met with the doctor. She answered our questions about what to expect.

We then met with the doctor one-on-one. She answered all of our questions and tried to reassure my husband, mother and mother-in-law that I would be okay. My husband is a bit obsessive-compulsive, so I was very impressed with how well she handled him and his questions. She really provided care for our entire family.

Following that we went into the examination room where they performed a sonogram to judge the baby's gestational age and determine his position. Then we went back in with the entire group for some more counseling. A little later we were taken back into an examination room where I was given a sedative. Our son was then given a shot to stop his heart and the laminaria sticks were inserted to open my cervix. After a little more counseling we were sent back to our hotel for the evening.

It was a long and stressful day, and I was exhausted. We ate dinner and I fell asleep shortly thereafter. The nurse called about 9:00 PM to check on our emotional and physical wellbeing.

The following morning the protestors were at the clinic again, but this time they had a huge group of kids with them. The middle to high school-aged kids stood on the street corner and hollered at us. Those children didn't have the slightest understanding of what we were going through, but they had been taught by someone that they had the right to judge us. It was really quite sad.

The guard checked us in and we met with the group again. This day was much shorter; just a quick ultrasound to determine the baby's positioning and some sedation for a laminaria change. We had a short counseling session and then were released back to our hotel.

The third day proceeded much the same as the second day except that at the end of the third day they determined that I might go into labor overnight so I should stay at the clinic. I was released only to get my things from the hotel and to grab dinner. I arrived back at the clinic at 9:00 PM. The attendant and the nurse greeted us and showed us to our beds. I was exhausted so I went to sleep pretty quickly. My husband (who is a bit of a night owl) stayed up and chatted with the attendant for a while. She was so great about answering his questions and making him more secure.

The next morning they gave me oxytocin to start my labor. A couple of hours later I delivered our son into the world. The drugs made me very amnesic but I do remember having a dream that my father-in-law and brother were looking down on me from Heaven with the baby. They reassured me that everything was okay. I think sometimes God gives us those little nudges to help us through the hard days.

Later that afternoon, when the drugs had worn off, we had a viewing of our son. I was unprepared for what I would see. During the two weeks since our final ultrasound the baby had developed severe hydrocephalus. Still I am grateful that we made the decision to have those few precious minutes with our son. I felt reassured that he was in a better place and that we had made the right decision.

It has now been five weeks. There are days when I am absolutely devastated. There are days when I almost feel like myself. I hate that my son is gone. I hate that I had to make the decision to end his life. I hate that my womb and my arms are empty. But I am strengthened in the fact that I made my decision by focusing on him and what was best for him. I am eternally grateful to the wonderful people that guided me through this horrible experience with compassion, love, and understanding.

Update: I find it hard to believe sometimes that those were my words but then this whole experience has changed me and caused me to grow. It's been two years now since I made my decision and while there are good days and bad days, the deep agony is mostly gone. I entered that pregnancy with my son with such an innocent arrogance. It was my destiny and I thought I was walking blissfully into its fulfillment, instead I walked through the most trying time of my life thus far.

In his ever-so-short life, my son taught me lessons that my previous 26 years had been unable to. Despite what I thought, I do not know until actually in a situation, how I will react. He taught me how judgment is wrong and how much it hurts the person being judged; I have learned how to express my disagreement with a decision rather than with a person. Mostly, he taught me how deep love can go. As hard as it was, as much as it hurts, I wouldn't change it. I am proud to be his mother, I am proud of the impact his life has had on this world and I wouldn't go back for anything.

If I could offer a few suggestions for those who are just starting their journey:

1. Seek wise counsel—be it from your pastor, a psychologist, a grief counselor, or anyone. Just don't let the sadness eat you up inside.
2. Your spouse will react differently. Do not allow that to become an issue in your relationship. Do not take it personally when one is crying and the other can't seem to stop "fixing up the house." We all grieve differently and no one way is right. You might want to consider joint counseling to assist you in keeping the lines of communication open.

3. Always remember that grief is a process. There is no set timetable on completion. That doesn't mean that it's healthy to wallow in it forever, but also don't allow others to make you feel bad that you're not "over it" within their defined time frame.

I wish you peace during your journey and pray that you find hope in the fact that the contributors to this book have survived similar losses. It can be done.

28

KerriAnn's Story "A Mother's Intuition"

I was always in love with the idea of being a mom. What a wonderful calling, I thought. What an awesome responsibility. I remember doodling the names of my future children over and over on my notebooks in school. I would fantasize about what my children would look like. I wondered if they would have red hair, blue eyes, or freckles. It all seemed like a dream that was not yet tangible, but I knew almost certain to come true. I would be a mother… some day.

I found out I was pregnant for the first time in May of 2000. I was 26 years old, and had been married for almost two years. My husband had bought a home pregnancy test and begged me to take it. My periods had always been irregular, so I really didn't think anything of not having a period for a couple of months. My husband thought otherwise, and he was right… there were two blue lines! After a day or two of disbelief we were thrilled. We began to plan for our firstborn child and imagine our lives as parents.

Almost from the beginning I had a "sixth sense" that something was just not right. I told my husband, my friends and my OB that I just had a feeling that something was terribly wrong with the baby. I really had no reason to be concerned. I was young, healthy, and had an uncomplicated first trimester. Everyone reassured me that it was just first-time mom nerves, but I couldn't shake the feeling of dread. I would later realize that my unexplained feelings of uneasiness were my mother's intuition. Unfortunately I was right—there was something terribly, terribly wrong.

As the pregnancy progressed, I wondered at every little milestone… feeling the baby flutter at 13 weeks, wearing maternity clothes at 18 weeks, and the anticipation of the 20-week ultrasound.

At 20 weeks I was scheduled for a level II ultrasound because I had refused the triple screen test earlier in the pregnancy. My husband and I arrived at the hospital for the ultrasound, and were adamant that we did not want to know the sex of the baby. We wanted to be surprised. How ironic! Surprised! We had no idea that a much, much bigger surprise awaited us. How innocent and naïve we were. Thinking back, I am almost embarrassed at how naïve we were.

I remember lying on the bed for the ultrasound when a friendly, upbeat technician came to greet us. She was chatty, pointing out different parts of the baby's anatomy to us. Then she became silent. She typed with such purpose and urgency. I tried to tell myself that it was just an important part of the ultrasound, and she really needed to concentrate and focus. She said not a word for what seemed like an hour. My husband and I never questioned her. I believe we were both intuitively afraid of what the answer might be. She told us the doctor would be right in to see us, and he was, right away. He did not have the same poker face as the technician. He tilted his head to each side as he performed the ultrasound and his eyes were full of expression and disbelief. He turned the monitor off, turned to us, and said, "I have major concerns about your baby. There are several very serious abnormalities. We may have to talk termination." With that he began scribbling on the exam paper sketches of kidneys, ureters, and bladders, and pointed out everything that was wrong with my baby. There were cysts on one or both kidneys, a keyhole-shaped bladder, and even the possibility of a cancerous tumor on the kidneys. I felt the room spin around me. I thought to myself, "This can't be happening, not to me. Please God. You can't be serious."

Within 15 minutes I was surrounded by several doctors, nurses and medical students as they performed an amniocentesis. During the amniocentesis they asked me if I still didn't want to know the sex of the baby. It seemed so trivial at that moment so I gave them the go ahead, and they told me I was carrying a little boy. My son—Ronan.

I was referred for further testing at a nearby hospital with a fetal surgery center. My OB thought that fetal surgery might have been an option for Ronan. It was a glimmer of hope, but a long shot I knew. Because I worked as a pediatric nurse practitioner, I knew that if both kidneys were truly affected there would be very little anyone could do to save my baby.

I had to wait for a week before I could be scheduled for the full work-up of testing. I was desperate to have an answer as soon as possible. My husband and I had already planned to go to Montreal that weekend and we went along with the trip as planned. I found Montreal to be an intensely spiritual city with many breathtaking churches. I think I lit a candle in each and every church. In some ways, it was the perfect place for me to travel to at that time. My husband and I are Irish Catholic and we turned to our faith during that time. I had never prayed as hard in my life as I did that weekend in Montreal.

I recall sitting in a sidewalk cafe and hearing the sounds of African drums coming from the speaker system. Ronan kicked and kicked to the music. I wondered if he would have been a musician like his uncles and great grandfather. I had already started to think of him in the past tense. I knew in my heart that the news to come in the following week would not be good, and that those days were likely the last I would have with my child.

We found a pregnancy boutique in Montreal, and my husband convinced me to go in and take a look around. There were two French Canadians behind the counter, eager to show me the pregnancy pillows that would give me an idea of how clothes would look on me in the third trimester. I stood in the dressing room and cried. Pregnancy was supposed to be a journey full of anticipation. But I knew that I was probably as pregnant as I was ever going to be at that point. My husband spent about $300 on maternity clothes in that boutique, which was so out of character for him, but comforting to me. We never discussed it, but we knew we would never need to buy clothes for the baby. The clothes for me were, in some way, a gift to our baby.

We arrived at the fetal surgeon's office for a day full of tests. We had a three hour ultrasound in the morning, then an hour and a half fetal MRI, an hour-long fetal echocardiogram, and then another ultrasound which took about an hour. By the end of the day I was emotionally drained. But we still had to meet with the fetal surgeon and a pediatric urologist. We met them in a conference room. They had a huge white board behind them, and they began drawing sketches of kidneys, ureters and a bladder. They discussed every possibility with us. They explained why fetal surgery would not work, why newborn dialysis was not an option, and how my case was one of the most complicated fetal obstructive uropathies they had ever seen. They finally told us the dreaded words "I'm sorry, there is nothing we can do." My son had multicysytic dysplastic kidneys. It was incompatible with life. We decided to terminate.

I went to see my OB the next day. He had not performed any of the ultrasounds, so he seemed a bit confused and shocked that I was coming in to discuss termination of the pregnancy. While I waited in the office he contacted the fetal surgeon by phone to confirm for himself the diagnosis and prognosis. We then discussed termination options. The fetal surgeon had felt strongly that we should be induced and deliver so that we could hold the baby. My OB thought that was a "terrible idea," and that women who were already in so much stress should not have to go through the physical pain of labor. So I chose to have a dilation and evacuation (D&E) procedure at 22 weeks gestation.

As I walked back to the operating room, I remember the baby kicking. I felt such guilt, but I felt I had no option. Either way, my baby was going to die. I was afraid that if I carried him to term he might suffer at birth. I was also afraid that I might suffer emotionally over the next few months if I did not terminate, only to deliver a stillborn baby. I knew there was no easy way out of it. Any decision I made would change my life forever.

When I awoke from the anesthesia I felt my abdomen immediately. He was gone. My baby was gone. I had no idea where exactly they took him No one offered me his body or his ashes, and I didn't have the foreknowledge to ask or make any kind of arrangements. I regret that I didn't ask about that. Why did I just leave my son to be discarded? Why didn't someone advise me to take him to be buried? I left the hospital and my baby behind.

I had the D&E on a Wednesday and was back to work as a pediatric nurse practitioner that following Monday. I spent the entire day seeing babies and children who were sick, but none of them were even close to being as sick as my baby. One mom was crying in an exam room because her newborn was constipated. I wanted to shake her and say "Do you really think that's a problem? Constipation? Come on lady, get a grip. Your baby is perfectly healthy. You have no idea." But I didn't. It took me every bit of strength I could muster to not break down in that exam room. I was leaking milk through my shirt, stimulated by all of the crying babies. Oh, how I wished that one of the crying babies was mine. I would have listened all day to him crying. And what a beautiful sound it would have been.

My family and friends were mostly supportive of our decision to terminate. My parents were on vacation in Ireland when I found out that Ronan was very sick. I did not want to ruin their vacation, so I didn't tell them that their grandson was not going to survive. They told me over the phone of the beautiful christening outfit they had bought for him. They had no idea that I had tears streaming down my face during that conversation. They arrived home the evening after I terminated.

My husband's family does not know that we terminated the pregnancy. My husband did not think his parents, who live in rural Ireland, could possibly understand that we did it out of love for our son. I think he underestimated them. Part of me feels a bit ashamed that I cannot be honest with everyone about what happened to my baby. The fact that some people will judge us negatively because of our decision infuriates me. I still feel a bit of regret from time to time. I wonder if I should have carried him full term and then let him die on his own. But in the long run I realize that the outcome, whether I carried him to term or not, would have been the same.

29

Kristi's Story "Did She Think I Wouldn't Love Her?"

There are certain words that can haunt you forever. Early on in my second pregnancy, I was having a conversation with a close friend. I had told her how I had not yet bonded to my unborn baby and how I was still getting used to the idea of being pregnant again. I had a healthy three-year-old son at the time. It was a planned pregnancy, it just happened sooner than I thought it would. I told my friend that I would easily give up the baby if there was a way to guarantee my son would grow up healthy. Those words will stay with me always.

I worked as a pediatric nurse, mostly in intensive care. I had seen so many parents grieve what were previously healthy children, lost to illness, trauma, or just some crazy, random accident. I just wanted some cosmic promise that wouldn't happen to me and my son.

My husband was able to take some time off from work to come to my second OB appointment with me. We were hoping to find out the sex of the baby. My OB started the ultrasound and said that everything looked great. Then he paused and said, "This is the hardest part of my job." Then I heard more haunting words, "It looks like the baby is anencephalic." We both knew immediately what he meant; my husband worked in the medical field as well. It meant that our baby's skull and brain didn't form completely due to a defect in the closure of the neural tube very early on in the pregnancy. I couldn't even cry at first, I was so shocked. How could this particular defect have happened? I had been taking prenatal vitamins with the recommended amount of folic acid.

My first words were "Do I have to go to term?" I thought the sooner I dealt with it, the easier it would be. My OB, likely in an attempt to make me feel better, said that because it was a fatal defect, it really wouldn't even be considered a termination. He said that he wanted us to get a second opinion and would call a perinatologist. When he left the room, I fell apart. My husband and I both cried.

Coming out of the exam room, my OB told us that he was able to set up an appointment with the perinatologist for the following week. I was almost 16 weeks gestation, but I knew there was no way I could wait a whole week to confirm my baby was going to die. Looking back, it seems strange to me that I never doubted my OB or his diagnosis. I didn't even feel a second opinion was necessary.

As soon as we left the office, my husband started making calls to friends in the hospital. He arranged for the perinatologist to see us that same day. Sadly, the perinatologist confirmed the anencephaly diagnosis.

The next day I received a phone call that the labor and delivery unit was holding a bed for us. I was completely speechless. I had assumed I would have a dilation and evacuation (D&E) under general anesthesia. I thought I would go to sleep and everything would be over when I woke up. I called a friend who offered to watch my three-year-old son, and I met my husband at the hospital.

The experience was so surreal. I, again, couldn't cry. I was hooked up to an intravenous drip of Pitocin and, aside from what felt like bad menstrual cramps, I was comfortable. My daughter was delivered after about eight hours of Pitocin-induced labor. We made the decision not to see her. Aside from the anencephaly, we knew a 16-week fetus would not look anything like a full-term baby. I had a picture in my mind of her, and that was how I wanted to remember her.

The placenta took another five hours to deliver. My husband and I left the hospital about 20 hours from the time we entered.

I was in a fog for several weeks after coming home. I had never felt such pain or emptiness before. It was truly like losing a piece of my soul. I kept asking myself if it happened because my baby thought I didn't want her. Could she have thought that I wouldn't love her as much as my son? Did my mind or body do something to reject her? Of course the rational part of me knows that bad things just happen; that it was just bad luck. I hope my daughter is in a place where I will see her again. I believe in reincarnation, and I like to think I just needed to keep her for a short while until she went where she was destined to go.

30

Liz's Story "Heartache Into Healing"

I think in the "Worst Day of My Life" category, I have two; the day I found out that our baby was very sick, and the day I left the hospital with empty arms and nothing but a few mementos.

My husband and I had been married almost four years, together almost eight. We were ready for a family. We found out we were pregnant after the first month of trying and said to each other how lucky we were when we knew so many people had trouble conceiving. We were already counting our blessings. We started making plans. We were going to take the baby hiking and camping and to baseball games. I was going to quit my job and be a stay-at-home mom. When the baby was older we'd go to amusement parks and museums. Oh, what a great life our baby was going to have! We had so much love and anticipation.

My first trimester was uneventful but full of morning sickness, a heightened sensitivity to smells, and fatigue. We had an ultrasound to date the baby's gestational age at around nine weeks. In hindsight, that might have been our first clue that something was wrong. My cycle dates and our baby's size didn't match up. In fact they were almost a week apart. My OB questioned me again as to the date of my last menstrual cycle and I was positive of when it was. She asked me if I was completely sure. She changed my due date and I'm guessing it is much more common that a woman miscalculates her cycle than it is that she's carrying a baby with a fatal chromosome problem. But at that point we were still blissfully naïve.

I had the AFP blood test done at around 17 weeks and a week later I got a telephone call at home from my OB. She said the blood test showed the baby was at an increased risk for having trisomy 18. I had never even heard of trisomy 18, and it didn't occur to me that the reason I'd never heard of it was because there are virtually no survivors. I remember scribbling down instructions while my head was spinning and I was choking back the tears. That was the moment my life changed forever. I couldn't reach my husband at work and I knew he wouldn't be available to get to the phone for another hour. Oh, the longest hour. I searched the Internet about trisomy 18 and sobbed as I read the words, "incompatible with life." No, this wasn't happening to us. My life was falling apart and I couldn't even get my husband on the phone! When I finally reached him he calmly said, "Let's not panic. We don't have clear answers yet. Let's just take this one day at a time." That actually helped calm me down a little bit until he got home. We spent most of that evening doing research. And praying. I couldn't believe that just 24 hours prior we had bought the first baby t-shirt and now the baby might not ever wear it.

The next day we went for our appointment with the perinatologist. First we met with the genetic counselor who informed us that our risk (based on the blood test) was a one in 10 chance that our baby had trisomy 18. Trying to be optimistic, we felt good since that meant there was 90 percent chance the baby was fine! We were trying to convince ourselves that the last 24 hours of agony would all be worth it when they declared our baby was indeed healthy and it was all a test error. My husband even said, "This is going to be a great story to tell the baby in a few years of how he/she gave us this day of panic, but everything turned out fine." He had almost convinced me it was possible. Next we went in for our level II ultrasound. We knew the soft markers for trisomy 18 so we were paying close attention to everything the technician was doing. Our hopes were dashed almost immediately. The technician started scanning at the top of our baby's head and, since she couldn't say anything to us, she was typing in what she saw: choroid plexus cyst, etc. It was all up on the screen for us to see. And she never said a word the entire time. It was just awful. It was the worst moment of my life. The technician kept typing in defect after defect on the screen without even looking at us. I sat there quietly sobbing, holding my husband's hand, still somewhat in denial, hoping against hope that all those defects were purely coincidental and not related to trisomy 18. My husband was a rock until the technician left the room, and then he burst into heaving sobs and I knew it was over. There was no mistake or coincidence; our baby had trisomy 18, which was "incompatible with life."

The perinatologist then came into the room. He looked heartbroken as he told us, "I'm so sorry. I'm so sorry." He went over the ultrasound again in great detail to show us the exact markers our baby had for trisomy 18. Our poor baby had every single marker that we'd read about. He was so sick. We decided to do an amniocentesis even though the evidence was overwhelming that he had trisomy 18. We just wanted to know for sure. The only good news we received that day was that our baby was a boy. Our baby boy. A "daddy's boy" who would never experience going to baseball games or riding his bike. The doctor talked with us about what our options were: continuing to term, termination by labor and delivery (L&D), or termination by dilation and evacuation (D&E). We were willing to hear about everything since we weren't totally sure what we'd do at that point. We were leaning towards interrupting the pregnancy, but we just wanted *all* the information we could get. We told him we'd call him when we decided. We were having such a hard time just wrapping our heads around all of it. Two days before I was a happy, blissfully naïve pregnant lady and that day left me feeling devastated and hopeless. I couldn't stop the tears from coming. We were in the office for several hours and yet it felt like minutes. It's funny how time gets distorted in the midst of such pain. We cried the entire ride home and all evening.

I woke up in the middle of night (still being 18 weeks pregnant I could only last a few hours before waking up to pee) and sobbed uncontrollably while I sat on the toilet. My heart literally ached. The reality of it all was starting to set in. What a horrible situation: our baby was very sick, but there was no surgery to fix him, no prayers that could be answered, and no medicine that could be given to cure him. Our baby had a small chance of making it full term to be born alive, but even if he did, he would die shortly thereafter. What were we going to do?

I tried to imagine both scenarios of continuing to term and interrupting the pregnancy. Since we knew our baby boy was going to either die in utero or shortly after birth, I tried to imagine how it would be to continue the pregnancy knowing that any moment we would get the awful news. How would I function every day knowing our baby could die at any minute? What if I was all alone at my doctor's office when I got the news? What if I went into labor early? What if our baby was born alive, but died alone in the bassinet while my husband and I slept? All these thoughts were racing through my head as potentially possible if we carried to term. I weighed that against the heartache of having to interrupt the pregnancy. Ultimately, the final outcome would be the same: our baby was going to die now or in the next few months. My husband and I agreed that interrupting the pregnancy at that point was the best option for us. Since we had no control over losing our baby eventually, I wanted to feel like at least I had a little control over how and when we said goodbye. I didn't want that moment to be a surprise. I didn't want my son to be alone in his last moment; I wanted his last moment to be in my arms. I wanted that moment to be full of love. I chose L&D because I wanted to see and hold our son. We called the perinatologist four days later and told him we wanted to schedule an L&D induction. He told us we could do it the next day, but we balked, that was too soon. We scheduled it for the following week.

I used that week to do research every day. Honestly, I think I was hoping for some glimmer of hope that somehow *our* son would survive trisomy 18 to be perfectly healthy. Sad denial. All my research did was confirm that our decision was the right one for us. We also used that week to prepare for the day our son would be born. We called a friend and asked her to make us a baby blanket and cap for our baby, and she broke down crying saying she would be so honored. Our friend, a Catholic deacon, offered to say a blessing/baptism over our son in the hospital. We got film for our cameras. My husband bought a stuffed animal bunny because he said all babies should have toys. We took 11 days from diagnosis to induction, which was probably longer than most people, but everyone needs their own time to prepare and that's how long it took us. I just wasn't ready to say goodbye to my baby boy yet. We got the results of the amniocentesis that confirmed our baby boy had complete trisomy 18. Any last hope was gone; we knew what we needed to do.

In that week before the L&D I celebrated my 34th birthday. My birthday will forever be a bittersweet time of the year for me. My angel and I have birthdays only three days apart. I spent that day taking pictures of my pregnant belly (the only pictures we have of my bump) and cuddling with my husband. And crying. Family and friends called to wish me a happy birthday and offer condolences to us at the same time. It was very surreal.

I was very lucky that there was an excellent women's hospital just four miles from our house, so I had the comfort of my own home before and after the induction. We went to the hospital at 7:00 on a Monday morning to have the laminaria inserted. The nurse came out from behind her desk when I was checking in and wrapped me up in the most protective hug. Like the kind you get from your mom when you're a little kid. She whispered, "I'm so sorry." The tears continued to flow. After the doctor inserted four laminaria I was sent home to rest for the day. I went back at 5:00 PM to have them removed and had five more inserted. My husband asked to hear our son's heartbeat through the Doppler since he'd never heard it before. When we heard our son's heartbeat my husband just lost it. Seeing him so devastated actually brought us closer. Then we were sent home again to rest, but I couldn't stop thinking that within 24 hours we will have met our son, and how on earth was I going to say goodbye to him? How was I going to give him back to the nurses, never to see him again? I wasn't scared of labor and delivery, but I was so scared of saying goodbye. I cried the whole way during our last trip to the hospital.

We arrived at the hospital at midnight. The nurses administered Cytotec to further ripen my cervix and bring on contractions. The moment I'd been dreading was here. My husband and I were so quiet; the nurses were so respectful and each person who came in our room offered their condolences which of course brought on a new round of tears. The contractions steadily got stronger every hour with more and more doses of Cytotec. Around 10:00 AM the social worker came to see if we had any questions or concerns. She handed us resource information on the loss of a baby. We said we wanted to see the hospital chaplain and she gladly arranged it. By noon the contractions were uncomfortable enough that I needed to make the room more calming. We turned the lights down low, turned on our George Winston CD's and I attempted to meditate and focus on my breathing. But I was still distraught at the idea of saying goodbye to our son. Around 3:00 PM, when I was really struggling with the pain, all of a sudden a feeling of complete calm swept over me like a wave. I looked up at my husband and I genuinely said, "I'm not afraid anymore. I'm ready." My husband said, "I know. Me too." It's as if our son had given us that peace to finally get ready to greet him. My gut feeling is that was the exact time that my son passed away. Less than an hour later our son was born.

The feeling inside of me immediately changed from anguish and trepidation to the feelings every mom has when her baby is born: pride, joy, happiness, and appreciation. I had just given birth to an angel who was born still. It's hard to describe, or even understand myself, but my husband and I didn't cry at all in the three hours we held him. It's like we weren't even sad while we were holding him. His face was so peaceful and I think that was truly a gift from our son; that we could see how at peace he was made us feel so relieved. He was our tiny sleeping angel. We took dozens of pictures, had him baptized, and sang a special song to him. I wish I had considered asking the nurse if we could have him throughout the night, but the thought hadn't even occurred to me at the time. After three hours we called the nurse in to take him away. I begged the nurse to take good care of our son. She swore she would. No one should ever have to give their child over to a nurse for the last time.

Immediately after we gave our son to the nurses I felt as if I were on auto-pilot. I was shell-shocked and sleep deprived. They switched our room from the birthing floor to the recovery floor. The sad tear drop which had been placed on my door (signifying that I had lost a baby) went with us. I forced down a few bites of food and asked for a sleeping pill. I drifted off to sleep. I awoke in the middle of the night and again I found myself sitting on the toilet unable to control the sobbing. Reality had set in again; my baby was gone. I couldn't believe my baby was gone.

In the morning the doctor gave me the all clear and we got ready to go home. The staff had prepared a lovely box with our son's footprints, some hospital photos, a crocheted afghan, and our baby's hospital ID bracelet. I would go through these things countless times in the next few weeks; it was all I had. Leaving the hospital was the other worst moment of my life. I was carrying my son's box of mementos, tears streaming down my face, and no one dared make eye contact with me. Everyone I walked past looked away. I felt so horribly alone; just a pitiful mom without her baby.

The next few days were the same routine over and over: look at the photos, cry, reminisce with my husband about how beautiful our baby boy was, cry, attempt to do some mundane task like laundry, cry some more. I took sleep aids for several weeks because I didn't want to wake up in the middle of the night anymore. I've never cried so much in my life. I couldn't believe my baby was gone. I couldn't believe such a tiny person who was here such a short time could have such a profound effect on my heart. I learned the hard way about the depth of parental love. I was in a state of despair. My heart continued to ache.

I took life one day at a time. My sister came out to stay with me when my husband went back to work. My sister offered to help me make a scrapbook memorializing the few things we had. It was a labor of love. And so very healing. I actually didn't want to finish it because somehow that was symbolic of me having nothing left. So I lingered on the last couple pages for several weeks, just so I could still be working on it. But eventually I was done with it and had to come to term with the fact that our son was gone. I met with a psychologist. I leaned on my husband. I took life day by day, sometimes hour by hour.

My emotions in the first few days after the diagnosis were definitely denial. It couldn't possibly be true that our baby boy wasn't perfect. I finally accepted the truth that our baby was never going to do any of the things we had envisioned; never going to start kindergarten, go on a first date, graduate from college, and give us our first grandkids. I wept so many tears that our son was so sick, because babies should never know pain or sickness. Then I had fear: fear of saying goodbye to someone I wasn't ready to let go of yet. After we lost our son my emotions quickly turned to overwhelming sadness. I stayed in that sadness for a long time, several months. I would see a pregnant woman and I couldn't escape the feeling of "That should be me." The burden felt unbearable. The days slowly got better. I went from crying every single day to only crying four to five times a week. That felt like such an improvement. Then only two to three times a week. Then only once a week. My husband held me countless hours while I sobbed. Sometimes he cried too, sometimes he just held me. But he always understood and he never made me feel foolish.

The longest-lasting emotion (besides the sadness) was the anger. I never really got angry at God or myself. I firmly believe that sometimes Mother Nature has a fluke moment and that's what happened at the exact moment our son was conceived. It wasn't anyone's fault, so there wasn't anyone to be angry towards. But I still had the anger. I directed it at all the people who didn't "get it," the people who I felt moved on too quickly, or said the wrong thing, or the ones who didn't say anything at all. I was mad that the entire world didn't stop the day my son died. I was furious at pregnant women who complained of benign pregnancy things like not sleeping well. I was angry at parents who complained about their kids. I wanted to scream at them, "Don't you know how lucky you are? I would give anything for a healthy child!" Mostly I was angry that the world did not consider me a parent because I didn't have any living children. But of course I refused to take that out on anyone, so I isolated myself, afraid I'd lose control and let people see I wasn't really handling things that well. I went back to work. I smiled, did my job well, but inside my heart was broken. Finally, the anger gave way to understanding. How can I be angry at people for not having the exact reaction/behavior I want them to when they haven't been though what I've been through? I began to realize that I expected too much of others. And that the people who did support us with quiet strength were truly amazing people. The kind of people I wanted to emulate. The kind of people who reach out to others in their darkest moment. From these courageous people who dared to hold me up during this time I learned sympathy, empathy, nurturing, and vulnerability like I had never known. All lessons learned only because I lost my son.

We initially did not name our son. We had called him "Baby" for the first 18 weeks of the pregnancy and we felt like that was the name he knew from us. We didn't want to change it to something he didn't know. So we referred to him as "Baby." But then two weeks after we let him go I had a dream that he had been born alive and healthy and we got to bring him home with us. And that he still didn't have a name. When I woke up the next morning I told my husband, "We have to name him." Initially my husband resisted, but I insisted even harder. We chose the name "Gabriel" because we think of him as our little angel. We talk about Gabriel all the time now.

Two and a half years later I cannot believe how far I've come. At the time I didn't think it would be possible to be genuinely happy again. It took a long time, but I am me again. Not the same exact me I was before, but a new me. I am profoundly changed. I no longer have the anger or despair. I am more empathetic of others, especially if someone is going through a difficult time, no matter what the reason. My husband and I are closer than we ever thought possible. We leaned on each other in our most stressful time and our reward is a stronger bond. I'm more appreciative of how precious life is. I don't sweat the small stuff as much anymore. I'm more likely to tell others how much I love them. I am constantly reminded about Gabriel, because of all these riches he has brought to my life. He is also in our lives daily because of the pictures and mementos we have. We have a shelf in our bedroom with his ashes, picture, an angel figurine, and a poem. We have a garden bench in our backyard with his name and date on it. Every year on the anniversary of Gabriel's birthday we release balloons in his honor. The memories are bittersweet now. I still occasionally cry, but it's a good-feeling cry, the kind where you feel so much better afterwards.

We've gone on to have a healthy son and we hope to add more children to our family. Every single day I am thankful for my living child's life and that, of course, makes me thankful for Gabriel. I think I'm a better mom now because I know how precious life is.

31

Louise's Story "His Big Brother"

Always the planner, the organizer, and the one in charge. That's how friends, co-workers, and family would describe me. My life was following an enviable path. Newly married to an amazing man with a very loving family, a soon-to-be homeowner of a lovely townhouse in one of the most sought after towns in New Jersey, and expecting my first child, which, of course, was a planned conception.

My husband always wanted children. Even before our engagement in 2004 he spoke of having a baker's dozen. I on the other hand wanted to make sure we were married, had a home to provide, were in a financial position to support a family, and had taken all the proper medical precautions before trying to conceive. In April of 2005, at 27 years old, all the stars were aligned and I knew it was time to begin that journey. I had been off my birth control pills for five months; I had begun a regiment of prenatal vitamins three months prior; was one month shy of finishing my MBA (Master's in Business Administration) and was in peak physical condition.

The conception journey was fairly easy. After only two months of trying we were pregnant! It was a very joyous time for our families. It was to be the very first grandchild on both sides. At my first prenatal visit my OB/GYN, whom I had just switched to since moving to the area, assured me that I was young, healthy and likely to have a smooth pregnancy. My weight was good, my blood pressure excellent, and everything was in working order!

Like many pregnancies, the morning sickness, or shall we say, all day sickness, kicked in at six weeks. Due to nausea I had to skip my cousin's wedding which was a five hour plane ride away. I missed a week of work and spent a lot of time on the couch eating pizza and napping. It was all worth it though when, at that first ultrasound appointment, we saw the heartbeat fluttering away.

Time went by, the nausea and exhaustion never ceased, but I was growing! Every four weeks I saw my OB and everything was normal. At my 16-week appointment, a Thursday, they did my alpha fetoprotein (AFP) blood work. I thought nothing of it, assuming it was like all the other random blood draws they did. That weekend I had some random spotting. Concerned, I called for an appointment that Monday. I saw the OB on call. Since I was alone and my husband was traveling, I didn't have anyone with me at the appointment. The doctor checked my cervix and everything looked normal, however, she insisted on an ultrasound to make sure the spotting wasn't a result of placenta previa. During the ultrasound the technician was quiet and kept checking me internally and externally with her wands. That was only the second ultrasound I'd ever had so I thought nothing of it. At one point I asked if she could see the gender and she said yes, it was a boy. My instincts were right! Well, at least one of them was.

After my scan the technician had me wait to see the OB again. Usually when you are called to see the doctor the nurse comes and gets you. This time was different. The doctor called for me. I knew something was up, but I thought maybe it was placenta previa. I went into her office. I sat in the chair across from her desk and she came and sat next to me. Not good. She began saying that our baby's head had what is called the lemon sign. 'Lemon sign?' Yes, that was an indication that the baby may have spina bifida. She told me that I should see a specialist since he/she might be able to better diagnose the condition since the hole in the back could not be found via ultrasound. I was shuffled off to the appointment room and given an appointment at the Maternal Fetal Medicine (MFM) department at our local hospital for the following morning. In shock, I went to my car and began to cry. I still didn't even know what spina bifida was, but it sounded pretty serious and very bad. I called my parents, who were away on vacation, and cried and cried. I tried to reach my husband but his phone kept going to voicemail because he was flying. I silently drove home and ran to the Internet.

There were so many links of information I didn't know what was exaggerated, and what was real. What I found to be consistent was that spina bifida, in its most severe form (what my baby presumably had) called myelomeningocele, was known to cause paralysis of the legs, incontinence, hydrocephalus (water on the brain) and was associated with multiple surgeries throughout one's life. When I finally reached my husband he rushed right home and all we did was read and cry.

Sleep was impossible but I somehow managed a few hours' worth. The next day, a Tuesday, we were at the MFM department. The wait was short. We met with one of the kindest perinatologists who explained what the exam would be like and what the condition was; everything we read on the Internet the night before. During the appointment we also received the results from our AFP, which were convincing that something was wrong. Based on my blood work, I had a one in five chance that my baby had a neural tube defect.

Putting into words the emotions my husband and I felt is impossible. The worst had happened. The baby I was nurturing inside of me was ill and there was nothing I could do about it. I must have been in the exam room for almost four hours. I had multiple ultrasounds, discussions with the doctor, and an amniocentesis was performed. My husband and I went home that afternoon with a decision to make. Do we want to bring a child into the world with so many disadvantages stacked against him? He may never walk, never finish school, never live alone, never marry, have children, and will probably be in and out of hospitals for his entire life.

Though a devastating idea, to my husband it was obvious to not continue the pregnancy. Most of my family felt the same. I felt like my head was in quicksand, I couldn't breathe, think, or rationalize anything that was going on. I felt as if we had to hurry and decide. I didn't want to continue nurturing the life inside of me just so it could end. I was almost 17 weeks at that point and couldn't imagine going into my fifth month of pregnancy not knowing what to do.

I decided we should terminate the pregnancy. My love for my son would be unconditional if we brought him into the world. But would my love sustain him through the rest of his life, when my husband and I were long gone? Who would care for him? Who would love him? Who would pay his medical bills? Where would he live? Children are easy to love and cuddle and care for. When we become adults there is an expectation that we should be self-sustaining, what if he never is?

With all of these thoughts in mind, after a follow-up ultrasound which finally detected the hole in his spine in the sacral region, we decided to terminate. It was the Tuesday after Labor Day. The doctor inserted laminaria vaginally to begin the labor process. The following day we returned for surgery. I had a dilation and evacuation (D&E). The whole surgery took less than a half-hour and by late afternoon my husband and I were home.

The few days and weeks following the surgery were when the real healing began. I cried like never before. I was completely and utterly inconsolable. Nothing in life mattered. I read a book titled *A Time to Decide, A Time to Heal* which was about other women who terminated for medical reasons. I joined online and in-person support groups. I researched and researched how it could possibly have happened to me. The support groups were phenomenal. I had an immediate connection with other ladies who knew how I felt. I know some who have had miscarriages, but this was not the same. You don't choose to miscarry, it chooses you. I chose to end my baby's life. He didn't have a say.

After a few months of reconciling everything in my heart and head, we were ready to try to conceive again. I was now taking four milligrams of folic acid every day, the only known way to help prevent neural tube defects, and a new prenatal vitamin which I researched and found to assist women who may have trouble metabolizing folic acid. Why my baby had spina bifida, we may never know. It occurs in one in every 1000 pregnancies and I was that one. Neither my husband nor I have any family history of birth defects and based on my genetic counselor's information, it was a "fluke."

A very long and emotional five months after beginning the conception journey again, we conceived our son. During those five months I switched OB/GYN's to one who was a friend of the family. I couldn't bear to go back to the other doctor, there were too many heartaches associated with the office and I no longer wanted to be a number. My new doctor was extremely hands on and took his time with every appointment. Every ultrasound was frightening. I didn't want to receive bad news again, and what would I do if I did?

My healthy son was born in November 2007. Not an imperfection to be found. He scored a 10 on his APGAR! The love for my son is incomparable and has been truly a saving grace in the healing process. My little guy would not be here if my first pregnancy had not turned out the way it did. I am not a religious person so I don't know if there are angels looking down on us but I do know that both my babies are where they need to be.

Soon after our loss, what I prefer to refer to it as, I was driving and the song "Tears in Heaven," by Eric Clapton came on the radio. It was written by Clapton to explain the grief he felt from the loss of his son. I broke down and cried. Each and every time I hear that song I am reminded of my first baby and sing along,

> "Would you know my name
> If I saw you in heaven?
> Will it be the same
> If I saw you in heaven?
> I must be strong, and carry on,
> 'Cause I know I don't belong
> Here in heaven.

Would you hold my hand
If I saw you in heaven?
Would you help me stand
If I saw you in heaven?
I'll find my way, through night and day
'Cause I know I just can't stay
Here in heaven.

Would you know my name
If I saw you in heaven?
Will it be the same
If I saw you in heaven?
I must be strong, and carry on,
'Cause I know I don't belong
Here in heaven."

Is there a Heaven? I don't know. But I do know that I must be here, mind, body and soul to provide for my current son and live my life to the fullest.

32

Lucy's Story "Lucy, James and Sevi"

Since I was a little girl I knew I wanted children—lots of children. I wanted a big, happy family gang of maybe five or nine children. Then all of a sudden I was 32 years old and people started referring to my "biological clock." I had lived through several meaningful relationships, had never been that keen with birth control, and fully acknowledged my luck in never finding myself with an unplanned pregnancy. My boyfriend James and I had been together for one year; one roller coaster, happy and drama-filled year, when I started gagging on my toothbrush and my nipples were so sore that I held my breasts all day at work.

I knew I was pregnant before I even missed my period. I was finally pregnant. I don't remember a single moment of dread in that discovery. I walked around the city patting my belly, and smiling the smile of the luckiest and most special person in the entire world. James and I had not been getting along well and during a heated discussion, I blurted it out. I blurted it out because I was not afraid of his reaction. I knew that I wanted this baby. I wanted it with all my heart and soul. I was ready for him to tell me to get rid of it. I was ready for him to run away. I was even ready for him to be overjoyed, which he was.

We reveled in sweet, sweet, cozy, intimate glee with our secret—our new life-affirming secret joy. We conquered doubts about money, time, and space and spent hours every night making lists and noticing baby-harming sharp furniture edges in the living room. We fretted about how to deal with owning only trucks that weren't appropriate for infant car seats. I dreamed about owning my own business after she was born; and how she would chill in her playpen while I wrenched on bikes (I worked as a motorcycle mechanic.) I dreamed about how James would rush home after work to hold us, and how we would raise her to be a strong, beautiful, and exquisitely loved child.

When we told our friends and family, they shared in our happiness. We felt so special, so worthy, and so blessed. My mother melted from her yearlong standoff with me, and I was now a jewel in her eyes and in her heart. My father cried with pride and love and for the desire, now sated, he had not allowed himself to believe in. James' mother swelled with the blessing of her first and only grandchild. They believed in us now. For all the years of ruining our lives in our parents' eyes, we were now something to be proud of, to treasure, and to place hope in.

I had some irrational fears about the baby. I had little daydreams of my baby and me in situations where harm would come her way and I would muster all of my mother power to snatch her from death just in the nick of time. I had disagreements with family members who argued against my parenting principles. James and I were concerned about how aspects of our relationship would affect our beautiful baby. We were trying to be confident about our abilities to provide the most stable, loving, and nurturing environment for our child. We decided she was probably a girl and we named her Sevi Delilah.

At what would become my last regular checkup around 16 weeks gestation, my doctor said to me, "Gosh! You're so skinny!" I was skinny. My breasts were gigantic, but my tummy was flat. My doctor scared me when she said that, even though she was trying to hide her concern in a compliment. I left her office and set out to get "unskinny." That night I dreamt that my baby didn't have arms or legs. I did manage to gain about eight pounds that week.

The appointment for the first big ultrasound was around 18 weeks gestation and we were very excited to get to see our baby. Even though we thought the baby was likely a girl, our deepest concern was that the technician would inadvertently inform us of the sex of our child.

Seconds into the procedure, the technician started sighing and seemed very, very frustrated. I felt her frustration and, getting nervous, I started asking her questions about the image I was seeing on the screen. I saw a spine and asked, "Is that the spine? Looks like a nice spine." James was late to the ultrasound appointment and I was trying to stay calm, but I knew something was wrong. When James finally arrived, we looked at a few more images while the technician huffed and sighed, and then she said, "Thank you, it's over. I have to go show these to the doctor." She left us in the darkened room all alone.

James would later say, "When your girlfriend tells you she's pregnant, she has a baby." No one thinks something could be wrong with their baby. People have babies every day. They have been doing it for lifetimes and lifetimes. Sometimes the embryos don't stick, but we NEVER imagined something could be wrong with our baby. Something wrong with her, some weird thing that we didn't even cause that would take her away from us. With our baby suddenly in peril, being left alone in that room was not okay.

What seemed like hours passed as we held each other; completely terrified of the unspecified peril. The technician came back in and said there was not much amniotic fluid. "This space here," she said, "is dark and that means fluid, but the baby is supposed to be surrounded by fluid. See how you can only see her spine? She is cramped in a little ball because there is no amniotic fluid. I'm so sorry."

The head technician came in and nodded her head yes, in corroboration, and said, "I'm so sorry." I wanted to scream at them SHUT UP! Stop saying you're sorry! Stop condemning my baby! Sorry is for when something is over and this is just beginning! What does she know? She's only the technician. She can only operate that machine. That machine has no power over my baby, over us, or over our lives. Get on with your "sorry!"

My will to deny continued through another appointment with the High Risk Department where the quiet, soft-voiced doctor gingerly explained the grave situation. I searched his eyes, his face, and his words for some hope and when I found it, I clung to it. I cleaved it and shut out all his other words. I came home and scoured the Internet for information regarding amniotic fluid disorders, kidney disorders, weak cervixes, saline injections into the womb, de-stressing the cervix, eating pomegranates, and drinking gallons of water.

If my baby wasn't making enough fluid then, "by God," I thought, "I am her mother and I will make it for her." Days went by while I tried to make amniotic fluid with all my heart and soul. I told my baby that I was her mother and it was going to be okay. I met again with the soft-voiced doctor but this time he described the situation to me as "PROFOUNDLY FATAL." All of the success stories, my inexhaustible will to deny, and the hope to bulldoze through the problem vanished in a silent and very un-profound instant.

James and I held each other for a very long time and cried. There were no words for us, only the deepest sadness of our lives. We knew some things: our baby would not live to grow up with us, that she would die minutes after birth; and that somehow we were now supposed to decide how we would not exalt our daughter's life, but rather how we would end it. There was sick irony in it all, and there was hopelessness because we couldn't even get angry at anyone. I tried yelling at the technician and I tried hating the soft-voiced doctor, but nothing satisfied me.

I remember just how difficult everything got after this very un-profound moment. I remember because I haven't been able to write much more into the story past that moment. I have found little journal entries and notes here and there that I wrote during those times, and they kind of seem like a different person wrote them. It has been exactly one year since we found out I was pregnant. It will soon be exactly one year since we lost our Sevi. Time is slowly changing some things, and every day I try to find ways to enable myself to go toward the pain instead of turning away.

Because of where I lived, I had the option to terminate via dilation and evacuation (D&E) or to induce labor and deliver my daughter. I also had the option to carry her to term, but in her case, she probably would not have lived to the end of the pregnancy. We chose to terminate via D&E. I feel embarrassed and guilty, and sometimes I wish I had induced labor so I could have held her for just a little while. Because we chose a D&E, we never had much of a chance for an intact fetus, but the doctor was able to get her footprint for us. Although I miss never holding or seeing her, the whole theme of this story is missing what I never had.

After the procedure, I stayed home for a few weeks. I honestly can't remember how long it was. We didn't write any appointments on our calendar. We didn't send anyone any e-mails and tell them when things were going to happen. James stayed home with me for a few days and then had to go back to work and I was all alone. I thought I would move back home and crawl in a hole and never ever get out.

I sat at home, cried, and wailed. I went to the beach, cried, and wailed. I longed for another person to wail with me. I dosed myself with prescribed pain and anxiety pills and I tried to do whatever I wanted, but all I wanted was nothing. I wanted to die and to be and feel nothing. My milk came in and I realized that I could feel the spot where Sevi used to be and I coveted that disappearing pain until it was finally gone.

James and I went to a counseling session once. We had talked about it for months prior, but never went. When we finally did go, we chose a generalized pregnancy loss group instead of a group specifically for those who terminate for medical reasons. The difference of our loss was stark, exacerbated my guilty feelings, and actually angered some women who had lost their children due to miscarriage or other pregnancy tragedies.

One woman stopped me in the middle of telling my story and asked me if I ever requested a second opinion. I then realized it never occurred to me to ask for a second opinion. She said, "Did you see a urologist?" Was she suggesting I had overlooked something? Didn't she know I would have cut out my own kidney with a spoon if it would have saved my daughter? Didn't she know I would rob any bank to pay for a miracle procedure that would have saved my daughter's life? Didn't she know I would have died for my daughter?

   We had shared our story with our family and closest friends, but to most everyone else we explained as little as possible. I tried telling one person how we found out our baby was going to die, and that we did what we felt we had to do. She tried telling me that sometimes it's just not meant to be (and feeling so devastatingly guilty, I took that to mean that I had failed my daughter). I realized that I could not expose myself to unsupportive people like her, not yet. I always thought I was a strong woman, and being sure about my heart meant that I could withstand when others didn't share the same view—but not about this loss, and not with this grief.

   I do not believe others understand an iota of what this kind of loss is unless they have shared the same misfortune. People with good intentions fill your head with a list of the most inappropriate responses. It takes a little time to realize they don't mean to be insensitive when they say that it'll be okay because I can always have another one, or that at least she hadn't been born yet, or not to worry because I'll get over it. I quickly realized that despite the pamphlets that warned of a grieving process, and the previous experiences in my own life handling disappointments and loss, nothing prepared me for the journey upon which I unwittingly found (and continue to find) myself.

   I grieved by alternately regressing to the point of adolescence and then piling on another layer of guilt for acting out. I have bouts of insane jealously where I view all pregnant women as devils and all newborns as stolen treasures. How many ways can one find to feel guilty? What a punishment! I felt that maybe I had exposed myself to too many chemicals at work, or had too much stress during the pregnancy. I felt I had cursed her by saying that I was the momma and it was my job to protect her, because I obviously failed. I did find comfort when someone suggested to me that trying to blame myself was really like trying to take control of an uncontrollable situation.

   My relationship with James stretched to the breaking point repeatedly. Our initial reactions to our loss were the same, and we found emergency comfort in each other in the immediate aftermath. However, we eventually drifted to different corners to grieve in our separate ways. I didn't understand at the time, and I just felt abandoned. I felt twice dumped and without a friend in the world. This is about the time I really started to lean heavily on the *BabyCenter* bulletin board for those who terminate for medical reasons. I found a group of women going through the same thing and I had never personally experienced a greater gift than the sisterhood of our shared grief. I don't think I would have survived without them.

33

Marsha's Story **"My Cross to Bear"**

To fully understand my story, you have to travel through my pregnancy journeys. Each experience helped pave the way to the next.

In November 1990 my husband and I got married. We were both 25 years old and wanted a family—but we wanted to have some "couple" time together first. After waiting about two years, we decided we wanted to start our family. It took us three months to become pregnant with our first daughter. We found out we were pregnant in November 1992, and she was born in August 1993.

Our first pregnancy was fairly normal. The only concern the doctors had was that I was not gaining as much weight as they would have liked. I stopped working in August, three weeks before my due date (August 18, 1993). I had only gained 19 pounds. In the three weeks I was off before my daughter was born, I gained another 10 pounds. I had been through five ultrasounds to monitor the baby. Finally, 10 days after my due date and nine hours after being induced, my daughter was born. She was beautiful and weighed seven pounds, 11 ounces, and was 19 and a half inches long. I was 28 years old. After giving birth I was crying and upset. My husband and I swore we would never have another child. It was such a traumatic experience. But we knew we wanted more children.

My first miscarriage (second pregnancy) happened one year later. In June 1995, we found out we were pregnant on Father's Day weekend. I had taken a home pregnancy test and saw the '+' sign. I then proceeded to go to the lab to have my blood tested. I did that without my doctor's consent, as I had a friend in the doctor's office that I had called to get me in. My husband and I were so excited. We told our family on Father's Day. Monday came and I went to work and started to spot blood. I was very nervous, called the doctor's office, and they said to come in. I left work and went to the office where they proceeded to draw blood. I was informed the next day that my hCG level was at 161. HCG is the pregnancy hormone in your blood. When you go in to get your initial blood work done, the hCG level is tested. Most women don't even know about hCG levels. They usually aren't mentioned unless a woman has had problems with past pregnancies, or if the hCG level is low, or has fallen, when compared with a previous level.

My doctors said that I should come in again and have the hCG level checked on Wednesday. I was still bleeding. After having more blood drawn, I found out that the hCG levels were falling. When hCG levels fall there is no way to bring them up, so if that happens you are miscarrying. I continued coming in and having the hCG levels checked until they fell below ten, which they did about a week later. I continued to bleed for about a week, just as I would have bled with a period. My doctors said that I was experiencing what so many women experience: being pregnant without knowing it (though I did know it), and then having their period and miscarrying.

I decided to start trying to conceive again shortly after my first miscarriage. My second miscarriage (third pregnancy) occurred in January 1996. That was just seven months after my first miscarriage. I started to spot a little and went to the doctor. I was very nervous since the bleeding during my previous pregnancy had resulted in a miscarriage. At six weeks, I was sent to have a vaginal ultrasound. We could see my baby and the heart beating. I was very relieved. But two weeks later, the weekend of the Super Bowl, I went in for another ultrasound due to continued bleeding. The baby's heartbeat had stopped. I was scheduled for a D&C because my doctor said that the baby was too big to pass on its own. I was so disappointed. That was now my second miscarriage, third pregnancy, and my hopes for a brother or sister for my daughter were beginning to seem as if they were just dreams. I went in for the D&C, which was a painless procedure, physically. Emotionally, I was tired and upset. It was all out of my control and that made me angry. I was more determined than ever to become pregnant again and have another child.

My fourth pregnancy occurred in February 1997. It had taken us 10 months to become pregnant that time, even though we had started trying to conceive immediately after my last miscarriage. I went in for my 18-week ultrasound in May. I was so excited! I figured this was it—I was finally going to have another child after trying for almost three years and having had two miscarriages.

I took my mom and my daughter to the ultrasound appointment. We were in the room and the technician was doing the scan. We asked her what the gender was and she said, "A boy." I couldn't believe it! I was finally going to have my dream, one of each! In that split second I felt so complete, whole, thankful, joyous, and shocked! When the ultrasound technician was through with her scan, she asked me to speak to the doctor. I had been through enough that I knew that meant something wasn't good. My mom, my daughter, and I went into the doctor's office. My doctor said that there was some type of extra skin fold on my baby's head. I was numb, so numb I wasn't even listening. I thought he had said it was under the baby's chin. I thought that maybe my boy was just a chunky kid. My doctor said to call a hospital in our area and get another scan—a more detailed one.

I went home and called the hospital right away. I got in for the scan in the afternoon. I went in and when the technician was finished, I met with another doctor. That doctor told me that my son had hydrocephalus (water on the brain) and possibly Dandy-Walker syndrome. According to that doctor, my son would be severely mentally retarded. Needless to say, I was in shock! I calmly asked if I could use their telephone to call my husband. I couldn't get in touch with him so I called my mother-in-law. I just broke down and started wailing into the phone. I was crying uncontrollably and was so crushed.

I still remember that day very vividly. I was devastated. Someone had come in and pulled the rug out from under me, pushed me off a cliff, and thrown me out to sea without a life raft. I was in a black hole and had nowhere to go. My mother-in-law tried to calm me down and talked with me about it. When I was through with my phone call, I talked with the doctor again. He said that if I chose to complete the pregnancy, he could help me. If I chose to end the pregnancy early, he could not because the hospital was a Catholic hospital and they did not do those types of procedures. I went home feeling ashamed and angry. I felt dirty and low, pathetic and lost.

When I arrived home, my husband was waiting for me outside. I went into the house and was crying to my mom and sister "What am I going to do?" I then retreated to my bedroom, and my husband and I just sat there and cried. Writing this down at this very moment I am crying all over again. It is a terrible thing to have to choose to end the life of your unborn child. You may expect to do that for your parents but never for your own child. To this day, it is still a very sad thing for me.

My husband and I chose to end the pregnancy. We went in to another hospital, a women's hospital, in the area. They performed a higher level of ultrasound. That doctor gave me an even worse diagnosis. They thought they saw a hole in the baby's heart. And, according to the doctor, there would be severe retardation. I know doctors are not God, but sometimes they seem to be as close as we can get. We trust them with our lives. I just couldn't believe it, but I knew that three doctors would never tell me these things without reason. We then met with a genetic doctor. We went over our options and researched the diagnoses made to that date. We decided to do the termination on June 11, 1997.

From the moment I realized that my son was not going to be with me much longer, I disconnected myself from him. I didn't want to feel him kick; I didn't want to look at my tummy. I was so upset with myself and with the situation. I was not angry with my son, I was angry at God. I never asked "Why me?" but I did want an explanation. I went to bed at night rubbing my stomach and apologizing over and over to my son why I made the decision I did. To this day, I still feel the need to justify my decision. I feel that is my cross to bear.

I went to the hospital and was induced into labor. I was given Valium and the doctors did an amniocentesis to check if my baby had spina bifida or Down syndrome. He did not have either of those conditions. A cordocentesis was then performed. This is where blood is taken from the umbilical cord. My son then received a shot, through my abdomen, to stop his innocent heart from beating. Even though I was on Valium, I clearly remember the moment when I looked across the room at my husband and thought to myself, "I am murdering my son."

I delivered my son on June 12, 1997 at 5:55 AM after 10 hours of labor. I felt him fall between my legs and hit my thigh. I told my husband, "He's here," and the nurse came in and took him away. The nurse cleaned him up and brought him to me. He was wearing a hat and a white bib with a cross on it. I held my son and we named him Sky, short for Skyler. We baptized Sky and the hospital took a picture of him. He was so perfect on the outside. I remember looking at his body, his penis, his toes, his hands, and his face. He looked so normal. All of his problems were on the inside and I did not want to look at the back where the extra skin was. I wanted to remember him just as he was. He was one pound even and was very purple in color because he was born so early. He actually looked bruised and fit into the palm of my hand. I eventually gave him to the nurse and had to have a D&C done because the placenta was not coming out on its own. We were discharged later that day and I had requested that an autopsy be done.

We went to a funeral home, had prayer cards made, and purchased an urn for Sky's ashes. We did not hold a service, I just couldn't do that. I didn't want my daughter to have to go to a memorial service for her brother. I was also embarrassed and sad. I didn't want to face anyone or anything.

We received the autopsy results and they were worse than what the doctors had told us. It turned out that my son was missing his entire cerebellum. It just never formed. He only had two out of the three parts of his brain. That's where all the extra fluid was, and the doctors and ultrasounds could never have known or seen that. My doctors said it was extremely rare. They couldn't find any documentation on it. I was relieved, but more saddened. The genetic doctor gave me risks of it happening again, if it was: (a) a fluke, a three percent chance of happening again, the same as the odds in the general population; (b) a recessive gene that my husband and I possessed that just happened to link up, a 25 percent chance (one out of four) of happening again; or (c) a trait that I passed on to my son, a 50 percent chance of happening again. In those instances moms pass to sons and dads pass to daughters. That means if it was a trait/gene that I passed, my daughters could be carriers of the trait, but would not be affected by it. If my husband passed a gene/trait to my daughters, they would be affected by it. I left the appointment with the genetic doctor feeling no better than when I started. I didn't know why it had happened, and I didn't know my odds of it happening again. I only knew that I was missing my son.

I waited the requisite two cycles before starting to try to conceive again. My biggest frustration was that I had been pregnant four times and had only one living child. I was very sad about my son, but I was determined to have a sibling for my daughter and another child for my husband and me. If God was saying no to me, then I was going to keep going until he said yes.

My fifth pregnancy took seven months to conceive, but in March 1998, it happened. I had a slight amount of spotting in the beginning. I was very nervous about it, but I just pushed it to the back of my mind. I had not only a miscarriage to think about but now I had to worry about genetic defects. I would not let it run my life, but boy did it run my head. I never let on that I was really scared to death it would happen again. My ultrasound was set for July 20th. I had to go to the same hospital that offered to help me if I chose to keep my son but said it could not help me if I chose to end my pregnancy. Going into that room again scared me. I think my heart skipped a few beats. It was all too familiar. I took my sister with me. They scanned me and my first words were, "Is everything okay in the baby's head?" The technician asked me to wait because she was still scanning. She finally said yes, "Everything looks great." I just couldn't believe her. I was stunned. I was asking her to check and check again. She said it was okay and that I was having a girl! I went to use the bathroom and just started to cry. I was relieved yet I was sad. It just brought back so many memories of my son. I walked out of that hospital feeling happy and relieved, yet sad and guilty, all at the same time.

I gave birth to my second daughter, my third child (fifth pregnancy), in December 1998. She was delivered quickly. I arrived at the hospital at 3:15 AM ready to deliver but had to wait for my doctor to arrive. I delivered her at 3:48 AM, 33 minutes later. She was eight pounds even and 21 and a half inches long. I was so scared when she came out. She was very quiet. She was sucking her thumb and she was blue. They had to give her a little oxygen and I was just holding my breath. She was okay though. As my husband held me, I heard her cry for the first time and I cried too. The doctor mistakenly thought he was hurting me but I said it was the memories of my son that made me cry. I was happy for my daughter but I was sad for my son. That pregnancy was the closest I have had to a textbook pregnancy. I measured well, gained weight fine and had no problems. If she hadn't followed my pregnancy with Sky and all that had occurred, it would have been a worry-free pregnancy. Believe me, though, there was a lot of worrying.

My third miscarriage (sixth pregnancy) was seven months later. I found out I was pregnant in July 1999. I went in at 12 weeks to hear the baby's heartbeat and we couldn't find it. My doctor was not too concerned. I had a tilted pelvis and he thought that might be why we couldn't hear the heartbeat. I thought that the doctor should be able to hear it, but he said not to worry. I went in on my own the next week, at 13 weeks, and the nurse again couldn't find the heartbeat. "Not to worry," they said. Well, I was worried. I called the office when I got home and set up an ultrasound appointment for the following week. I left a message for the doctor that if he had a problem with it to call me. He did call me but said it was okay if that was what I wanted, although he personally didn't see the need. I went in to hear the heartbeat the day before my scheduled ultrasound. Again, no heartbeat was found. I just knew it wasn't there. I went for the ultrasound the next day and the baby had stopped growing at eight weeks. My doctor was shocked. He had no idea. My hCG levels were great, and the baby looked good at the eight-week ultrasound. He said the baby must have died that day or the day after the ultrasound. I was scheduled for a D&C the next day.

I went in for what I thought would be a routine D&C. When I awoke it was three hours later. My blood pressure was 87/12. I asked my nurse if I was still alive and he chuckled. I was weak and had lost two liters of blood. Apparently, when the placenta was being removed, my doctor noticed that the placenta had grown into, and become a part of, my uterus. When it was being removed, a hole was created in my uterus. This is a condition known as placenta accreta. A balloon catheter was inserted to try to get the bleeding to stop. I stayed overnight at the hospital. The next day my balloon catheter was removed and the bleeding was under control. I was relieved. My doctor had stated that if the bleeding did not stop, a partial hysterectomy would be necessary. At that moment, I was all for it. I was tired of doing the pregnancy thing and of losing baby after baby. When I got home, I was very weak and it took about two weeks to regain my strength.

My doctor had the tissue tested from my D&C. It turned out that my baby had triploidy. Triploidy is when there are three sets of chromosomes instead of two. My baby, a boy, had 69 chromosomes instead of the normal

46 chromosomes. I found out that it was maternal triploidy, meaning that my egg didn't divide as it should have and the extra set of chromosomes was from me.

The doctor was frank and told me to rethink having any more children. I was not happy to hear that. I didn't want a doctor or my body to tell me when to stop having children. Two months after my D&C I met with a high-risk doctor. He was very supportive and said he would be willing to take me as a patient if, and when, I became pregnant again. He was willing to work with the possibility of a placenta accreta. I met with him in October 1999.

In June of 2000, I found out I was pregnant again. I was very happy but also nervous. I cried when I found out because I was scared that I would lose that pregnancy, too. I had already told myself many times that no matter what, whether I carried to term or whether I miscarried, that would be my last attempt to have another child. I was 34 years old at the time. I would be 35 if I delivered full-term.

I had many ultrasounds throughout the pregnancy. I took extra folic acid and extra iron in case of blood loss during delivery. I took baby aspirin to thin my blood to deal with clotting. I refused the amniocentesis because my level II ultrasound looked good as well as the results from my AFP test.

I asked to be induced and in February 2001 my second son was born. We named him after his father and his grandfather. I cried during labor because I was so scared to push. I just didn't know what to expect, since there was a possibility that I would experience placenta accreta. My water broke at 7:15 AM, I had the epidural at 8:15 AM, and by 9:00 AM I was dilated to 10 centimeters and ready to push. He was born at 9:21 AM. There was no tearing, no episiotomy, and nothing went wrong. I hardly bled and my high-risk doctor said I could have intercourse two days later if I wanted. It felt like I didn't even deliver a baby, if you can believe that. My son was eight pounds even and 20 inches long. He was beautiful. I was very thankful for him.

I have been pregnant seven times, have had three D&C's, and have given birth to four children, three of whom are here with me. I know the sex of five out of seven of my pregnancies. My son Sky's condition was rare (one in 25,000), my placenta accreta was rare (one in 2,500), and my son's triploidy was rare. I have to say that I am tired of being told that my experiences are "rare." How "rare" can one person be?

To be honest, when I first began having miscarriages I was very sad about them. When I had to decide the fate of my son Sky, it really made the miscarriages pale in comparison. You see, I was one of those people who always said, "No way, not me, I will never do that." I had said I would never get an abortion. By the way, I HATE that word. I prefer the terms "terminate," "let go," or "release." I never had an AFP test with any of my pregnancies until my last daughter, my fifth pregnancy. I vowed I would never terminate a pregnancy because of a defect. I was wrong. When put in that position with my son, I chose that route, for quite a few reasons.

My feelings afterward ranged from feeling hypocritical, embarrassed, angry, deprived, cheated, depressed, spiteful, regretful, sad, and happy. Yes, happy because my son Sky is not here living with pain. He is our angel in the sky watching over us, and one day I will get to see him and hold him.

I know that not everyone agrees with the choices others make. I cannot ask anyone to accept what I decided. Everyone is different. You really can't say what you would do until you have been faced with the same situation. You have no right to judge me or anyone else for that matter. It is a very individual choice; something that is thought out and many things are considered. You do what is best for yourself and your family. I chose what I thought was the best option. That does not mean that I am always okay with it. My head says, logically, that it was the right thing to do. My heart? It's sad and makes me think I am a quitter, a coward; I didn't do enough for my son. My heart really hurts, and I will never be over my son. That is the cross I bear in my life. I wish there was some way to bring this issue out. Some people do not choose to have abortions as a way of birth control. Some do it out of love, out of health issues for themselves or their child.

I want women to know that they are not alone, if faced with this experience. Whatever choice a woman may make is her choice, based upon many things. It isn't easy. Try to choose what you can live with. Believe in yourself.

It's also important to remember to be careful what you think or say about others. I am a firm believer that those thoughts will come back to haunt a person in the future. Try not to judge others because, one day, you may be judged as well.

34

Mary's Story "Because We Loved Her—The Story of a Late-Term Termination"

We're expecting number two!

Finding out that I was finally pregnant with our second child was a joyous moment in my life. My husband and I had been trying for some months to get pregnant, and the evening when I finally got that positive home pregnancy test I was elated! So was my husband when he came home and I shared the news with him. We wanted very much to add to our happy family and to give our beloved son a brother or sister. One of my fondest memories of that pregnancy is of my son, on his second birthday, announcing to our family and closest friends, "I'm gonna be a big brother!" We had been coaching him for days on saying it clearly. Everyone at the little birthday party was overjoyed, jumping up and hugging us. It was great.

The pregnancy progressed fine. I was not feeling well, but nothing out of the ordinary for early pregnancy. I was 33 years old, and would be almost 34 at the time of delivery. We had one very healthy son, so we opted to forgo any invasive testing. Having suffered a miscarriage at 16 weeks with my first pregnancy, I was concerned about the risks of invasive tests. Moreover, my husband and I felt that whatever was in store for us, we would happily and gladly accept it. While we had both always considered ourselves supporters of a woman's right to choose, the idea of terminating a pregnancy of our own because of a poor prenatal diagnosis was simply "not for us."

Our initial blood work tests all came back fine, as well as our early sonograms. We had rented a Doppler, and frequently listened to the baby's heart beating away, feeling that all was well in there. At our 18-week sonogram, however, the baby was measuring a little small—about a week off for dates. My OB reassured me that everything was probably fine, and said that "Unless they are three weeks off, we don't worry." I was sent on my way and assumed that everything was fine. The worry about Baby being small did nag at me though. I knew I wasn't as big as I had been with my son and it just kept lurking around in my brain. Everyone around me assured me that everything was fine, too. "It doesn't matter how big or small your baby is, only that everything's in place!" I remember one person saying. Still, as all pregnant women do, I did worry. In hindsight, I so wish they had asked me to return for a repeat sonogram to check for growth, but I did not have another sonogram until 28 weeks. That's when everything started to unravel.

Why is this baby so small?

At the 28-week sonogram, I was anxious to see that everything still looked good with our baby, and to hopefully hear that he or she had begun to catch up with growth. Unfortunately, that was not to be. Sure enough, at that sonogram, our baby was measuring a full three weeks behind in growth. I was sent to a perinatologist for a detailed sonogram and to rule out IUGR— intrauterine growth restriction. At the perinatologist's office, we had yet another sonogram which only served to confirm our baby's small stature and the diagnosis of IUGR. We talked with the perinatologist at length about my health, my family history, our previous pregnancies, and then he ordered a very large panel of blood work on me to begin to rule out less common reasons as to why our baby was not growing properly. At that visit he did offer to do an amniocentesis, but said "It's really not going to change how I care for you, so if you don't believe in invasive testing, there's really no point in doing it." We of course never imagined what kind of horrible diagnoses existed, thinking that the "worst" thing you could hear back from an amniocentesis was that your baby had Down syndrome. Again, we felt that we would be able to deal with a condition like that, and so we decided against an amniocentesis at that point. I was put on bed rest and told to begin drinking protein shakes to try and entice our baby to grow. I was to see the perinatologist for sonograms every two weeks.

Instantly, our family, friends, and extended support system kicked into gear. People brought us breakfasts and dinners, offered to care for our son, clean our house, and do anything and everything we needed so that I could rest. I stopped working and we extended our son's days at pre-school. My mother traveled from out of state to stay with us for several weeks. Our best friends came over to paint the bedroom that our two kids would share and to help put up the crib and get things ready. Meanwhile, we continued to see the perinatologist. The baby continued to measure consistently three weeks behind.

It's a girl!

Finally, at one of our many sonograms, yet another technician asked if we knew what we were having. I couldn't stand it any longer—I had to know! My husband gave in too. She zoomed in on the baby's "important" parts and asked us if we knew what we were looking at. Even at that point I thought "boy?" but my husband guessed correctly that he was viewing female anatomy. We were having a girl and we were ecstatic! We were over the moon! We both cried tears of joy at that sonogram.

Things continued to progress much the same until, at one of our sonograms, the perinatologist suggested that they do an amniocentesis to rule out the one possible condition that had come up and not been ruled out as to why our baby could be so small. Some of my blood work came back positive for a virus called cytomegalovirus (CMV). This is a very common virus with which most people in the world have been infected. However, there can be complications and birth defects if you become infected with it for the first time during pregnancy. My blood work showed that at some unknown point in the past, I was infected with CMV. An amniocentesis would let us know if I had gotten it during pregnancy, and if our baby was infected as well. I was 35 weeks along at that point. We obviously were not worried about the risks of a miscarriage from an amniocentesis, so we figured we should go ahead. We assumed that after we got the results from that, we could breathe easier through the final few weeks, knowing that we were just having a small baby. If the amniocentesis showed that our baby did in fact have CMV, the perinatologist said that there were drugs that could be given in utero to stop the progression of the disease. Going forward with the amniocentesis at that point seemed like a no-brainer. The perinatologist did it right there at that visit, and told us that we would have the results in a few days.

Good news and a sigh of relief!

Our wait for the amniocentesis results lasted over a weekend, but on the next Monday I got a call from the genetic counselor at the perinatologist's office. She said she was calling with good news! The initial results from our amniocentesis were back and the baby was all clear for CMV as well as the most common chromosomal anomalies, like Down syndrome. I vividly remember hanging up the phone and weeping out of relief and joy. Our baby was simply a small baby—whew! She would catch up after birth with lots of care and breastfeeding and nurturing, which I was so excited to do! I don't think I could wipe the grin off my face for days. We spread the news to all our friends and everyone joined us in the wait for the scheduled c-section that we were to have in two weeks.

A few days later, I was on my way out to a doctor's appointment. I had just dropped my son off with a neighbor, and had only come back into the house to get my jacket when the telephone rang. I was literally closing the door and almost decided to let the answering machine get it and head out, but I didn't. I went back and answered the phone. It was a phone call that would change my life forever.

Things fall apart

As soon as I picked up the phone and heard my perinatologist's voice on the line I knew something was wrong. There was no reason for him to call me—supposedly everything was fine. And in a single instant of hearing his voice, I knew that if he was calling, it was because things weren't fine. He asked me to sit down and told me that the news he had to share was not good. At that point, my mind raced—the worst I could imagine was a baby that needed lots of surgeries, or maybe one that had some growth problems related to IUGR. Unfortunately, what he had to explain to me about our precious baby was far worse than a growth problem, and one that all the surgeries in the world could not fix.

Our baby had a very rare chromosomal deletion on her 4th chromosome. This deletion is referred to as 4p-, or Wolf-Hirschhorn syndrome (WHS). The initial amniocentesis tests do not test for such rare chromosomal problems. They only look for the most common trisomies, which is why we were able to receive the "happy" telephone call from the genetic counselor a few days before. After testing for the more common genetic anomalies, the amniocentesis sample was tested further for other problems, and that was when our devastating diagnosis was made. As my doctor read to me from what I now know to be the standard medical literature that describes WHS, I was in complete and total shock. He was using words like "severe mental retardation," "difficult-to-control seizures," "non-verbal," and "feeding problems, often requiring in a G-tube insertion." These were not images and concepts that I could connect in any way with the baby I was carrying and expecting to meet in only a couple of weeks. The literature quoted frequency statistics of WHS as one of every 50,000 births. How could this possibly be happening to us? I did not cry. I felt nauseous and I had no words. I explained that to the perinatologist and told him that I needed to get off the phone to call my husband. When I hung up I just sat there, alone in my house, paralyzed with shock and fear. Finally I thought to look up the diagnosis online. What I began to read left me open-mouthed and aghast. My mind was reeling. I called my husband and finally began to break down and sob uncontrollably as I tried to tell him what I had just learned. He told me to sit tight and that he was on his way home.

Making decisions

The next few days were a blur of telephone calls, e-mails and Internet searches. We talked with genetic counselors and a geneticist at Children's Hospital, and all of our regular doctors numerous times. I remember feeling completely nauseous during those days—tense with worry and desperate to figure out how we could help our baby. We had been thrust into a very scary world and had no knowledge of how to navigate. It was terrible. The geneticist was the only person we found who had actually worked with patients with WHS. In his 30+ years of practice, he estimated that he had worked with about 20 of these patients. I remember his exact words as, "This is a fairly severe condition to live with." This was from a man who spends his days caring for patients with genetic anomalies. I shuddered to think what "fairly severe" in his language would mean in our everyday lives.

The information we read online was absolutely horrifying. It portrayed children living on feeding tubes and having up to 100 seizures per day and then dying at age two or three. It was painful to read. Even worse, however, were the few patients I read about that survived into adulthood with WHS. They still suffered from all of the childhood symptoms, with the exception of the seizures, which seemed to subside with age if the patients could survive them. As teens and adults, they were still non-verbal, often unable to walk, and lacking bowel or bladder control. As terrifying as it was to imagine a very sick and suffering baby and young child, the idea of my daughter living that kind of existence into her teens, twenties, or thirties was truly unfathomable. And then it dawned on us—if that happened, she might outlive *us* and require round-the-clock care in an institutional setting. I remember feeling like I thought I would die or have a nervous breakdown thinking about those things.

We had no idea what to do to protect or help our very sick baby. Our young son's life was about to be changed forever as well—how would this kind of intense care for our sick daughter impact *him*? What would happen to our marriage? How much would all of this cost? We were able to make ends meet, but we had no savings and often fretted over run-of-the-mill extra bills like life insurance premiums coming up due. The idea of non-stop staggering medical bills was frightening. Of course we were willing to *do anything* and *pay anything* to care for our baby—but the prognosis that was being laid out before us seemed to outline an existence for our child that no amount of money or care could help.

At some point, the perinatologist and genetic counselor mentioned terminating the pregnancy. We initially discounted this out of hand. We were shocked and appalled at the idea—for crying out loud, we were only two weeks away from our c-section! Terminating was unthinkable. We had no idea that terminations were even possible at such a late gestational age. It was just not something that seemed like an option. However, as days went on, and we had more conversations with doctors and read more online about Wolf-Hirschhorn syndrome, the idea of being able to spare our daughter *and* our son from the life that would lie ahead seemed more and more humane. I remember praying for God to please take my baby. I remember sobbing and sobbing and telling my husband that I didn't know what to do and that I was incapable of making these decisions. I remember feeling like an overwhelmingly crushing weight was on my chest, and there was nothing I could do to get it off. I remember wishing that I myself could somehow die, only to escape the hell I was currently living. Neither option was a good option for us. All roads led to suffering for all of us. What was the best way for us to be loving parents?

Back in my blissfully naïve days of thinking that a pregnancy termination was something I could never do, I remember being of the mindset that whatever God, or fate, or the universe bestowed upon us, I was strong enough to handle it. Having worked in the public schools, I had seen and taught many disabled kids. "I could do that if I had to!" I thought. The noble and self-righteous bits of my ego carried that banner high and proud. But you see, when you become pregnant—when you become a mother and are ultimately solely responsible for the welfare of the life within you—that ego has to die a good bit. You come to realize that what is noble and righteous and what *you* can do or handle really is not the point anymore. Your only goal in life is to protect your child.

It is often said that all babies are blessings, and how true that statement is. But what about a family's obligation to the *baby*? Is it a blessing to a child to welcome them into a life where they will only know physical struggles and mental incapacitation? Would I have been protecting my daughter by knowingly giving birth to her when I knew full well that she would suffer and struggle throughout her life? None of those questions was easy to answer. I never wanted to have to figure out what my real answer would be. But there we were, forced to make impossible decisions in a matter of days, with so much hanging in the balance.

Ultimately, after many days of crying together, talking to our parents, praying, going over best and worst-case scenarios, and generally tearing our hair out, my husband and I opted to do the unthinkable and terminate the pregnancy. We were going to say goodbye to our beloved daughter before we ever even got to meet her. At such a late stage of pregnancy, there were only two options for doing this. Our perinatologist made the calls for us and arranged for us to be in touch with a clinic in Kansas. We called and made an appointment for the following week. We made plane and hotel and rental car reservations. We arranged for our young son to stay with my mother for a week. Although everyone we talked to over the phone at the Kansas clinic was compassionate and loving I was absolutely, indescribably, terrified.

Going to Kansas

Watching my mother drive away with my son in her car the night before we were to fly to Kansas, I thought my heart would break. I was having panic attacks that something would happen to him while we were gone, or that our plane would crash and he would lose both of his parents in this tragedy. I carried pictures of him with me constantly and looked at them several times each day. I cried packing my suitcases. How does one pack for a trip like this?

My in-laws drove us to the airport on a sunny Mother's Day Sunday morning in May. I remember riding in the backseat thinking that I was going insane and that this was the end of life as I knew it. The trip was ridiculous. We went through security and read magazines on the flights and even engaged in inane conversation with other passengers on occasion. The absurdity of doing these things with the knowledge of where we were going was so painful. At times I wrote in a journal a letter to my daughter, trying to explain to her what was happening and why we were doing this. And I cried more.

In Kansas, everybody is friendly and talkative. We learned that quickly as we checked out our rental car. The smiley clerk wanted to know what brought us to Wichita, where we were staying, and what we planned to do while we were in town. I started feeling a sense of panicked paranoia that everyone knew why we were there, and that they were all on a mission to somehow stop us, even if that meant harming us. I felt unsafe and scared—all in the friendliest Midwestern town one could imagine.

That night in the hotel I once again brought up information about WHS on our laptop computer. I forced my husband to read it again. We sobbed and asked each other if we were doing the right thing. I have no idea how we ever fell asleep.

Monday morning we reported to the clinic at 7:00 AM. We had to pass by a couple of protestors to get into the parking lot and walk through security to enter the clinic. We were ushered into a separate wing from those who were terminating an unwanted pregnancy. There were five other couples in our room, and you could have heard a pin drop in there as we all sat filling out our paperwork. The doctor came in and gave his sympathies to us all. He acknowledged that it would indeed be the worst day of our lives, but also affirmed that he and his staff would help us get through it.

The morning was spent getting detailed information about the medical procedures that we would go through, finishing paperwork, and paying for the procedure upfront. We had a sonogram and then they brought in pizza for lunch. It is the little things like the silliness of eating pizza for lunch at such a dire moment in my life that still sends me reeling. As the day went on, we got to know the other couples a bit more. They came from all over the country and one came from Canada. During the last week we had all shared in the experience of receiving devastating news about our babies. One lady was a medical student in New York. She had gone in for an extra ultrasound from a friend, "just for fun," only to see and recognize with her own eyes that her baby was having severe brain hemorrhaging. Two other couples had received the news that their babies had spina bifida. Yet another couple had a complicated genetic anomaly that they did not even have a name for. The last couple, the Canadians, spoke very little English. What we could make out in their thick Russian accents was that their baby too had a genetic problem of some kind. We came from different places and from very different walks of life, and we were being united there in Wichita in a way that none of us ever wished for.

Next, a very kind lady doctor met with us for over an hour. After hearing me sob and carry on for so long, she was hesitant to even provide us with the necessary documented referral, suggesting to us that maybe we should go out and meet some families with WHS kids and then decide. It was a very logical suggestion. In that moment, though, I knew in my heart what we had to do. I could not bear the thought of leaving that clinic, that town, that ugly hotel room, only to return in a week to endure the same horrible fate.

Finally, after the payments were made, the papers were filled out, and all the doctor meetings and exams were done, we were ushered into an exam room where I was given "twilight sedation." This drug apparently worked great on me because I don't remember a thing. It was more like "pitch black of night sedation," for which I am very grateful. A lethal injection was made into my belly, which ultimately stopped the heart of our beloved daughter. Then the doctor inserted laminaria, which are actually seaweed sticks, which expand slowly to dilate the cervix.

After the sedation wore off, we returned to the group room and sat once more with the other couples. The doctors and nurses and the clinic chaplain were in and out and offered words of support and healing. Their compassion was wonderful. But the doctor was right—it was the worst day of my life. Around 4:00 PM, as we were sitting there in the group, my husband happened to have his hand on my belly, and we both felt our daughter kick for the last time.

The next day we returned to the clinic for exams and re-insertion of the laminaria. Each night in our hotel we were called by a night nurse who checked on us. We were also given "homework" to review some materials on grief and to decide how we wished to handle our baby's remains, whether or not we wanted to view her after her birth, and whether or not we wished to have handprints and footprints made, and to have her baptized.

On Wednesday we returned for the same thing. The doctor determined that I was dilated enough that I would deliver that day, so we stayed at the clinic. I changed into a hospital gown and they began to give me chewable pills that would start contractions.

I labored in a room with the other women and their husbands. One-by-one, as we progressed, we were taken back into a delivery room. I was the last to go. The contractions were incredibly painful and I was shivering and shaking uncontrollably, apparently a side effect of the pills. The doctor was sitting by my side during labor, monitoring my progress. By our third day there, we had developed quite a respect for this doctor who was willing to risk his own life each day in doing a job that has spared so very many sick babies. His compassionate and caring manner, along with that of everyone at the clinic, made us feel so cared for during our darkest hours.

At a moment when the doctor was out of the room I knew it was time for me to be moved back to delivery. I needed pain medication immediately and I sensed that things were progressing. The next bit is a blur to me. I was taken into a recovery room en route to delivery and waited there alone for what seemed an eternity, in excruciating pain from the contractions. Finally, I was wheeled into the delivery room where I saw the doctor, his nurse, and my husband. I remember saying "I need to push!" The nurse checked me and agreed, "Oh, yes you do, honey." Then she gave me a sedative and the next thing I remember is waking up in the recovery room. It was done. A mix of incredible relief and dread washed over me. The unthinkable thing we came there to do was over, but my precious baby would never be with me physically again. I already missed her.

Later that afternoon we were able to view our daughter. The chaplain and the doctor were in the viewing room, and candles were lit. Our baby was brought to us in a basket, wrapped in many blankets. We opened the blankets and saw her tiny body. We caressed her face and head, held her tiny hands, and looked at her feet. We cried. We told her we loved her. The chaplain read the prayers that we had requested. From her physical appearance, it was clear that she had many problems. I remember feeling the need to get out of that moment. In hindsight, this is one of my biggest regrets. I did not want to leave my baby there, but I was feeling incapable of simply existing in that room, with those people, with my poor baby who was already gone… So, after some pictures and telling her many times how much we loved her and that we were sorry, we got up and left. Not until many days later did I realize that I never picked my child up to hold her in my arms. I still ache to hold her and can only pray that she knows how much I regret that. I don't know if it was the sedation or the exhaustion or the emotional toll, but I just simply did not pick her up out of that basket. I still hate that fact.

We returned to the clinic on Thursday to have a final exam. On Friday, we packed our bags, returned the rental car to the smiley clerk, and got on a plane to come home. In a very small way, our ordeal was over, and in a very big way it had only just begun.

Surviving

It has been almost a year since we said goodbye to our precious baby girl. I cannot believe it. I still cannot believe that those events actually occurred in my life. I have gone to therapy, both individual and group. I have done acupuncture. I have listened to tapes and read self-help books and books on grief and loss. I have taken anti-depressants. I have taken walks and written in journals. I have looked at her blanket, her footprints, and her pictures. I have cried, and cried, and cried. There have been moments when I have thought that I would *not* survive this. But somehow, the days have passed one by one. My amazing little son and wonderful husband have been my saving graces, along with a strong support system of friends and family.

The guilt has been the hardest to deal with. And why wouldn't there be guilt? Even though I know that my decision was based out of love for both of my children, terminating a pregnancy is contrary to every instinct one has as a parent. There is still a nagging that sometimes surfaces, wondering "What if it would have been different for *our* daughter?" Over the course of the last year I have come to be much more at peace with the decision, but I honestly don't know if this is the kind of thing one can ever really be "at peace" with. The majority of my everyday colleagues, friends, and acquaintances know only that we "lost our baby," not that we chose to terminate out of love and a desperate desire to spare our child from a sad life trapped in a broken body. There is shame in not being able to tell the truth. I am coming to realize more and more, though, that I made the right decision for *my* family, and that what others know or think is really of no consequence. I did not make the decision hastily or without an inordinate amount of thought and consideration. I judge *myself* for my choices and actions. I do not choose, at this time, to invite the negative judgment of others into my life. Some day in the future I hope to reach a place where I am ready to publicly put a compassionate name and face on pregnancy termination, in the hopes of changing many people's preconceived ideas about this taboo subject. For now, I am still grieving and healing. I am happy to take any of this guilt, shame, sadness, and suffering, as any parent is glad to do in order to spare their children, and that is what I hope I did.

I pray for my daughter every day and give thanks for the short time that she was with me. I give thanks for the blessings she brought to our family, such as a greater appreciation of each other, and the desire to never waste one minute of our precious time here together. Because of Evie I know what an extraordinary honor it is to be a mother and to love a child. When you have a "normal" child you know it's an incredibly special and wonderful experience. However, when you have a very sick child and choose to say goodbye early, your entire perspective on life, death, and parenthood is altered. Because of the lessons my daughter taught me and continues to teach me, I am able to be a better mother to my wonderful son. I strive to honor her every day through my thoughts, words, and actions. Thank you, Evie. I love you.

35

Michele's Story "Why I Go On"

My day started like any other. I woke up, felt our baby move and kick, showing me how alive it was ("it" because we didn't know at that time whether it was a girl or a boy), and began my day. My husband and I prepared for the morning drive to downtown Denver, as we had an appointment to see a perinatologist for a level II ultrasound. I was nervous; we had debated for weeks whether or not we wanted to know the sex of the baby and had finally decided we would wait until our baby was born. This was to be a routine ultrasound, just to make sure the placenta was okay.

I remember every detail so clearly: the drive, parking, checking in, showing my nearly three-year-old daughter the many buildings from the waiting room window, and meeting the ultrasound technician.

We had no idea anything was wrong until the perinatologist came in and started pointing out all of the details. He was using medical terms which I understood all too well since I am a physician. "As you can see here, the nuchal fold is enlarged. We see this with chromosomal problems like Down syndrome and Turner's," he said matter-of-factly, like he was discussing a case with a colleague. "Do you see the chest here? Your baby has intestine in the chest which is displacing the heart—a diaphragmatic hernia. When we see hernias at this young of development, the lungs do not form properly. Your baby will not be able to breathe when it is born."

I understood each and every word and felt the bottom drop out of my world. As the perinatologist left the room for my husband and me to talk, he said he was sorry. His comment cinched my fear. I sobbed uncontrollably, trying to explain to my husband, who did not understand a word of all of the medical jargon, that our baby would not live. My daughter watched anxiously as Mommy cried, having no idea what was going on.

The rest of the day was a blur, as I knew our baby would not survive, and as I knew we would have to decide whether or not to continue the pregnancy.

We spoke with a genetic counselor. Was this because of our in vitro? Was this something that I or my husband carried? What was the next step?

I immediately had an amniocentesis later that morning. It hurt and I was terrified. I remember the doctor saying, "Be careful, I don't want to touch the baby's arm with the needle." I thought, "Why does it matter? My baby won't be born alive."

We spoke to my OB/GYN, who confirmed the bad news about the survival of our baby and tentatively booked a labor and delivery room for us for the next week. We had a second ultrasound just to confirm the findings of the first. I held a tiny seed of hope that everyone had just made a big mistake, but that seed disappeared in a puff of smoke as the second opinion was the same as the first.

I don't know how I survived those days. I went through the motions of a normal life, but felt like someone else was in my body. It was five days of pure hell. I cried constantly, screamed "no" multiple times to God, asked "Why me?" I couldn't sleep and needed a sleeping pill. I could not go back to work as a doctor, seeing patients, trying to function when my life felt like it had just ended.

I hated that my baby was still kicking, was still alive, yet here I was, contemplating her death. I did try at one point to cherish her last movements, as it would be my last connection to her. The night before my induction, I did manage to talk with her and tell her that I loved her.

I knew at that point that we were going to have a daughter. The chromosome analysis was back—she had a ring chromosome of 15, a rare genetic disorder that is usually random, but can sometimes be passed on from a parent.

My parents, in-laws and sister-in-law came to be with us as we entered the hospital to deliver our baby.

We took pictures in the hospital bed—my husband, me, and our three-year-old daughter—our last pictures of me pregnant. I hated that we were trying to smile and be happy despite the upcoming nightmare, and then trying to capture it with a camera.

The night before her birth was the most horrible, as I had many painful procedures, enduring the worst pain I have ever had. Would this ever end? Would anything go right? Why did everything seem to go wrong?

The induction went slowly. I needed a slow induction because I had a risk of rupturing my uterus from a previous classic c-section. I couldn't eat any solid food. The procedures were painful: an epidural, a second epidural because the first one failed, a Foley catheter to help dilate the cervix, and laminaria. They were all horrible.

My state of mind was calm; I cried a little, was very nervous, but I was going to be strong. I didn't want to show emotion to my family because they couldn't handle the pain. So I cried by myself or with my husband.

We planned her birth, her baptism, and her cremation, all while in the hospital, all while she continued to kick and tell me how alive she was. Each kick a stab in my heart that was shattering into millions of pieces.

My baby girl, Faith Celeste, was born and died on January 18th at 3:00 AM, three and one-half days since the whole process started. It was also my dad's birthday. She was born with one push. Is that all? This is it? All of my pain and sadness, for this tiny moment?

She was alive when she was born and moved a tiny bit. I didn't think I could handle that, but finally realized the best place for her was in my arms, so that I could love her as she died.

We held her for hours, cradled her, and loved her as best we could in that short time. We took as many pictures of her as we could with each of us, with each of our family members, and with her stuffed animals that we had bought just for her.

You see, I didn't want her to have a hand-me-down toy, but one of her own. So we had shopped for toys and a blanket, just for her, before going to the hospital. That trip to a major chain of baby stores was the most difficult for us, seeing all of the healthy babies, seeing healthy pregnant women, knowing what horrible fate lie in store for our baby.

She had my nose, ears and chin, and seemed to look like her older sister. Oh God, she would never know her sister, they would never play together, grow up together, or fight together. Can my heart shatter into smaller pieces? The answer was yes.

Eventually, her body did become cold. I hated that her skin was cold, that I couldn't keep her warm, and that she had an odd smell. She did not have a sweet baby smell like the one I remembered with my daughter. I didn't like her smell, but I held her anyway, because she was my baby. We kept her with us for nearly eight hours, having wonderful support from the hospital nurses.

I sang to her my favorite song, "You Are My Sunshine," just as I had sung it to her while I was still pregnant. I actually sobbed it, as it hurt so badly to think that was the only time I would be able to sing to her.

I will never forget those few, precious, fleeting moments we had with our daughter. I prayed that she knew love, that she would never be cold, that she would always be held and comforted, and never be alone and scared.

We dressed her and wrapped her tightly with her new blanket and her monkey toy, which was just as big as she was. Having the nurse take her away was one of the hardest moments I have ever had. I knew she was going to the morgue, that she would be cold, and that she would be alone. The nurse covered her face. I was shocked, but immediately knew what it meant: our baby was dead. I barely stopped myself from running down the hall to yank back my baby, wanting so badly to have her in my arms again, to never let her go. I managed to eat, dress, and with great difficulty, go home. All without my baby. I had never dreamed this could happen to me. My arms were empty as we left for home.

My life after our heartbreaking choice has been difficult. Everything in my world stopped on the day of that awful ultrasound that shattered my heart. I could not believe that people were still working, playing, living, while my life was so ugly and hurtful.

My world was a big, black pit of despair. To this day, I'm not sure how I survived. I think a primitive part of my brain took over my basic functions. Somehow, I still woke up in the morning, played with our daughter, ate food, had conversations, watched television, and went to bed, but I don't remember anything except horrible sadness, hopelessness, grief, gut-wrenching sobbing, and agony.

My life was a thick fog that could not be penetrated by any light, by anything other than my tears.

My husband and I were scared to be alone, so we asked my parents to stay another week with us, since they lived in another state. We didn't think we could handle our grief by ourselves. It turned out to be a very good decision as I ended up needing a D&C for retained products five days after the loss of our baby. I remember feeling acutely aware of the pain my mom was feeling for me. I could read it in her eyes, seeing her unshed tears as she watched her own child struggle to function. She wanted so badly to help me feel better, to take away my anguish, yet she was as powerless to stop the pain as I was. She was there for me as only a mother can be, and offered a shoulder to cry on when I needed it most.

Nearly one month after our loss, I suddenly felt like the fog had lifted. I had moments of happiness that weren't forced, I enjoyed playing with my daughter, and I remembered there was a world around me.

There is a film effect that describes my feelings of the world stopping—one person in the center of the screen, standing still or in slow motion, surrounded by people rushing by. When my fog lifted, I gradually started moving, slowly rejoining the world around me. My life stuttered, stopped, started again, and finally I rejoined those people, who were, after all, moving at the normal pace called life.

I was by no means over the loss of our baby, but I could at least appreciate the sun, so to speak. I took seven weeks off from work before I felt that I was ready to go back. It was difficult, and that's putting it lightly. In a medical clinic of more than 80 employees, most of them knew I was pregnant and that I had lost the baby. I have a practice of more than 1,500 patients, many of whom knew I was pregnant. Most everyone wanted to express their sympathy and that terrified me, because I knew I would cry if someone told me they were sorry. There were a few who had no idea I had lost the baby and wanted to know why I was out of the office. Some simply looked at me with a sad look, and some just gave me a hug. It was so stressful, as each expression of sympathy made my loss more real, and made me wonder if I could handle any more condolences. I kept silently praying for someone to not know of my loss, so that I didn't have to tell my story again, so that I didn't have to hear "I'm sorry" yet again.

But I made it through and I soon realized that each person who was sad for my loss was not trying to torture me on purpose. I was finally able to appreciate that not all people know what to say or do when someone is grieving, especially the loss of an unborn child. I forgave people for their blunders, realizing that we are all human and that we all stick our foot in our mouths at some point.

I just passed the three month anniversary of our loss and as cliché as the phrase is, time really does heal the pain. Each day I get a little bit better, but I will always have a scar on my once shattered heart.

I now divide my life into "before I lost my baby" and "after I lost my baby." I so want to go back to my life before I lost my sweet baby girl. But that is not my life. My life is here now and I cannot live in the past. I still struggle with the things that "should've been" and anticipate that my upcoming due date in May will bring back many of the emotions I had in the beginning. But I am here now, I am alive now, I am breathing now, I am me now. I keep repeating these words to myself, my new mantra, to remind me to live for today.

My life has been difficult since our heartbreaking choice, but knowing that my baby girl is in God's arms, that she never suffered, and that I was able to make this sacrifice for her, is the reason I go on.

36

Nicole's Story "Lightning Strikes Twice"

My partner and I had been together only 10 days when we knew that we were soul mates. We decided we wanted to have a baby and get married. So nine months later our first child, a little girl, was born. When she was four months old we walked down the aisle. We thought it might take awhile to fall pregnant again so when our first child was six months old we started trying for another. I fell pregnant straight away and our second child was born 15 months after our first. That time it was a little boy. My husband and I had said we would like four or six children so we knew that there would be more.

In 1997, I was pregnant with our third child. For whatever reason, I knew there was something wrong with the baby I was carrying. I had an ultrasound at 14 weeks, but nothing abnormal was found. Four weeks later I went for my routine 18-week ultrasound. I was told that our baby had spina bifida (SB), and to go home and ring our family's general practitioner to talk about a termination.

I was in shock. I had heard of spina bifida, but did not know what it was. I told my husband, who also couldn't believe it. I rang my doctor, who suggested we terminate and referred us to a specialist who said he did not believe in abortion/termination but would support us doing it.

My background was a religious one. I went to church every week, and because of my beliefs I could not think of terminating. We did talk about the options, otherwise we would not have been true to ourselves. After four weeks of deliberation, we told the doctors that we could not terminate and that our baby would come into the world when he was due.

We had months of tears, which would turn into years of more: but also lots of joy and soul-searching. He was born in August 1997 with a huge hole in his back. He is now nearly 11 years old and has had 16 different surgeries with still more to come. With our other children to care for, it put a lot of strain on our family at times. It has also meant time out of work, affecting our financial stability. He has partial paralysis from the legs down, bone deformities, a ventriculoperitoneal shunt, is incontinent, suffers from pressure sores which turn into ulcers (which can take up to six months to heal) and has a type 1 latex allergy.

In November 1998, I became unexpectedly pregnant with our fourth child. I was in a panic. I had been cautioned to take folic acid before trying to conceive again because there was a chance we could have another baby with spina bifida. Since the pregnancy was unplanned (even though we wanted more children) I had not done those preparations for that pregnancy. I had ultrasounds with the specialist, as before, and things looked okay. Our fourth baby was born in July of the same year: a healthy baby boy.

It was April 2000 when we uprooted our family and moved from the country to the city so that my husband could work at The Royal Children's Hospital. We lived there for two years and toward the end of those years, we decided to have another baby. I started taking folic acid four months before I got pregnant. Due to our increased risk for spina bifida, I continued to take it three months into the pregnancy.

Being pregnant again and finally wanting a place of our own we decided to make the move back to the country. We had always rented, but figured with baby number five on the way it was time to look ahead. I had my eye on a piece of land which was up the road from the hospital and across from a school so we went to the bank for a loan and started building our house.

It was the day we were loading the truck to move when I received a phone call from a very dear friend who was pregnant with her second child. She began to tell me that her baby was dying. I was devastated, not that I knew exactly how she felt, but I did know what it was like to find out there was something wrong with your baby. I would not wish it on anyone. Her 18-week ultrasound showed that the baby had no kidneys (Potter's syndrome), so when she reached full-term there would be no chance of survival.

They had to have him early due to the added strain on other organs as she got closer to her due date. They decided to wait until 29 weeks so if the doctors were somehow wrong there would be a higher chance for his survival. Sadly what they were told was true and they said goodbye to their little boy.

In my first trimester of my fifth pregnancy, my daughter came down with German measles, which meant there was a possibility that the baby I was carrying could be born with fetal anomalies. It was something we would not know for sure until after the birth, and it was an added strain to the pregnancy.

I was due for my 18-week ultrasound and was nervous. We knew we had a higher chance of having a child with a neural tube defect, but thought "It can't happen to us twice; we can't be that unlucky."

Lightning does strike twice. We saw it before they told us. We were having our second spina bifida baby. I cried because the diagnosis in itself was a loss. I was grieving for the "normal" baby that I would not have.

The following ultrasounds showed the baby's condition was getting worse. We made the decision to have our baby early. There were other factors, including our other children and that our boy with SB was to have an operation at the same time that I was due. I told my husband that if I were to have the baby early that no one was to know until we had him. They knew he had SB but that was it. I could not cope with explaining my decision to others. My friend knew we were going to have him early, but that was all.

I had our case heard before the ethics committee of the hospital because if I was going to end the pregnancy, it would have to be past the point when it became a moral/legal issue with gestational weeks. That was because the cut off time was the same week as the birthday of my other child with SB. I could not have one child and lose one child with the same condition in the same week. If it were a different month even, I thought it would sit better in my head. The committee agreed.

I went into the hospital at the start of September and Joshua was born on the 3rd of September. He lived for about an hour and a half. It was horrible. I was in labor knowing I was ending my baby's life.

Nothing will ever be the same in my life, how could it ever be?

The look on our other children's faces when they came to see him and thought he was asleep, and were told he was dead, was absolutely awful. I did not comprehend what it would be like after the fact. I was so naïve. The mental pain afterwards was excruciating. I kept rubbing my tummy for what I was missing. I knew only a pregnancy, not a child that played, smiled, and laughed.

I needed to be pregnant again, not to replace him but to help heal me and to help our other children. I did not want that to be their last experience of a baby. My husband had said "no more children" before we had Joshua, but he agreed to discuss it later. He could see my pain and felt his own and wanted us to have another. So we started trying for another. I had started taking folic acid the month after Joshua died. I did not care if I had to take folic acid for years; I was going to take it until I became pregnant again.

After about five months we talked about another child and decided to try. It was a hard decision to have another baby. We knew that emotionally, and for me physically, it would be hard. On my 30th birthday, my husband announced to the family that I was pregnant. Most of the family was not happy. That began another episode of unhappy times. It was seven months after Joshua's death and it was a shock for them all as I was just over two months pregnant by then. There was pressure from everywhere. People kept expressing their views and how they felt and would not let me express my views. I could not breathe.

Our sixth baby was born healthy in November 2004. He is gorgeous like our other children.

My husband wanted to go and have a vasectomy but I was still unsure if that was the end of our story. We talked about it and I spoke of how we had six children in all but we only had five with us. Our last child would miss out on what the others all had; a sibling close in age and who they got to spend time with at home for a few more years than our last would due to a bigger gap because of Joshua's absence. I also said that I didn't want another baby if he didn't. A few months after our talk, he came to me and said that he wanted to have another child. To make our circle complete our last baby was born on our angel baby Joshua's due date. All our dates through the pregnancy were the same. It was a bittersweet time but I knew that our last baby—another boy, had a part of Joshua with him.

So here I am six years later, at times still grieving and still living with the loss of Joshua. Through the hard times of fetal diagnosis and making two different decisions, I can only hope that our family is stronger from being in those situations.

37

Renee's Story "Protecting My Boys"

In December 2005 I started wondering if I might be pregnant. My birth control pills usually made my cycles like clockwork, but this month my period was late. My husband and I had two healthy boys at the time, and although I had always wanted three children, my husband was happy with just two. I stayed awake most of the night of December 18th, in fear of what my husband would think if I told him I was pregnant. I was worried he might leave me. He came into the living room and asked if everything was okay. I started sobbing and asking him not to leave me, then told him that I thought I might be pregnant. He told me not to worry and that we would figure it all out when we knew for sure.

I went out and bought a home pregnancy test. Immediately the test strip turned positive, as I had suspected. I was both overjoyed and scared. It didn't take long for my husband to be excited and overjoyed as well and we told our two sons, who were five years old and seven years old, that they were going to be big brothers.

Everything with the pregnancy progressed as usual and looked great as far as we could tell. Even so, I was constantly worried that something was wrong. I tried my best to push the negative thoughts to the back of my mind. In the days leading up to my ultrasound appointment I confided in my best friend that I was worried about bringing my boys to the ultrasound. I was very protective of them and didn't want them to witness anything upsetting. She said that she understood my fears, but that only I could decide what would be best.

I woke up Wednesday, March 29th, 2006 and got myself and my boys, Zachary and Zane, ready for my ultrasound appointment. My husband, the boys and I arrived at my OB's office and had to wait a bit because the couple with the appointment ahead of us had just found out that they were having twins. I was on the edge of my seat with excitement and worry. I walked into the exam room and the nurse finally came in to start the ultrasound. She measured the baby's head first. Zane kept asking, "Is it a boy or a girl?" He was so excited. I noticed as she scanned across the baby's abdomen that she measured and moved over the area several times. Of course I had *no* idea what she was looking at. The nurse jumped up from her chair and said, "Something looks wrong with the kidneys, let me get Dr. M in here."

My worst fears had just come true. I feared that my boys would witness something horrible if they came with me, and now they had. I had never felt so helpless and scared in my entire life. I was trying to hold it together so my kids wouldn't see their mom in complete despair, but it was difficult. I was devastated. Another nurse came in and asked us to go across the hall to another room. Sympathetically, Dr. M told us that our baby's kidneys were severely enlarged and polycystic. He told us that usually was a sign of other problems and that the outcome for our baby would be grim at best. He tried to make an appointment for us to see a perinatologist, but they couldn't see us until Monday, April 3rd. That meant five days of waiting for more information.

Those five days were pure torture. I had to go on living life as normal for my sons. They were involved in activities that required us to drive them. I had an acquaintance come up to me and say, "So you are having another one?" I just dropped my head and said that I didn't know, that things weren't looking good, and left it at that. I was fortunate that my husband was by my side the entire time. He was very worried about my mental wellbeing. I had suffered from depression in the past and had actually weaned myself off my antidepressants after finding out I was pregnant.

On April 3rd we arrived at the perinatologist's office. The ultrasound technician came into the room and asked if we knew what gender our baby was. We said that we didn't because our last ultrasound had ended so abruptly. She showed us that we were having a boy. She was very quiet while taking the measurements. She gave me a picture of the baby's foot to take with me. She left the room and Dr. R came in and took some more measurements. Then, with tears in her eyes, Dr. R told me that she couldn't give our baby any chance for survival. She showed us his kidneys on the 4D screen and it was very easy to see that they were so enlarged that they took up his whole abdominal and most of his chest wall. I had almost no amniotic fluid left since his kidneys weren't working to produce urine, and there was no visible bladder. She said that his lungs would never develop due to the lack of amniotic fluid for the baby to swallow and because there wasn't anywhere for the lungs to grow. She said that I had two choices and neither of them would be an easy choice. I could choose to induce labor and terminate my pregnancy or I could carry him until I went into labor on my own. She couldn't tell me when that would be, but it might have been soon since there is an established link between a lack of amniotic fluid and preterm labor.

She left us alone for about 20 minutes or so while I cried. I knew almost immediately what I needed to do. I didn't think that I could carry to term knowing that the end result would be a dead baby. How could I go on with life as usual with my sons? I was concerned not only for me and my baby, but for my family as well.

Dr. R came back into the room and told us to go home and think about it. She let me know that since my regular OB was going to be headed out of town in two days that if he couldn't assist me with a termination she could.

It was basically a no-brainer for me. My husband told me that it had to be my decision because it was my body, but that he would support me no matter what. We discussed how either situation would affect our living sons.

I made an appointment with my regular OB the next morning to tell him my decision. He scheduled my induction to start that night, Tuesday, April 4th. Both he and Dr. R had told me that an induction usually takes from eight to 24 hours, but could go as long as two days. Since he was going out of town, my OB told me that his on call partner would start my induction at 6:00 PM. During that time I had arranged for my mom to fly in from Alabama to be with me. I needed her support. I didn't know what to expect and just knowing my mom would be there was a blessing.

My mom arrived on the afternoon of April 4th. I got to the hospital just before 6:00 PM. In a cruel twist of fate, I had to walk past the baby nursery to get to my room. I sobbed while I changed into my hospital gown. I started to calm down a bit as an amazing nurse and my mom held and comforted me. My husband had gone to register me and when he returned another nurse came in to tell me that the on call doctor had refused to assist me with my termination due to moral reasons. While I understand that we all have our own moral beliefs, mine wasn't a decision that was made lightly. My baby was going to die anyway. I was his life support at the moment. I honestly felt at the time that *no one* was feeling my pain. My baby was moving less and less with no fluid to swim around in. My OB called me from a convention he was attending in Dallas to speak to me about his partner. By 6:30 PM we were back in our van on our way home. We would call the perinatologist on Wednesday.

On Wednesday, I called and spoke with the nurse at the perinatologist's office. She had talked to Dr. R, but the earliest their office could begin my induction was Friday, and Dr. R's partner, Dr. P, would be the one on call that day. Dr. P was out of town, but the nurse was pretty sure that Dr. P would have no problem helping me with my termination. The nurse told me that if there were any issues, the office would call me on Thursday.

I struggled through another few days of just getting by—of getting up and moving through the motions for my boys. They didn't know what was really happening. They only knew that they weren't going to get to be big brothers to a new baby brother after all. We told them that the doctors were going to help Mommy to deliver him and that he would go to Heaven with their grandma and great-grandpa. I sobbed every day in the shower. I read the book *Empty Arms* that the nurse from the first hospital had given me. Reading it helped me to realize that I wanted to see my baby and have him blessed.

On Friday, April 7th, 2006 at 10:45 AM, Dr. P inserted two doses of Cytotec in my cervix. Four hours later she inserted another two doses, then four hours later another two doses, and then I asked for my epidural. My cervix was refusing to thin and wouldn't dilate at all. After six doses of Cytotec they started the Pitocin. After 16 hours and four bags of Pitocin, my cervix still wasn't dilating. The doctor tried the Cytotec again, and then started talking about sending me home for a couple of days and I would come back and try again. Hearing that, I started to get nauseated and upset. I didn't want to have to go home and come back. Dr. P conferred with the head of OB/GYN of the hospital and he suggested something my husband called "Voodoo medicine" (the only thing I could laugh about in the situation). They put a balloon catheter tube into my cervix and forced saline into it to inflate it about three centimeters. That was sometime Sunday night. I'm not sure exactly what time it was as the hours and days seemed to blend together by that point.

I had called the anesthesiologist in about every two hours to put more medicine in my epidural line. I was in a lot of pain and my contractions were pretty much nonstop for two days. Around 5:00 AM on Monday I had asked for more medication. I also asked my husband to help me to turn over since I had no feeling at all in my right leg and very little feeling in my left leg. I told my husband that I didn't know if it was just a sensation from the medication or not, but something felt warm between my legs. He lifted the sheets and they were covered in blood and fluid.

Dr. P must have spent the night at the hospital because within five minutes she was in my room. She removed her sweater and put on a surgical gown. The nurse could see my baby's head, so I pushed twice and it was done. It was 5:15 AM on Monday, April 10th, 2006. My baby boy, Zeb Michael, was delivered an angel. They wiped him down and pulled the amniotic sac off of him. They wrapped him in a warm blanket and gave him to me. I unwrapped his blanket and was astonished that he looked perfect in every way. Everyone had encouraged me to hold him, and now I know it was the right thing to do. He had 10 fingers and 10 toes. He even had his boy parts already. Because babies' skin is still transparent at 20 and one-half weeks gestation, I could actually see his kidneys. A chaplain from the hospital came in and said a blessing for Zeb. My mom, my husband and I held him for about an hour.

I was released from the hospital around 1:30 PM that same day. It was definitely the longest four days of my life. We had Zeb's remains cremated, with the hopes of spreading his ashes on my mother-in-law's grave in Alabama. She passed away in October of 1992. Her birthday was the day before Zeb's, on April 9th. I was so scared that Zeb might be born on her birthday.

My heart will never heal, but I know it will get better. I have faith that with each day it will get easier. I am thankful that I am healthy and I know that I have to be here for Zachary, Zane, and my husband.

It's been two years now and I haven't had the strength to spread Zeb's ashes on my mother-in-law's grave. He is wrapped up nicely in a box that my father-in-law had made with Zeb's name on it. Maybe someday I will be able to part with him, maybe not. I'm fine either way.

I've since gone on to have a healthy baby boy, who we named Zeke. Although the pregnancy with him was littered with problems and several issues showed up on the ultrasounds, everything turned out fine. Our family is now complete. I have four sons, although I only have the honor of raising three of them here on Earth.

38

Sara's Story **"Indelible"**

On Friday May 12th, 2006, the phone in my office rang. It was 4:11 PM. It is strange how some details will always remain in our minds while whole days become lost. 4:11. I was breathless. I kept thinking "Just hurry up. Call us so we can let people know on Sunday, on Mother's Day." We were waiting for our amniocentesis results.

In our case it would be Mothers' Day as we were two over-the-moon mums-to-be. Lesley and I had been through so much to get to that point and yet, despite the increased risk due to my age (over 40), I had never been so joyous in my life. I felt I was born to pregnancy. Each time I threw up, gagged, and every single night of insomnia (which was since conception) I felt so happy. I wished on every star, said prayers and sang loudly every day driving home from work. This was our secret miracle. There was not one day I wasn't thankful. Lesley, the first person who glimpsed the fluttering heartbeat at the first ultrasound, was equally excited and ready to yell from the rooftops. I was just 18 weeks pregnant with our "elf."

"Sara? It is Andrea. Your results revealed a male trisomy 21. The amnio result was positive for Down syndrome. We would like you to come in to discuss these results next week." Out of habit, I blindly wrote on a yellow Post-it "Trisomy 21." I don't remember hanging up the phone or calling Lesley but the sound of hearing her whisper a despairing "No!" will remain in my memory forever. When I hung up the phone, my whole body shook as though I had been plunged into ice water. My knees were buckling. I left my office and, after being steadied by a dear co-worker who knew of our pregnancy, I somehow drove to pick up my partner. We couldn't speak. We were in shock. A neighbor waved happily to us in our laneway. As I put the car in park, I felt all control fall away. An unearthly loud wail rose from my deepest core.

It was as if we had been pulled underwater. We clung to each other during the days that followed. I slept little. It seemed easier to just *stay* in hell than to descend over and over again. Each time I awoke I was whipped sharply with despair. It wasn't a bad dream. It was my life.

In between waves of raw emotion, when we no longer had the breath or physical strength to cry, we studied and read everything we could on the Internet. There were so many sources—both heartwarming and heartbreaking stories revealing such vastly different experiences. I knew this as I had known people with Down syndrome earlier in my life. We needed to learn as much as we could. I would have died for the loving smile and kindness of our sweet son.

As I felt the early stirrings of our son inside of me, I prayed for guidance. At my darkest moments I asked the Creator to make the choice for us. I felt I would have to choose either a life marked by our son's sacrifice, or choose to let our son go in peace.

I wanted to die.

Lesley saw this and feared for me. She called the hospital of our obstetrician to try and get some psychological support for me. In light of our circumstance, the obstetrician on call tracked down the director of the Genetics Department and asked if he would call us. He was attending a conference. He called us as soon as he received the message. He spoke to Lesley and gave us all of his phone numbers and said to call him any time. I will always be so very grateful to that man.

When we met with him and one of his counselors the following week we felt very supported. I was unable to look at anything but the carpet. I couldn't look at anyone in the face. I could not let anyone in to my feelings. They were too dark and too strong.

After reviewing our genetic family history for the counselors' statistics, we went over the medical findings and issues that had come to light. I will always remember the first statement "People with Down syndrome have been known to be especially kind." The counselors made a point of offering every support we needed no matter what our choice would be. There was never an assumption of termination, or of carrying to term. I realize, in retrospect, that we were very blessed to have the well-rounded counseling we had. We were not influenced in either direction, either by slanted information or by the way in which the information was worded. I barely spoke although I heard every detail and remember it verbatim. I asked as well about fetal pain research as it related to terminating a pregnancy.

With breaking hearts we decided to book the termination, but I needed the promise that at any moment, if it felt remotely wrong, even walking right into the operating room, I could change my mind. That was important to me. I needed to hold on to that. It was felt that, given my emotional fragility, a surgical procedure would have been better for my mental health, especially since I still hoped to give birth in the future. As I was one day past 18 weeks our obstetrician would not terminate the pregnancy. There was only one doctor who would do the termination at 18 weeks and beyond. She is a remarkably special person. She met us and explained what she did in the procedure that would ensure that the fetus passed peacefully. I have always been actively pro-choice. However, I never expected to make that choice myself. Our pregnancy was so wanted and there I was choosing to end it. It was cruelly surreal.

We were sent to see the perinatal psychiatrist at the hospital. She was very concerned with my lack of sleep. I couldn't have cared less if I never slept again. Surely, if I was rested it would feel even more real. I was given a prescription but when it came time to take it, I couldn't. I was concerned that it might be unsafe to the fetus. I held tight to the fact that I could change my mind at any moment, so I was not going to harm our elf in any way. I left a message for the psychiatrist, crying, "I can't take this if it would hurt the pregnancy. I could still change my mind." She called me to assure me that it had been taken safely in the second trimester. I remained wary.

With the surgical termination scheduled over a week away, Lesley and I went up to the cottage to be with my parents. I sat in the chair overlooking the lake, feeling tiny fluttering inside, and tried to hold on and treasure each tiny sensation. I was being swallowed by sorrow. I still prayed that somehow we would not have to make a choice.

I struggled with my faith. I whispered to my mother that I was afraid of how God would see our decision and bring retribution. My parents are devout. She first asked me where I had dug up that Old Testament God. Then without hesitation my mother said, "You know, God's gifts are often very complex. You may have learned of the baby's condition in order that you can act upon it out of compassion and love. That you have the strength of heart and courage to make such a selfless decision is a gift from God."

As time grew closer to our termination, I could feel myself retreating further behind a shadow. To step out of the house was incredibly hard for me. I was beginning to show and I couldn't risk anyone asking me when I was due. On our last day at the cottage, Lesley and I walked along the beach. I was glad she had this chance to speak aloud to the elf. Then we stopped and I looked across the waves. I asked the lake to safe keep my heart. I looked to the horizon to safe keep my faith and my hope, for I could no longer believe in joy. I asked for the waves to carry my grief so that when I needed to feel it would ebb and flow in a healing way. Lastly, I asked for the wind to startle me and remind me that I was alive.

Lesley and I prepared to leave for the city. Once the car was packed, my mother said to me something she had said before but in a completely different context. "Let go and let God." This was such a different context than I knew this phrase in the past. Releasing our beloved boy was the letting go. God would take on the journey from there. I knew her words, as clear as the tears on both of our faces, were heaven-sent.

The next day my sister drove us to the hospital for the insertion of laminaria to dilate my cervix. I sat in the chairs waiting. Pregnant couples on the obstetric floor surrounded me. I stared again at every fiber of the carpet. I felt numb. We were met by a social worker who spoke with us for some time. She went over the procedures and forms as well as how to arrange a cremation with a funeral home.

I couldn't eat past midnight. It occurred to me many times that a simple sandwich could derail the whole procedure. I fasted, aware that each minute carried with it the will to choose a different path. Yet with every moment of revisiting our choice I knew even more sorrowfully that we were making the right decision, one made out of profound love for our child. I found no comfort in that. There was nothing that would catch my heart in free fall. That night and the next morning at dawn, I wrote a letter to our elf. I described the many dreams we had for him, and why, as his mums, we felt we couldn't make any other choice.

On the morning of the termination, after showering, I took an indelible marker. I drew a small heart and wrote on my skin where I thought the doctor and nurses would see it, "This boy is dearly loved." I sobbed uncontrollably in the hall before the day surgery door was open, in the waiting area, and in the patient area. Poor Lesley was not allowed to come in to the patient area. Thankfully she was with my sister and my dearest friend during that whole time. I can't imagine how difficult her wait must have been. I wept going into the operating room. I desperately tried to tell everyone—anyone—why we had chosen to end the pregnancy. As I lay on the table, I was gasping for air, feeling my ears fill up with my tears. Before the anesthetic began, I needed everyone to understand how much we loved our son and to care for him. The doctor leaned in from behind me, against my cheek, and gently whispered something softly to me. As I lost consciousness I knew that she understood the love behind our decision.

In recovery, I awoke still choking on sobs. I tried to speak to a nurse. She looked down at me and said, "I can't talk to her." I was shaken. Another nurse, a volunteer named Sheila saw that and immediately came to my side. She stayed beside or circled near me for the remainder of my time at the Day Surgery Department at the hospital. Sheila was an angel to me. At one point we had to check my bleeding. I was feeling faint and was steadied by her hand. I noted she wore a native bear paw silver ring with turquoise. "That is lovely." I said. She paused. I saw something pass across her face "This was my partner's. She died last fall." I looked at her. She knew loss. "You will feel like you won't make it through, but remember that you will." she said as she squeezed my hand.

Whenever I think of our termination, I give thanks for Sheila.

The following days I was crushed by the stillness inside me. Had I passed by a mirror and seen no reflection I would not have been surprised. I didn't know there were even deeper levels of pain. At the encouragement of the psychiatrist, we tried to keep up distraction, yet slowly the crash of hormones wrapped me in a fog I can't describe. It was like tar weighing me down. The free fall seemed endless. Would the ground never come? Minutes passed so slowly. Why is it that joys are so fleeting and yet sorrow lingers?

I think the worst moment for Lesley was filling out the funeral home papers for the cremation orders. The coroner's form stated plainly "Baby Boy." Up until that time we weren't sure we would name our elf, for he wasn't born. He didn't ever come into being except in our hearts. Seeing the starkness of those words "Baby Boy" we began considering names.

We were given a shoebox-sized box from the funeral home. Baby Boy and my last name. Date of cremation. Lesley and I headed up to the lake.

All I could think of when I saw the box was when a friend's teacup poodle died. The poor owner was sent a box that must have contained the ashes of at least a few great Danes. This seemed so large. We didn't know what to expect inside. We unwrapped the box and then another, like Dr. Seuss with boxes in boxes, and then a black recycled plastic box. We had to call the funeral home as the box wouldn't open. They told us we needed to pry it open with a screwdriver. There they were in a clear plastic bag—silvery fine ashes, such a tiny amount with a slight shimmer to them. So small and light. Fairy dust.

We wanted to sail and release our boy's ashes from a kite high above the beach where he would have played. Upon arriving at the cottage we had consecutive days of no wind—barely a leaf fluttered. We valiantly ran back and forth trying to get him to fly.

We gave our son a traveling name of Raphael—Raffi for short—the laughing archangel of healing. We wanted him to have the option of using our name or being free to accept whatever name he is given by the Creator, or perhaps his next birth, or he could chose to be with us as we are with him.

As we stumbled trying to raise our kite, I imagined him, grabbing his toes rolling back and forth laughing at the silly women thinking they could make enough wind. The kite was thrown up, frantic running would commence as the kite smashed down and skittered behind us. Perhaps the lake was a crystalline mirror for a reason. On Tuesday we decided we would have to do it differently.

We waded out to one of the rocks I named as a child "the Tiger Rock." If, as a child playing in the water, you knew where that rock was, you would be able to gauge where all of the other diving rocks were situated. No matter how choppy the lake would be this Tiger Rock served as the bearing for all the others.

It was a hazy, still day. The horizon was obscured. It was very hot, around 30 degrees centigrade (86 degrees Fahrenheit). I played my Tibetan singing bowl, which I had played on my belly since conception. The tone was different this time. It was higher. First Lesley and I released some sand. I have a bowl in which I have collected sand that people have brought me from all over the world in their travels. We wanted Raffi to know the world was his. He was free to follow a grain of sand to anywhere. Then we began to release his ashes.

Lesley made a beautiful arc with her hand. The ashes hung in the air briefly, like a silvery mist. We told him of our love and dreams for him and that we would always be with him no matter where he was, with the Creator or wherever his soul is free to soar.

I rinsed my bowl in the lake as it had some ashes in it. I poured the water from it away from me to the horizon, envisioning a sense of opening and releasing that someday I would feel, but can't just yet.

We walked up from the beach. We got in the car to go home and we went to look at the lake (we always call it saying goodbye to the lake but didn't this day). Within the brief time of walking up from the lake and putting the dog in the car something happened. Rolling in toward us, there was an incredibly thick white mist. Unlike the hot day, it was cool. The lake was completely obscured and we felt this white air envelop us. I would like to think the heavens came down to guide our Raffi. Lesley and I were both silent. By the time we got in the car and drove up the driveway and further down along the road we looked through the trees to the lake and there was no sign of fog or mist.

My milk came in during that time. I followed the doctor's advice and wore a tight sports bra all the time, including in the shower. I so wanted to share that milk. It expressed to empty arms. I was desperate for something good to come from our loss and wished I could share the milk. I even looked to see if there was a program of wet nurses for babies. But Lesley was right. I had to let my breasts stop producing. There was no infant. There would be no feeding. My body was no longer a place of life, no longer a garden, no longer part of a miracle. My breasts were just one more part of me emptying.

I wondered if at one point I would be utterly hollow—too hollow for even an echo. It was a most complicated grief.

I couldn't focus on anything. Five days after our termination, I was being encouraged by family members to return to work. They meant well encouraging me into some normalcy, but I was far from ready. I tried to return the following Monday. I walked into my office. There was the yellow Post-it "Trisomy 21." I lost it. I sobbed uncontrollably. In that office I first heard I was pregnant. I hid crackers in my drawer and warm ginger ale when I was queasy. Then it was 4:11. Everything was frozen in a different time with a different me. It would always be 4:11 when my voice was excited and hopeful. How did I get here? How did this happen? Where did our dreams go? My co-worker helped me escape down the hall when no one was walking through. I realize I hadn't listened to my heart and had come back too soon. One week later I was able to return.

I also ignored my intuition regarding my physical healing. I was bleeding heavily intermittently for weeks. I asked my OB and was told that if I wasn't soaking over a pad an hour it was just my body likely returning to normal. Unfortunately while it ebbed and flowed there were times when my bleeding was extreme and then it would slow down. In the end it became critical. I was bleeding well over a pad an hour when I was taken to Emergency. After three days on induction medications to try to dislodge the tissue, it had to be removed through emergency surgery. Another memory I will carry with me is the look on Lesley's face when I had multiple intravenous tubes everywhere in Emergency. I could not leave her.

Around that time, something else remarkable began to occur. During moments of despair, bright color would suddenly flash across my face. Butterflies followed me. Whenever I saw only thick, bleak, gray fog, when I couldn't draw a breath, when I could not feel anything but sorrow (or worse: nothing) suddenly a bright butterfly would fly across my path, often in an unusual place. I was at a baseball game at an inner city stadium, wondering if anyone else among the 33,000 in attendance was grieving, when a stunning swallowtail flew up to me. One day Monarchs came in huge numbers. On another, one was simply waiting by my back gate. A white butterfly went right into my face when I was bitterly thinking there was no hope. They were constant. To some, butterflies are the souls of passed children; to others they are powerful transformative creatures. I feel whoever they are, they were messengers coming from a very distant land—a land of the living, a land where there is joy and color and hope. They are from a foreign place. I would like to think Raphael was their sender or was among them. They were reminding me there was life. Joy waited.

Their meandering path slowly led me back. Indeed, the path of grief after a heartbreaking choice is much like that of a butterfly. The journey doubles back on itself. Just when I felt I began to get my footing, something would throw me back. As time passed I could gauge my healing in only two ways: I would either stumble less often or I would be able to rise more quickly.

Lesley and I kept returning to the lake and Raffi's tiger rock. It all looked the same except, like me, it wasn't the same at all. The wind and water that caught the ashes of our angel had drifted far away. Our running and turning footsteps (that were left in the sand from our doomed kite flying) had long since been covered over by little feet running with bright plastic buckets filled with captured minnows and confused frogs. Small footsteps were everywhere of children running to show Mum what they caught in the creek. The cedars were heavily laden with golden buds.

This most singular grief can be so isolating. We told very few friends that we made a heartbreaking choice. We were neither ashamed nor hiding, but felt it was very private. How could anyone fully understand the depth of love from which our decision arose unless they too had been through the same intense circumstance? From the early days after deciding we had to terminate our pregnancy I turned to a community of women I met through the Internet who also had to make a heartbreaking choice due to a poor prenatal diagnosis or endangerment to the mother. To describe these women as having been my lifeline would be no exaggeration. I owe so much of my healing and moving forward to them. In my times of greatest sorrow they were there. One of these women may have even saved my life, insisting I go to Emergency in light of my increased bleeding. In the nearly two years that have passed since I first met this community, our friendships have only deepened and broadened. They have been a true gift to me. Some women I will know and treasure for the rest of my life. We have shared so much and continue to comfort new members, who are fresh in their grief, with the same gentle care that welcomed us.

One of the significant milestones in the grief process of a heartbreaking choice is the estimated due date (EDD) of the lost pregnancy. I felt something was emotionally and perhaps physically suspended until that day passed.

On October 16th we would have had our little boy in our arms and be reeling with exhaustion and joy. I would have been sneaking a lovely long sniff of that baby head smell I love, while my cheek would have felt his impossibly soft skin.

I wasn't sure what to do for that day. Lesley was able to take the day off work and be with me. I was so grateful.

We needed to honor Raphael and give thanks. He was such a gift to us. In the depths of grief I asked a friend, "How will I ever be able to love again?" She said, "Your capacity to love will always be greater because of him." This was true.

I knew I would never lose Raffi in my heart and would always picture him with me but I didn't want my love to tether him or keep him earth bound. I felt he needed to move on and become. In light of this, it seemed important that whatever we did on his day it had to be a continual act of releasing and giving.

My thoughts turned to the future sorrows of other women. Next year those same butterfly messengers that had visited me would need to lead others out of the fog. If one woman could look up from the ground and see a magical flutter of color, Raffi would be honored.

Women would need to wish too.

When I was pregnant, I sang lullabies and dreamed and dreamed. I have started singing lullabies again, so far for others, but it is a start. I wished on every star, or 'Santa Claus', on everything that could technically generate a wish. I feel that the more we wish or pray, the better we can see beyond where we are, to where we could be. By our due date I had begun wishing again, sometimes for me, and often for friends.

In honor of Raphael, Lesley and I took the ferry to the island by our city with many milkweed pods bursting with ripe seeds. Monarch butterflies need milkweed. When the seeds fell down to gestate, the fluff would have risen and offered Santa Claus wishes to anyone who caught them (or spots them—in my rule book). They would have flown across to New York or across to Michigan or back to my neck of the woods. Wherever they went, they would have given a chance to hope and dream once again to someone.

The summer was long gone. There had already been a frost and even very briefly snow. Times were getting a bit dark. Butterflies had flown to warmer places. The air on the island was crisp. We could hear the rustle of drying leaves on the trees. A few trees were still aflame with color. Bright orange berries weighed down branches. We walked past the place where we were married and further along a well-worn path. We listened and watched. It was a beautiful day.

Then, despite the wind and chill, there he was. A perfect Monarch butterfly crossed our path and alit on a plant. I went right up to him as he posed for a close-up. He wasn't the least bit skittish. After I took a picture of him he followed us down the path for a bit and then flew up past the trees. What a gift on that cool day.

We released many seeds around the island, making wishes and prayers as we went. We had a picnic on a beach. I looked down and saw many perfect flat skipping stones. I began skipping stones along the lake. In my mind I was showing Raffi how it was done. You have to be gentle, light, yet strong and fast. Like so much in life you can't get eight or nine skips unless you just naturally let go.

As my stone leapt across the water, a milkweed seed went by. I wondered whose wish it would carry.

39

Shari's Story "An Atheist's Perspective: Allegedly Pregnant"

Prologue: On July 5–6, 2006, nine days after finding out about a chromosomal abnormality in my first pregnancy, I sat down to write this journal. I needed to sort out my thoughts because I hadn't been sleeping well, so I told my story to my computer. I never knew that it would be shared.

First Trimester

We found out we were pregnant on April Fool's Day of 2006 when I was 34 and Paul was 33. Because conceiving had taken so many months without success, we didn't really believe the home pregnancy test. Can they play pranks on you? In truth, we believed the science of the test, but the idea of being pregnant didn't sink in right away. For the first week, we spoke to one another using the term "allegedly." We also decided not to tell people until May 1st.

Despite the doubts, I did take Paul to the bookstore that very day, and we purchased two mom-to-be books and one dad-to-be book. Then we spent the whole afternoon reading about what to expect during the upcoming nine months and happily discussing our future.

On April 6th, Paul sent flowers to me at work with a note saying, "Allegedly? Definitely." I loved his commitment, but wasn't quite there myself. However, I had already scheduled a doctor's appointment for the following Monday.

I guess I started believing in the pregnancy during our trip to Dallas from April 13th through the 16th. I felt nauseous and gassy the whole trip, and realized that my morning sickness had started. However, I still didn't think of it as a baby: just a pregnancy.

I had an OB appointment on April 24th. Paul joined me in order to see the ultrasound. Basically, we saw a lima bean with an asterisk for a heart. When we got home with the lima bean pictures, I brought up the topic of Down syndrome because of my age, and we decided that doing a first trimester screening was the route we should take. Because I had yet to grow attached to the baby, I verbalized that we'd still have to abort the pregnancy if bad results came back. Paul surprised me by mentioning how that decision might bother him, because he'd seen the heartbeat. I think that was when I started to think that I would need real reasons for terminating a pregnancy, instead of just thinking that a Down syndrome pregnancy would automatically mean abortion.

After another uneventful but nauseous week, we called our parents on April 30th to announce the pregnancy. Obviously, both moms were thrilled and siblings offered their congratulations, too. We also decided to tell people at work about the pregnancy on May 1st. We're planners, and that was the plan. I still didn't have too much of an attachment to the baby, but I had nausea and huge, painful boobs, so I was sure that I was pregnant.

On May 23rd, I went to the perinatologist's office for my first trimester screening. First, I had a meeting with Randi, the genetic counselor. I was very confident when telling her about my healthy family and good genes. I even told her that I was sure the screening would just be a formality, but I wanted to hear from an official source that I was low risk. Randi was very friendly and I liked the one-on-one attention. When she was talking about the implications of high-risk testing (amniocentesis), I asked her about the chorionic villus sampling (CVS) test. She told me that a doctor from Durham came in occasionally to do CVS procedures upon patient request. Since I was secure in how healthy I had always been, I figured we'd just do the amniocentesis if needed.

Next, I met Steve, the ultrasound technician at the perinatologist's office, who spent almost an hour doing an ultrasound to look at the baby's measurement of fluid behind its neck (the NT measurement). Although he was very friendly and even showed me the 4D imaging of the baby, I didn't get a confident feeling that everything was all right. As he was leaving, I asked, "Did everything look okay?" and he replied, "For the most part." Then Dr. D came in to do the same measurement. She made comments about the cute baby, and even made a guess about it being a boy. I saw a measurement for the NT at 2.5 mm, and asked if that was the measurement she was looking for. She indicated that it was, but didn't say if it was good or bad. At the end of the appointment, I had blood drawn, which would measure some pregnancy proteins and check for cystic fibrosis.

When I got home from the appointment with the printed pictures from the ultrasound, Paul and I did get a little excited about the baby. We looked through our ever-increasing pile of pregnancy books, and found one that said an NT measurement of up to 3.0 mm is low risk. That same book said that some new tests check for a nasal bone in the first trimester, which many Down syndrome babies do not have. I felt even more confident then, because Dr. D had pointed out the nasal bone while doing her ultrasounds. Because of the good results, Paul and I started to think ahead about our baby boy. (I was more convinced about the boy thing than Paul.)

During that next week, Paul and I told friends and neighbors about the pregnancy, and even started to choose boy names with a points game that Paul made up. It was, I now know, my most positive, happy week of the pregnancy.

On Wednesday morning, May 31st, I got a message from the perinatologist's office that my screening results were in. On the afternoon of Thursday, June 1st, Randi and I finally got to talk. She started by saying that my risk for Down syndrome had increased from one in 300 to one in 97 based on the NT measurement and the readings from two proteins in my blood. I took notes as she explained that my free-beta protein level was 3.99 and my PAPP-A protein was 1.5. The average for each of those proteins is about 1.0. The 3.99 reading seemed extreme to me, and she did admit that it was very high, but she also said that a Down syndrome baby should have a low PAPP-A measurement, and mine was high. (That only reassured me a little bit.)

My confidence was gone. In hindsight, I realize that my bad feelings came from the fact that doctors had always told me that I was average or above average in all health areas. Now, I was reading at three times WORSE than average. How could I be sure of a healthy baby when I was worse than average? Rationally, I knew that one in 97 was good odds, but my heart didn't feel it. I just wanted to get the amniocentesis done to know some definite answers. Randi mentioned that since I was ending my 13th week of pregnancy, it was too late to do a CVS to know immediately, so I scheduled an amniocentesis for Tuesday, June 20th, at the beginning of my 16th week. The waiting game had begun.

Obviously, Paul and I had a lot to think about. Our e-mails the next day helped us make our decision in advance.

I wrote:
"I've been thinking all day and last night about reasons to keep a child with Down syndrome. I really can't think of many. The main reason would be that we've told everyone that we're

pregnant, but that's not a real reason. The negatives of a DS child would be so much greater... Struggles with the child's intelligence and health, our expectations of what parenthood involves, responsibility for a whole life (rather than 18 years), our knowledge of how others treat people with DS, etc."

Paul replied:

"I can't think of any either. It would be hard, especially after it took us so long to conceive, and the sickness you've been going through, but it would probably be the best for our family and for the child in the long run. Maybe that makes me a bad person, but I just don't think I could enjoy being a parent like that, especially if we know that we could have prevented it... but then what? Are the odds any better next time? You'll be older, so the risk goes up because of that...I'm just going to try and be optimistic that we don't have to make this choice, but if we do, I think the right one is to end it."

After the news from Randi, I stopped talking about the pregnancy with colleagues unless they brought it up. I did share with my class during the last week of school, since I figured it was only fair to let them know what to expect in the fall, but my excitement about a baby was no longer forefront in my mind. All I could think about was the risk of Down syndrome.

I also wanted reassurance from some source (preferably a doctor) that I had nothing to worry about. I wished the doctors would be more positive, like, "Oh, don't worry...we see this all the time and you're in good shape." However, any doctor or online resource I found could only offer statistical analysis, and nothing reassured me.

Somewhere during the next three weeks, I had an appointment at the OB's office and I heard the heart again, but I really felt like I was faking excitement about being pregnant. Paul and I had a trip to visit his family planned in early July, and I knew that I wouldn't be able to share his family's excitement without good news from the amniocentesis before the trip. I even put off finding a long-term substitute for school and starting to plan for the baby's room because of my worries. I had made it through the first trimester, but that didn't really make me confident about anything.

Maternal Instinct

Finally, on Tuesday, June 20th, Paul and I both went to the perinatologist's office for the amniocentesis. The appointment started with a long, targeted ultrasound, where Steve looked for many of the baby's features that would confirm or contradict the Down syndrome risk. Steve found the baby's pinky finger (good sign), a four-chambered heart (good sign), a new NT measurement (he said it was normal), a closed spine (good sign) and all necessary leg and arm bones. He also confirmed that our baby was a boy. Afterwards, Dr. B came in to take the very same measurements, and she discussed with us that, based on the targeted ultrasound, we could now see our risk as one in 194 instead of one in 97. She said that 50 percent of Down syndrome babies do not pass the test we just had, so our risk could be cut in half.

Upon hearing that, Paul and I both questioned whether the amniocentesis was necessary, considering that it carries a one in 200 risk of complications. (Steve did tell us that this perinatologist's office's risk is more like one in 500, but the official number is one in 200.) Dr. B explained that we could go home to discuss the results, and if we changed our minds and decided upon the amniocentesis, they could probably fit us in within 24 hours. With that news in mind, Paul and I left to go out to lunch, a bit more confident than when we'd gone in.

That was the point where my heart truly started debating my brain. I pictured a bag of 193 white marbles and one black marble. I knew that reaching into the bag would NEVER result in my picking the black marble, but I also knew that I didn't feel confident that our baby would not be the black marble. Upon arriving home from the appointment, I put 194 pennies in a bag and Paul put a black X mark on one of them. We played the "penny game" repeatedly that day, and we never drew the bad penny, but I couldn't sleep that night.

My thoughts that night were about having a child with Down syndrome. If we didn't get the amniocentesis, and I delivered a baby with Down syndrome, could I hold it in my arms that first moment and love it right away? I didn't think so (and still don't). But why did I have this fear of Down syndrome? I thought about how even mentally retarded adults intimidate me. I don't know what to say or how to act around them. I know that's MY problem, but is it a fear that I need to face. I thought about how a Down syndrome person is automatically going to have at least mild retardation, and I pictured how frustrating it was for the child in my class who has the lowest IQ. I wouldn't want my child to be that one. I also considered whether the child would know that he is mentally retarded. I still don't know that answer, but I do know that I would be aware of the problem, and it would change my life.

Upon discussing my concerns with Paul the next day, he explained that he deals with odds at work all the time, and one in 200 is pretty much a sure thing, so he wasn't worried at all. He was looking forward to having our baby boy.

But after a second night of not sleeping, I decided that I had to do the amniocentesis. Here are our e-mails from June 22nd:

> *I wrote:*
> *"I truly think that knowing for sure will give me back my confidence for the whole pregnancy. I spent about two hours online yesterday evening while you were watching your movie, lurking on bulletin board web sites about prenatal testing and chromosomal abnormalities, and I'm not alone in needing this reassurance."*
>
> *Paul replied:*
> *"I've always said and I believe that we should do this if you need to know for sure. Even if you come up with another concern later, at least we'll know that all of the things the amnio checks for will be okay, so it kind of pushes into more exotic problems that have even lower risks. If you want me to agree that it's necessary and that I need the reassurance too, I just can't, because I don't. But I'm not opposed to it at all, and if you do need that, then there's no question we should do it."*

I knew that I didn't need Paul's agreement about being concerned, but I did want his support to do the amniocentesis, and he gave me that support unconditionally (even knowing the risk involved).

Both of us were more nervous going into the perinatologist's office on Friday, June 23rd than we had ever been for any doctor's appointment. However, the amniocentesis itself went very smoothly, and Dr. D and Randi assured us that our FISH results (preliminary results) would be ready the next day, even though it was Saturday.

Physically, I felt fine after the amniocentesis, but I didn't sleep well again, because I was awaiting the results. Disappointingly, but not surprisingly, the lab didn't get the results done on Saturday, and Randi promised a call before 10:00 AM on Monday morning.

Heartbreaking Results

Now comes the part it hurts to write about: the call from Randi and the ensuing events. I was awake and downstairs on the couch by 6:30 AM on Monday, June 26th, and though I thought I would nap, I was wide-awake when my phone rang around 9:35 AM. Randi first apologized for the lack of results on Saturday and then said, "And I don't have good news to report this morning." I immediately assumed that the results weren't yet ready, so I was about to ask, "Okay, when will they be in?" when Randi informed me that the results showed a male with trisomy 21, Down syndrome. I understood and since the word "okay" was on the tip of my tongue from my planned next sentence, that was what I said. I do not remember the conversation we had, but I do know that I wanted to see the results and gave her Paul's work fax number. I did inform her that we would probably terminate, and asked her what to do next. She said she'd call my OB's office. At some point in the conversation, I said, "Now I feel like I'm in a dream. I just want to confirm. The results show that our baby DOES have the extra chromosome and therefore has Down syndrome." Randi confirmed for the second time that I was correct. I do remember telling her that I understand how hard that type of call must be for her to make, and she said that most of her job's phone calls are good news so she has learned to take the bad with the good.

According to my phone, the conversation lasted about six minutes. I didn't cry because I knew I had to call Paul and I then had some arranging to do, but I know my voice was getting that choked-up sound. As soon as I ended the call with Randi, I called Paul at work, and I think I did have tears by the middle of our conversation. I started the conversation with, "You're not going to believe this, but the results DO show Down syndrome." I don't remember any of the rest of our conversation except that Paul said he'd come home right away, and I mentioned that he should expect the fax from Randi.

It took about 20 minutes for Paul to get home. I think I cried the whole time, and it got worse when Paul came in and he cried too. The next hour included a call from my OB's office to say that the perinatologist's office would arrange the termination, and then me leaving a message with Randi to say that we would come down there to see the faxed results, and that she shouldn't worry about faxing anything to Paul. I think it wasn't until about 1:30 PM that we actually spoke to Randi and she told us to come right over to the office and we could talk about what was happening.

We cried again in the car on the way to the perinatologist's office, and again in Randi's comfort room. She told us about the results where 50 cells were analyzed and all had the extra chromosome 21, and she told us about the dilation and evacuation (D&E) procedure. Actually, I think she mentioned the option of inducing labor, but assumed that we'd go for the surgical procedure (she was right). I know that I was quite insistent about doing the procedure as soon as possible. We agreed to do the surgery at Duke University Hospital, regardless of the expense.

I have no idea how long we were at the perinatologist's office, but the whole time, Paul didn't say anything at all, except to respond to questions. I asked him if he was debating our decision at all, and he said he wasn't. I actually asked him that numerous times over the next few days, and he never had any question in his mind. The most confident thing he said about our decision was to remind me that he didn't feel comfortable around children in the first place, and this would make it worse.

As we were leaving the perinatologist's office, Randi said that she'd call with our scheduled times at the hospital. I thanked her for taking the time out of her schedule to talk to us, and she said that our situation was the important one at the moment.

I don't remember what Paul and I did when we got home. I know he was absolutely distraught, and I know we both left messages for our parents (who each called back within a few hours), but that Monday and the following day are still a blur in terms of what I did with my time.

A few hours after our trip to the perinatologist's office on Monday, Randi called to say that our appointments at Duke Hospital would be on Wednesday and Thursday, June 28th and 29th. I was relieved that this whole thing would be over within the week.

Sometime that evening my close friend Kara called, just to say hi, and I told her the story. It had slipped my mind until I spoke with her that her brother Patrick had Down syndrome, and had died at four years old. Kara was supportive of our decision to end the pregnancy, and I hope she really meant it. She did say that of Patrick's pre-school playgroup of six children, only one is still alive today.

Monday night, I spent time online looking for information about D&E and researching Down syndrome and FISH testing. Nothing I saw made me rethink our decision to terminate.

Here's an e-mail exchange Paul and I had on Tuesday while he was at work:

> ### I wrote:
> "I know that when you're sad, you are quiet and like to think things over yourself, but if you're questioning the decision (not wanting to change it, just questioning), I'm curious about what you're thinking."
> ### Paul replied:
> "I guess it's just the suddenness of this time yesterday everything was fine and today it's totally the opposite. There's a half-finished e-mail here that I was writing when you called and it seems so pointless now what I was saying and worrying about yesterday morning.

No, I'm not questioning the decision. It's just hard for me to go from being so excited and looking forward to the baby to deciding that we're not going to have it after all. I guess I was more optimistic than you were that things would be okay and I never prepared myself for this eventuality. I'm sure that I'll start to feel better in the days after the surgery, but right now our baby is still alive and growing inside you and I'm having trouble thinking of it being gone."

Grieving Stages

All through Monday night and Tuesday, I could do nothing but think about everything that happened. In no real order I think I went through the stages of grieving, modified in that I don't believe in God. Now, when I'm writing this a week later (it's Thursday, July 6th right now), I still think these same thoughts, although probably only about 50 percent of my daily and nightly thoughts are about the pregnancy instead of 100 percent.

The grief stages are: denial, anger, bargaining, depression, and acceptance.

I think my denial is about the whole pregnancy, and it might be good that I have that sense of denial. By Tuesday, I was able to verbalize my thoughts and explain to Paul that the termination was just ending the pregnancy, and not killing a baby or ending a life. I know that I was pregnant for four months, but I deny that I ever grew attached to the boy inside me. I read that some people like to have funerals and say goodbye to their fetus, but I don't need that. My fetus would not have lived without me (it still had about seven weeks until it could have had a chance of survival outside a mother's body), and therefore I don't believe that it was a child. It was always a group of cells growing inside of me, and yes, I had high hopes for that group of cells, but now I have high hopes for another pregnancy.

I've been angry, in the "Why us?" way. When I see or think about friends or strangers with healthy pregnancies or children, it makes me think about how unlucky we are. I think about how hard it has been on Paul, and how he will not be as excited about another pregnancy because he will have his guard up like I did this time. Paul told me that he got over the "Why us?" phase quickly because it's one that will never be answered, but I think it's the stage I've focused on the most.

My bargaining is more of a questioning of religion. At first, I wondered if this was some type of punishment for not believing in God. I wondered if praying would have changed the result. I tried to make myself feel better with the thoughts that both of our mothers prayed and I tried to use my own old argument that an evil/punishing God who gives out bad pregnancies to people who don't believe in him is not a God I want to believe in. Neither of those theories was making me feel any better. Somehow, I have now come to the realization that IF I were a believing/praying person, and IF I spoke to God about the pregnancy beforehand, I would have said, "God, if you give me a Down syndrome child, I will end the pregnancy." IF there is a God, he is aware of the way I think, and still gave me a trisomy 21 pregnancy, so it was God's choice to have this pregnancy end in abortion. (I can say that word now. I didn't say that word before the D&E.) Now, I feel better about being a non-believer. I still don't believe in God, but I think that I can better handle my decision because I know how to explain it to people who do believe.

Depression is more of an underlying feeling than an overt emotion for me. I've been sad for the past 10 days. I can't deny that. I still get choked-up at least once a day (more while I'm typing this), and I still don't like that this whole thing has happened to us. However, I tend to deal with depression by talking/thinking through my problems, and this journal and the e-mails I've sent to friends have helped me through the depression. I know it will continue, but it will get better as time goes on. Paul mentioned how he would like to be pregnant again by the original due date (December 3rd), and I agree. Even if that doesn't happen, I really think another pregnancy, whenever it happens, will truly be the end of our depression. Actually, we now know to have the CVS at 10 weeks (or whenever is the earliest time it's offered), so after we have a good result from a CVS on another pregnancy, I think we can both permanently move on past this experience.

Although the official last-stage of grief is acceptance, I think I got there first. I knew that I had a lot of the business end of termination to take care of, so I accepted that I had work to do to move on with my life. I made the necessary phone calls to set up the D&E, I informed friends and family of the bad news, I came up with a way to explain what happened to acquaintances (I'll tell them that there were complications and the baby died), I cancelled flight tickets for our July 4th trip, I cancelled my enrollment for classes during the week of the D&E, and I've continued to live my life just as I normally would during the summer. I know acceptance took longer for Paul, because he originally didn't think he could do anything for his birthday, and wasn't sure about attending a July 4th party, but I know he is at the acceptance stage now.

Medical Procedure

Back to the events on the days following the bad news:

On Wednesday morning, we left for Durham around 10:00 AM for our appointment with Dr. B. I was glad that I knew the doctor we'd be seeing, and I was just anxious to have the whole two-day D&E process over with. Dr. B was as nice as could be, and never gave any judgment about our decision. She didn't say anything like, "You're making the right decision," but somehow I got that feeling from her. (Probably just my imagination, but it helped to feel that way.) At one point, she mentioned that she was surprised by the results, and I guess that's because she had seen/done the targeted ultrasound.

Dr. B explained the D&E procedure, and it was just as I had read online. She would insert laminaria into my cervix that day; the cervix would dilate overnight, and a surgeon would remove the tissue from the fetus the following day. She made Paul and I feel better by confirming our guess that the umbilical cord would be cut first during the surgery, so that the baby would not be alive for any of the procedure.

From reading bulletin board comments online, and from my experience with an HSG test before I got pregnant, I expected extreme, painful cramping on Wednesday night. Dr. B gave me a prescription for some Motrin (I don't know why she had to prescribe it, since you can buy it over-the-counter) and also a prescription for an antibiotic to take before the surgery. It turned out that I was quite crampy on Wednesday evening, but nowhere near as bad as I had expected. I was able to sleep for a few hours, but since I wasn't allowed to eat or drink after midnight, the cramps were at full force for much of the night. I guess they were a little worse than the worst period cramps I've had, and I could not have gone to work feeling that badly, but they were bearable knowing that there was a light at the end of the tunnel.

We had to leave early on Thursday to arrive at the hospital by 9:15 AM. I took the antibiotic pills around 7:30 AM, and I threw up in the car (into a cup) around 7:55 AM. I vowed to make sure that every nurse/doctor that I saw at the hospital would find out that I might not have the antibiotics in me as I should have had. Somewhere on the drive to Durham, I noticed some pretty yellow flowers all facing toward the rising sun. I don't know why, but those flowers made me angry. I'm still feeling bitter toward yellow flowers that face the sun.

Paul and I had to wait in the hospital waiting room for over an hour, and I think around 10:30 AM I was called to change into a hospital gown and then go to surgery. Paul came in to help me change and took my clothes. When we were given time to say goodbye, we hugged and kissed, but when Paul went to rub my tummy to feel the baby, I pulled away. I still feel badly that I did it, but I just wanted to get into surgery and get the whole thing over with.

Again, all of the nurses and doctors I met at Duke were very professional and non-judgmental. I don't think everyone knew the exact surgery I was having, but certainly the anesthesiologist and the surgeon knew, and both of them were friendly and positive. I do remember being given some IV pain medicine and the cramps went away. I remember a lot of questions, and I remember reading my whole medical file while nobody was watching me (but I don't remember anything that the file said because this was after I had the IV pain medication). Someone came in to tell me that she would give me more of the IV medication, and I have no clue what happened after that. I don't even remember feeling tired or laying my head back on the pillow, but I know that an operation took place.

I wish I had a videotape of when I was waking up after the surgery. I know that I was moaning from the pain of the cramps, and I curled my legs up to my side to try to alleviate the pain. I know that I kept scratching my hair, and I know that I kept complaining about my cramps and asking for water. Whoever was there was telling me to breathe into the oxygen mask, and I know I was trying, but the whole waking up experience was a blur that could have taken hours or could have just been a few minutes. I still don't know.

By the time I really woke up, I know that I had been given something for the pain of the cramps because I was feeling fine, although weak. Paul was allowed to come in and I was somehow in a chair, not a bed, when he got there. I think a nurse helped me move. They gave me some Diet Coke and crackers. I asked for water, but for some reason they wouldn't give it to me. I think the nurse said something about how I would drink it too fast. Paul helped me change into my regular clothes and a nurse went over some post-op directions with us. (I'm glad Paul was there, because I don't remember what was said.) When Paul went to get the car, they called for a wheelchair and someone pushed me to the elevator and then out to meet Paul at the car.

I got a McDonald's chocolate milkshake on the way home, but the drive home is a blur. Paul dropped me off and I went right to sleep while he went to get my prescription for codeine filled. By the time he got back, I was feeling weak, but well enough to go downstairs and watch television, and the cramps never came back. I still have a full bottle of codeine pills in the bathroom drawer, next to the prescription Motrin and the prenatal vitamins that I haven't begun taking again yet.

Physical Recovery

On Friday morning, I realized that the whole pregnancy was over, and was sad for a few hours. To keep my mind off of it, I went to Home Depot to walk around and look for a birthday present for Paul, but felt a bit dizzy so I went back home to lie down. My only concern was that I felt a bit like I had a urinary tract infection. (I constantly felt the need to pee, but little was coming out.) I called Duke Hospital, and was told to drink cranberry juice and call the perinatologist's office if I was still concerned in a few hours. Paul and I had pizza for lunch, and he said that he wasn't as sad anymore because the whole thing was now over. Right after lunch, I called the perinatologist's office, and a nurse named Pat told me to come right over and she would give me a urine test to check for bacteria.

Again, as always, the staff at the perinatologist's office was wonderful. Not only did Pat see me right away and give me a prescription for something to help even though she didn't see any bacteria, but Dr. D stopped into the nurse's office to give me a hug. I didn't know how to respond except to appreciate her time and friendliness.

Within a few hours of taking the first of the antibiotic pills from Pat, I was feeling a bit better, urinary tract-wise. With the exception of feeling weak over the next few days (the surgeon told Paul that I had lost more blood than he'd expected), I didn't have any symptoms. I've been spotting on-and-off for the past week, but all of the web sites say that "irregular bleeding or spotting" is normal for the first two weeks.

Emotional Recovery

The night of the D&E, Paul and I were sitting in our family room watching television. It just seemed like a normal day, where we would watch television and read and go to sleep. When I mentioned to Paul that I felt a weird sense of calmness, he said that he was feeling the same thing. Our lives were back to normal. For five years, we'd hung out together without the possibility of a child coming, and now after three months of knowing about a pregnancy, we were back to our previous routine. I didn't feel like there was anything wrong with that, and neither did he. After weeks of worry and stress, our lives seemed normal again.

However, my sleep pattern didn't return to normal for the first few days after the surgery. Even though I am completely confident in the decisions that Paul and I made, and I'm looking forward to trying again for our next pregnancy (I'm even feeling promiscuous again, unlike while I was pregnant), I didn't sleep well on Wednesday through Monday nights. My tossing and turning and thinking about the pregnancy and the abortion made me decide to write this journal. Oddly, on Tuesday night, the night before starting to write this, I actually slept soundly for eight hours, but I had committed to putting this all down on paper, and I'm glad I've done it.

Three days after the surgery, trying to stay active and move on with our lives, Paul and I decided to go to a Durham Bulls game. Through what I thought was an evil twist of fate, Paul and I ended up sitting in a section at the stadium with a group from the Special Olympics. My initial instinct was that we should move, and avoid seeing happy people with Down syndrome, because it would make me debate my choice. However, I wanted to be strong and see what would happen, and I'm glad we stayed where we were. These were adults with special needs (not all Down syndrome), and every single one of them needed a personal assistant. Each special adult had a companion to help him/her go to the bathroom, order a soda and hot dog, and even put on a hat that was provided for them. Seeing the extent of the needs that Down syndrome people may have makes me sure that I wouldn't want to bring a child into the world with this disorder. Paul and I would never have the life we expected to have, and neither would our child.

At the baseball game, I also thought about whether our child would have been low or high functioning. I've read that some people with Down syndrome have only mild mental retardation and can even go to college with accommodations. However, I also thought about how mild mental retardation would put our child with the lowest IQ of the kids I teach, and that is just not fair to have a child performing so much slower than his/her peers. I remember a girl from the Manlius Little League when I was growing up who always got to be the 4th out of an inning. If that is the accommodation a Down syndrome child needs to participate in normal activities, the child is truly not living a normal life. So it turns out that sitting where we did at the Bulls game ended up being quite good for me.

On the other hand, we also saw plenty of happy, healthy children and pregnant women at the Bulls game. Each family depressed me in its own little way, and the ones that affected me the most were the dads with their sons at a baseball game. I really want Paul to have that experience with a son someday, and it's sad that we'll have to wait a little longer than we expected.

I *do not* regret anything, and I will always know that we made the right decision for us, but I also would like to avoid conflict. If a parent of one of my students from next year hears about our choice and disagrees, he/she may treat me differently as a teacher. I think it would be easier for me if people didn't know. I will never lie about our decision, but I will avoid telling people in order to make my life easier.

Regarding the future of this journal:

The remaining issues to deal with are when I will commit to taking my prenatal vitamins again (I think that will happen when I stop bleeding all together) and when Paul and I can have sex again (Dr. D will answer that on Monday, I hope). From now on, my journal entries will be dated with when they are written, instead of telling a whole story at once. And if I'm truly getting back to my normal life, I know that I won't write anything else at all. That's me.

Epilogue: I never wrote any more in my journal. It took us six months of trying to conceive and one round of Clomid to find ourselves pregnant again. Because of my trisomy 21 experience, I never grew attached to my second pregnancy, even after a perfect CVS. I faked my way through decorating a nursery, baby showers, and nine months of discomfort, each day expecting my world to crash down again. To my delight, Maggie is perfect and is a smart, happy five-month-old. We would like to have another, and I am prepared for another scary pregnancy. I can only hope for the best.

40

Suzanne's Story "Change of Plans"

My husband, JA, and I have always been good planners. We always worked well together, thinking about how to make short term goals get us closer to long term goals. It's an ability that carried us through graduate school and medical school together. And we just always took for granted that when we worked hard on our plans, things would work out in the end. Maybe it wasn't a smooth road, but our destination would remain the same.

Of course we had all kinds of plans for our family. We would start having kids once we finished with our education and had stable jobs. We planned on having three kids, each about two to three years apart. Things were progressing right on schedule. We got pregnant fairly quickly with our beautiful daughter, MJ. The pregnancy and delivery were free of complications and major worry. MJ was healthy and strong and became the light of our lives. That isn't to say adjusting to parenthood was easy. It was actually quite a struggle to realize how little you control when it comes to babies. MJ was never a good sleeper so the physical and emotional recovery was slow. And it took me many months to feel comfortable in this new identity as "Mom."

About the time MJ was 18 months old and my husband and I were feeling more confident as parents, we figured it was time to start trying for baby number two. So we ditched the birth control and found ourselves immediately pregnant. At first, we had some mixed feelings about it, a little overwhelmed by what we had started. But we felt proud of our loving family and wanted to welcome more members.

When I was about seven weeks into the pregnancy, I had a sudden bout of stomach cramping, diarrhea, and spotting. We were at my in-laws' house and I immediately got on the telephone with my mom, my sister, and my midwife. I could tell they were trying to be reassuring but couldn't really give me any promises. They all knew the risk of miscarriage with early spotting.

My sister had experienced a miscarriage a couple years earlier and understood all the fears that immediately arise when you're pregnant and spotting.

My husband and I went to the midwife's office the next day, terrified and expecting the worst. Instead we saw the little bean floating around inside me. No heartbeat was visible, but the midwife said that was common at just under seven weeks. We were relieved and counted our blessings. We even started telling family and friends about our good news.

I was feeling really good in the pregnancy, less nauseous and tired than with my daughter. Sometimes I worried a bit about miscarriage, but I reassured myself with the memory of our little bean at the ultrasound. At 12 weeks, I finally told people at work. JA and I were making plans for how to fit the baby into our lives. Plans to change bedrooms and move MJ to a "big girl bed." Everything seemed right on track.

I went to my 12-week midwife visit on my own, expecting another uneventful series of visits. However, when the midwife put the Doppler to my belly, the only heartbeat we heard was my own. She tried the transvaginal ultrasound as I got nervous and scared. When she still saw nothing, I started panicking. She went to get the OB to do a level II ultrasound to "double check, though things aren't looking good." I immediately started to cry. I called my husband to tell him my uterus looked empty and I'd be getting another ultrasound. The OB silently pressed on my belly with the ultrasound probe, measuring and documenting. I could see there was no one in there. The tiny bean was gone. The OB finally spoke to me, pointing out the empty sac that measured about seven weeks. I burst into tears. The nurse hugged me and the OB patted my knee saying she was sorry.

I was overwhelmed with sadness and disbelief. I called my mom from the parking lot, sobbing. My husband left work to meet me at home after picking up our daughter from my friend who'd been watching her. When we met at home and put MJ down for a nap, I just sobbed and sobbed for hours. JA was so supportive and gentle. It was a loss for him too.

The miscarriage ended up taking weeks to complete. We just let things happen naturally, no medications to induce cramping. My mom came to be with me and help with MJ. I didn't start really bleeding for a couple days. Then the bleeding went on and on for almost three weeks. I went in for weekly tests of my hCG levels, warned that sometimes your body doesn't expel everything on its own. I hated the sight and smell of that blood. It had that familiar sweet smell I recognized from postpartum bleeding after MJ was born. It was a constant reminder of our loss. I hated telling people about it, hearing the efforts to comfort by saying "You'll have another…" I just wanted to get over the miscarriage and move on. Looking back, I realize we never really took time to grieve.

I felt incredibly betrayed by my body. I mean, I always knew miscarriage was a possibility; many women have them at some point. But I'd been so falsely secure that my body would always be able to make a baby whenever we wanted. I spent years on birth control pills, celebrating each period as we avoided pregnancy. And then when we were ready emotionally, financially, professionally, etc., we couldn't make it happen. I was really in disbelief.

JA and I really wanted to get pregnant again right away after the miscarriage. After our initial ambivalence about that pregnancy, we realized that we really wanted another baby. We were in "baby mode" and wanted to stay on schedule. After all, that was all part of our master plan. So we waited for my period to come and go and took a chance at trying again. We figured it'd take a couple of months. But again, we were pregnant immediately. I remember being so nervous to take that pregnancy test, not really able to believe that we did it.

We were thrilled to be pregnant again. In fact, it worked perfectly into our plans. We were due in July, when JA could take several weeks off from work. Plus we'd have his mom available since she wouldn't be teaching in the summer. And now we could join the "baby club" that was forming among some of our newly pregnant friends. We started talking to MJ about the baby growing in Mommy's belly. She named him/her "Coco" and would talk to him/her from my bellybutton.

But the thrill was quickly followed by fear and anxiety. I was constantly monitoring my pregnancy symptoms, now aware that I didn't have many last time because my hormone levels were low due to the pregnancy not progressing. So I welcomed any nausea, dizziness, and breast tenderness. Still, I couldn't shake the feeling that we were really vulnerable. Unlike in our first uncomplicated pregnancy, I now appreciated how fragile pregnancy can be. I found myself always expecting the worst.

About eight weeks into the pregnancy we took a trip to visit my sister and I felt the pregnancy symptoms lessen. I wasn't feeling nauseous anymore. I gradually became terrified awaiting our first midwife visit. By the night before the appointment, I'd had myself convinced that I was going to miscarry again. I just didn't *feel* pregnant. I tried to prepare JA for the worst. I called my mom in tears yet again, scared and sad. On the drive to the midwife's office, I talked about how we'd wait longer to try again this time. And maybe we'd wait less time in between for our third.

At the midwife's office we immediately told her our fears. She said she had four miscarriages herself before getting pregnant with her eldest. She decided to skip the preliminary questions and go right for the ultrasound. To my enormous relief, we saw our little bean in there with that tiny heart beating away. No question about it. This baby was alive and growing! I cried yet again.

We left that appointment laughing about how scared I'd been. It was clearly time to stop obsessing about pregnancy symptoms. I needed to take it easy and try to enjoy the pregnancy. Of course, taking it easy became necessary when I came down with a wicked case of the flu shortly thereafter. That was followed by a sinus infection and a vaginal infection. I felt run down and sick for a solid month. It didn't help to hear JA talk about the dangers to the fetus when the mother has a virus or is taking antibiotics. I felt vulnerable and worried again. And I was just so tired, I felt like I wasn't being a very good mom to MJ either.

I went in for my 12-week appointment feeling nervous again. I had to bring MJ with me this time. When the midwife couldn't hear the heartbeat with the Doppler, I started getting really nervous. But I had to keep it together in front of MJ who could just sense when I was upset. I watched the midwife (my least favorite midwife in the group practice) fumble around with the ultrasound equipment for several minutes before finally getting a technician to help out. She pressed the probe to my belly and we saw the baby again. MJ got close to the screen, commenting about how the baby in Mommy's belly was upside down. This little one appeared fine on the office ultrasound equipment. It was reassuring.

The pregnancy progressed and my belly started to pop out. My 16-week visit was again uneventful, though I seemed to still struggle with various infections and exhaustion. But I wasn't really gaining weight like I had with my daughter. The midwife reassured me, saying I didn't really need to gain 40 pounds with MJ anyway. I did the quadruple screen blood work at that visit, not expecting anything troubling to come from it. In fact, I was reassured by feeling the baby's movements inside. Little flutters were happening more often by the day.

About a week later, I got a fateful telephone call with a message from my midwife saying that she wanted to talk about the results of my quad screen. After several telephone calls and waiting painful hours, I finally heard back from the midwife on call who looked at my chart and explained that the quad screen indicated a one in10 chance of trisomy 18. What? I didn't even know what that meant. JA and I got on the Internet and looked in his medical textbooks for everything we could find on quad screens, false positives, and trisomy 18. The midwife called later to check in on us and schedule a level II ultrasound for the next day. She confirmed that false positives can happen and that trisomy 18 is a dreadful diagnosis. The babies usually don't survive to term and rarely live more than a few weeks.

We didn't sleep much that night. We tried to tell ourselves not to worry until there was something definitive. But it was hard. My mind jumped to the worst case scenario all over again. Although, I really didn't even know what our options were. We went to the ultrasound appointment full of dread. Sitting in the waiting room with all the pregnant mamas was so uncomfortable. I wanted to be invisible.

The ultrasound technician started her job of measuring and documenting. She'd tell us what she was doing "I'm measuring the head circumference now," but was often silent. She didn't offer to tell us the baby's sex and we didn't ask much. Laying there holding JA's hand, we could see there was something wrong. An arm didn't look right and the technician sure spent a lot of time measuring that heart. Finally, she went out to get the fetal medicine specialist OB who gave us real information. He explained that the quad screen indicated a very high likelihood of trisomy 18 and that they did indeed see a number of physical markers. He calmly pointed out defects in the heart chambers, organs growing outside the abdominal wall, clubbed hands, short leg bones, curved feet, and even facial problems. Trisomy 18 is a fatal disorder, he said.

I laid there silent, holding onto JA. Finally, the OB stopped with all his information and suggested that it was a lot to take in at once and maybe we needed a little time. I nodded, silent. When the doctor and nurses left the room I started sobbing. JA held me and talked about how the baby just wasn't going to make it. "It's obvious from the ultrasound, what's the point of doing an amnio?" I cried until the doctor came back in the room. He recommended the amniocentesis for definite results. I agreed, feeling like I just wanted to be sure and to know what we were dealing with for future pregnancies. That procedure wasn't very comfortable, but I was feeling rather numb at that point.

We talked about our options for terminating the pregnancy. The doctor told us we could go to an outside clinic for a dilation and evacuation (D&E) or we could have the procedure done at the hospital. Of course, he recommended the hospital option so we'd have all the medical support, if necessary. He explained how he usually inserted laminaria to dilate the cervix overnight, and then induced labor with prostaglandin suppositories. He expected it would take about eight hours after the first suppository. Before we left the office, I asked what the baby's sex was. JA said we didn't need to know since it would just make it harder to say good-bye. But I wanted to know. The nurse leaned toward me with a hand on my shoulder and said, "It's a girl."

The next two weeks were surreal. We actually were getting ready to take a vacation to Mexico with some friends. We'd been looking forward to it for months. In fact, we made the plans after our miscarriage, figuring we'd be able to take our annual winter trip since we wouldn't be having a baby in March anymore. It turned into our "babymoon" when we discovered we were pregnant again. But now it was something else. It wasn't celebratory or relaxing. For me it became a time to say good-bye to our baby.

I really struggled during that time to feel comfortable in my body. At 18 weeks I had a noticeable bump that I tried to hide under loose clothes. Though there was no hiding it in my bikini by the pool. I also could feel her movements growing stronger. She was alive and real inside me. There was no denying that for me. I initially tried to emotionally distance myself from our little Coco. I stopped talking and singing to her as I'd regularly done before. But that just made me sad. I decided that I had to continue to treat my body gently, since I was still pregnant and full of hormones. And I needed to continue taking good care of Coco. I resumed our conversations. I told her over and over again how sorry I was that it was happening. I actually urged her to just go to sleep, drift away on her own. I remember swinging in a hammock one day on vacation, singing a lullaby to her in my head. It felt good to care for her that way. But it was still so, so sad, carrying what felt like a doomed pregnancy.

JA and I talked a lot during that time. He encouraged me to just blurt out whatever popped into my head whenever and wherever it happened. We couldn't just pretend like everything was fine. We couldn't pretend it was a normal vacation. He listened to all my random thoughts and held me when I cried. Over and over again he said that we were going through it together and he would be with me throughout. I was really afraid. Once I mentally accepted that we were going to terminate the pregnancy, I started dreading the actual process of labor and delivery.

During a layover on our trip home, I got the call from the OB's nurse saying the amniocentesis confirmed the trisomy 18 diagnosis. I told her we had decided to terminate and wanted to schedule it to begin as soon as possible. She set up our initial appointment right then. We'd spend the weekend home with MJ then begin with the laminaria on Monday.

My mom came to help us out. She stayed home with MJ that Monday evening while we went to the OB's office for the laminaria insertion. The OB showed us the amniocentesis results and reviewed all the information about the genetic anomaly, assuring us that it was a rare, random occurrence and that we had very little chance of it happening again. The actual procedure was more painful than I had imagined. The doctor said it would be similar to a pap smear. It was not! Physically, the pronged instrument used to stabilize my cervix was very painful. And that was followed by the slow, progressive insertion of the laminaria. I listened to the doctor debate over whether to use large or medium sizes, hoping he'd always opt for small. Emotionally, it was also the point of no return. After months of willing my body to hold onto the pregnancy, I was now forcing my cervix to open. It felt so wrong.

I went home that night. The doctor had warned me to expect some bleeding and cramping, though I never experienced any. Instead, I focused on taking care of my body and saying good-bye to Coco. My mom had made a decadent steak dinner with a giant spinach salad, to boost my iron stores. Then after we put MJ to bed, we began a ritual to let go of our baby. My mom is such an amazing, unique person. She'd been working for the past week to develop a ritual to help us through the process. JA and I lay next to each other on the bed with incense and nice music playing. My mom guided us through a silent process of acknowledging our feelings, expressing love toward our baby, and allowing her to go. She kept repeating the phrase "You are safe within the arms of love and soon you will be free." It was perfect. We all quietly cried. JA and I held each other for a long time afterwards.

It snowed heavily that night. Actually, it snowed throughout the day creating a beautiful blanket of sparkling white, icing all the trees I saw on our way to the hospital that morning. My mom took me while JA got MJ ready for the babysitter's. It was so sad walking onto the maternity unit. The very place I was wheeled to two and a half years earlier when we had MJ. I had to ask for directions, explaining we were there for a procedure. I walked by the nursery, trying not to look in, knowing I'd be leaving with empty arms. I saw the clear, hospital cradles outside the rooms, knowing ours would be empty. It was just so incredibly sad. Then I started to feel mad that they put me through this added insult. Couldn't I have gone to a medical unit instead? It was never presented as an option to me.

We settled into the room awaiting the doctor who was running late due to the snow. That was a theme all day. All the local schools and colleges were closed due to snow. Our nurse managed to arrive on time and stayed with us throughout the day. She was a quiet, calm presence. She tended to me gently and talked about the baby I'd be delivering. In sharp contrast, the OB kept referring to the fetus I'd be aborting. Seriously. Like my husband, I think he had the idea that if he took a clinical approach I'd be less emotionally attached and, therefore, less emotionally distraught. I found that insulting and cold. One of the midwives was there too. Unfortunately, it was the one midwife that I didn't like in the practice. I found her more annoying than helpful. She'd never been there for a procedure like we were going through since it was a new OB with different techniques.

My mom asked a lot of questions I hadn't thought to ask. As a former OB nurse, she knew more about the process than I. Would we be able to hold the baby? The nurse said she would wash and dress the baby and we could have her in the room as long as we liked. What happens to the body?

The midwife said that at 19 weeks the hospital can "dispose" of her or we could have her sent to a funeral home for cremation or burial. What should we expect with the prostaglandin? The doctor said I'd have some cramping (like intense menstrual cramps) and maybe some nausea. In fact, my mom asked so many questions that my doctor made some comment to me about her being "very inquisitive" after he had asked her and JA to leave for the laminaria removal. I wondered if they needed to leave during that time or if the doctor just wanted to stop answering questions. After all, JA had been with me when the laminaria were inserted.

Anyway, it turned out that the doctor's answers weren't all that useful anyway. Within five minutes of the prostaglandin insertion, I started feeling very woozy. I had diarrhea and nausea, dragging the IV with me to the bathroom while I got sick from both ends. I was also having intense cramping, like the labor pains I recognized from my unmedicated labor with MJ. I was vaguely aware of my mom and JA telling the nurse to get me the anti-nausea medication and narcotics immediately. I think it took a solid half-hour before they gave me any medications, something about having to go to the pharmacy to get the medications since they aren't kept on the floor. It was about 20 minutes afterward that I started feeling some relief.

I was in a sort of twilight-like state throughout that morning. Dozing on and off in the fog of the drugs. I saw my mom snoozing on the couch and JA typing away on his laptop computer. We'd smile at each other now and then. Around noon the cramping started getting stronger again and I was bleeding heavily. I could see my belly tighten with each contraction. I had a forlorn feeling that it wouldn't be long. The OB checked me and found I was about six centimeters. He said that if I didn't "abort" by 2:00 PM, he'd give me another prostaglandin suppository. I hoped my body could do it without another dose of that awful stuff.

Alas, 2:00 PM rolled around and my water still hadn't broken. The nurse made sure to pre-medicate me this time with the anti-nausea drugs and narcotics. When the OB checked on me, he found the amniotic sac was "hour-glassed" through the cervix. He couldn't even get the suppository to stay in my vagina and had to insert it rectally. By the time he left the room, I felt the contractions intensify to the point that I could not speak. The nausea returned too. My mom and JA held me, demanding the nurse get the doctor back for more medication orders. I was overwhelmed. I felt like my body was being torn apart. I used my labor breathing techniques but had such a dry mouth. My mom gave me wet wash cloths to suck on. JA held my legs which were aching with pain as my pelvis spread. The physical pain and trauma so closely matching the emotional pain and trauma I was experiencing.

The three of us were alone in the room when I instinctively started to push and felt the baby finally slide out. We called for the nurse, the doctor, and the midwife. In the meantime, we were all sort of frozen. I lay back with the relief of the pain dissipating. JA and my mom held my legs as I watched them look at the mass I had just expelled. My mom rubbed my leg and encouraged me to push a bit more to make sure the placenta came out too. I felt more tissue slide out. The nurse and midwife came scurrying in and scooped up everything from the table. My mom and JA let go of my legs as we watched them examining the tissue.

The midwife turned to me "The baby is still inside the amniotic sac. Do you want me to open it?" I nodded. It hadn't occurred to me that she could be born with the amniotic sac intact. All I knew was that I wanted to hold her. And I rather liked the idea that she'd been cushioned the whole way. They quickly cleaned her, cut the cord, and handed her to me.

I was shocked at what a littler person she was. She was whole. She was pink. Her skin was tacky and tight. Her eyes were closed, peaceful. I immediately noticed her little hands and feet with tiny nails. How perfect her feet were. Here was the person we created. My mom took a little water from a cup and baptized her. I smiled as I teared up. It was such a relief to finally hold my baby. JA was silent but near.

Then we started focusing on all her anomalies. The midwife pointed out her upturned nose and low ears. Her left arm was clubbed. And she had several organs in an enclosed sac outside her body that I hadn't even noticed at first. Her legs were bent and her feet slightly curved. But they still looked perfect to me. We handed her back to the nurse who dressed her and wrapped her. I kissed her tiny head. She was so light, like holding one of MJ's tiny baby dolls. I gave her to JA who was finally crying. He held her and talked to her then quickly passed her to my crying mom who had asked for a turn. JA tried to swallow his tears as he rubbed my shoulders. It was finally as real to him as it was to me all along. We were together in this great, overwhelming sadness.

When I could finally speak, I thanked JA and my mom for being there with me. I was so grateful they could join me in this saddest of all moments, just as they had as my birth coaches in the joy of MJ's arrival. The two tragic and joyful experiences so interlinked in my body and mind.

The hours after that dragged on in tedium at the hospital. JA left to pick up MJ and perhaps grieve on his own a bit. I just wanted to get home, too. The OB finally arrived an hour or so later, commenting on the completeness of the placenta so we wouldn't need to go in to remove anything. He went on and on citing the anomalies in her anatomy but finally saying she looked quite good, considering. I didn't even know what to say to him. When he finally turned to my healing issues, talking about giving me medications to induce uterine contractions without narcotics because he wanted to avoid further bleeding, I finally got the nerve to tell him how he vastly underestimated the physical experience I just underwent. I told him it was nothing like menstrual cramps. It was full on labor and delivery. He was defensive, saying he had warned me it might feel like labor at the end. But none of us recalled hearing that depiction. I was just glad that I let him know how rough it really was. Maybe he'll better prepare the next unfortunate woman in his care.

I went through the following days in a fog. I wanted to be with my family and no one else. I communicated with friends and more distant family through e-mails and occasional telephone calls. I was crying all the time. The sadness was a constant, although I was also surprised to find I could still feel happiness and gratitude. I still enjoyed moments of joy with MJ. Her two-year-old antics are always entertaining. And she serves as a testament that we can make a healthy baby. She's our symbol of hope. She also keeps me a mom. I want to have more kids because I so enjoy being a mom to her. I love watching her grow and learn and become her own person. Plus I love parenting with JA, who seems so at home as a dad.

As I write this, it's been exactly two months since our baby Coco arrived stillborn to this world. While I've gone through so many stages of sadness, anger, resentment, and sadness again, I know much healing is still ahead of me. I try to hurry the process sometimes. I found myself cleaning the house like never before and trying to tone and tighten my body back to a pre-pregnancy state. I even tried changing to a completely organic/natural diet, avoiding certain plastics, and wearing gloves whenever cleaning in efforts to reduce my risk of future genetic problems. But I realize these are futile efforts to find a reason for what happened and to exert control over the future unknowns. I remind myself that I did nothing different in that pregnancy than when I created the healthy little MJ who is again growing out of all her clothes.

I'm struggling to find meaning in all this suffering. One of the blessings of this experience has come from allowing others to help and support me. I feel especially fortunate to have such incredible friends and family in my life. I appreciate them so much more these days as they patiently listen to my feelings and ask how I'm doing weeks later. I still cry now and then, especially when I see pregnant women with toddlers my daughter's age. I still envy others' healthy pregnancies. But I've stopped imagining my parallel life of "how things would be now if I were still pregnant…" It's too much torture.

I'm also struggling to accept that life doesn't always work out as I had planned. I feel this is a lesson I've needed to work on for a long time. I can still find happiness and be myself outside that perfect picture of where I should be by age 35. I am grieving the loss of that perfect family image with our children perfectly spaced. I am grieving the loss of trust in my body and the innocence of expecting a healthy pregnancy. I am grieving all those lost plans along with our lost baby. And I'm working on being patient with this grieving process. I can still be me. I can still be whole in this process of loss and healing.

There are still so many unknowns before me. I figure this is a rough part of the road to our goals. Because, when I think about it, our real goal is to have a rewarding family life. We always knew there would be rough spots along with the happy times. And during any given day, I can slow down enough to realize that I'm actually happy for the moment. JA and MJ are wonderful parts of my life. I still don't feel we are finished with this process of creating our family, but I can be okay with where we are right now. I guess I've learned to appreciate my blessings and loosen my hold on plans that are beyond my control anyway.

41

T's Story "Autosomal Dominant Genetic Disorder"

My wedding day was the most carefree and happy day I had over the last three years. That was before I knew what "autosomal dominant" meant or how having such a genetic disorder would change my life forever. That was almost three years ago. Six months after we were married we decided to get pregnant and start our family. This is our story.

<u>Pregnancy: Odds say that you have a 30 percent chance of getting pregnant your first month trying</u>

My husband and I decided that in December of 2004 I would stop taking the birth control pill and the fun of making a baby would begin. We had discussed waiting for three months to let my body adjust to not being on the pill before playing out our version of the Olympics, but neither one of us could help ourselves when the ovulation predictor kit said "Go for it!!" Neither one of us truly thought we would nail it on the first try, but nonetheless I refrained from more than one glass of champagne that New Years. On January 12th, I had not started my period. Not really paying attention to how many days I was late, I took a home pregnancy test. I about jumped off the toilet seat when the second line appeared. "What? This is too soon. Don't we get a few practice months to fully live out our Olympic dreams?"

<u>Pregnancy One</u>

We beat the 30 percent odds; we got it on the first try.

I called my husband at work immediately; I just could not contain myself to wait to surprise him after he got home from work. We were both excited and immediately stressed about where we were going to live, but really happy with the anticipation of adding a baby to our family. We started looking for a house immediately. All of our friends were in the middle or at the end of creating their families, so we felt we were right on track. The pregnancy was going along great. I was also right on track with all the pregnancy symptoms according to *BabyCenter.com*, which I read religiously everyday along with five or so other web sites.

We had seen the doctor for an ultrasound at around seven weeks gestation and saw a heartbeat. She told us that we had a less than five percent chance of miscarrying now that we had seen the heartbeat. My husband and I were thrilled. That meant we had a 95 percent chance of having a baby, but we did not pay much attention to the percentages. We would never fall into that five percent range, not us. We were on cloud nine for all of a week and a half. Life was good until February 18th, the day I started spotting. I rushed alone to my OB's office where I was told that the baby's heart was no longer beating and that I should schedule a D&C to remove the remains. I was almost 10 weeks pregnant by that time. I remember that I did not speak a word for about two minutes, and then I drove home and sobbed the entire way. The D&C was performed the next day, on February 19th.

Pregnancy Two

Could we beat the odds again?

It was Good Friday weekend, and we decided to go and meet my brother and sister-in-law in Santa Barbara for the weekend. She was about seven months pregnant with their second child at the time. I was not all that upset to see her pregnant since the loss of pregnancy one was, in my mind, a minor bump in the road. After all—I was only 10 weeks along. I knew I would be back on track soon enough. It also turned out that I was ovulating that weekend, so my husband and I went for it again. This was the first cycle we tried to get pregnant after pregnancy one.

I could not believe it when two weeks later a home pregnancy test was positive. I thought proudly to myself that we must be really fertile to get pregnant so easily. I felt lucky.

Our Gem

I was just finishing up my final semester of law school when the bleeding began. I was so stressed out about exams and about the possibility of losing another pregnancy to miscarriage. We finally figured out that I have a very sensitive cervix, and that all vaginal ultrasounds cause me some sort of bleeding. This was of course after my OB had scared me into believing that I was miscarrying again. We changed OB's soon after the bleeding scares.

After two separate scares with bleeding from ultrasounds, we thought we were finally on our way to having our precious little baby. That small bump in the road was not stopping us. We made it to the second trimester with flying colors. We were told at a 14-week ultrasound that the baby was a girl, and we decided to name her Grace Elicia. We were busy, but we were happy with how great the pregnancy was going. All was well again at our house, and according to *BabyCenter.com* I was right on track, just like before.

We went to Cedars-Sinai Medical Center at 20 weeks gestation to have a level II ultrasound done. We opted to have the level II ultrasound because my husband's sister died at three months of age due to a heart defect. The doctor who performed the ultrasound for me happened to be the skeletal dysplasia specialist at Cedars-Sinai. We were happy to find out from her the reason for my own weird thumbnails and funny knees, which I had been trying to figure out for many years. I had asked my previous OB if genetic counseling was something I should consider since many relatives on my dad's side of the family had the same weird afflictions. She told me to calm down and take it easy and that there was nothing wrong with me. We were happy to find out from the skeletal dysplasia specialist that my condition was real and had a name—Nail-patella syndrome (NPS). I was not all that shocked or surprised. Really, I just wanted to know about my baby. I wanted to know if she would have my funny knees too. At the time I had no idea the full scope of what NPS was and how horrible it could be. I was lucky and I was innocently naïve.

Those two minutes of silence that I experienced during pregnancy one when the doctor told me my baby had died felt nothing like the two minutes I experienced at this ultrasound appointment. I felt like I would die when the doctor said that our baby most likely had NPS because she had some severe deformities that were normally associated with NPS. "What? Did I hear you correctly? Deformities?" Then she said, "Oh yeah, and it is a baby girl." She was so matter-of-fact about everything, like it was no big deal.

I remember my mind racing, telling me that everything would be okay, that this woman did not know what she was talking about, and that this baby was fine. I was normal. I was not deformed, so she must be wrong. I laid there as she frantically tried to get our daughter to move for a better view of the feet. I laid so still. I remember feeling like that was the thing to do to help the doctor see her mistake. Our daughter wasn't moving. She never moved much on any ultrasound I had. No one ever told me that was not normal. Then a second doctor came in, and he agreed. There was no mistake. We had about a million questions, and we were told to see a different specialist who had experience with NPS—Dr. P. They rushed us out of the room. "What just happened? Are you kidding me?"

We went to the nicest doctor on this earth, Dr. P, and he spent four hours with us using 3D and 4D imaging to get a good look at our baby's feet. He explained a lot to us about what NPS was and how it was inherited. Basically, it is an autosomal dominant genetic disorder, which means that there are no unaffected carriers for the disorder. It only affects one in 50,000 people, and it affects all races. If you have the mutation for it in your genes, you have a 50/50 chance of passing it on to your child. If you do not pass it on to your child, your child will not pass it on to his or her children.

One of Grace's feet was turned outward, but the other foot was turned under itself. It was like her legs were on backwards with her feet pointing behind her instead of in front of her. She was not moving correctly, so we were also told that there was a likelihood of intellectual disabilities. Intellectual disabilities are not a problem in NPS, but due to her foot deformity and lack of movement, it was suggested this too was a possibility. So not only was this sweet girl of ours going to be in a wheelchair due to the NPS, she would most likely be intellectually disabled too. We had decided we could handle the wheel chair, but when we heard mental impairment was a high possibility, we did not know what to think. Since there was a good chance that she had NPS based on the ultrasound findings, we learned she could also have severe kidney problems and vision problems. NPS not only involves the skeleton, but also the kidneys and eyes. The full extent of her problems could not be known for sure until after she was born. We were devastated.

We went home and agonized over what to do in silence. I searched the Internet for everything I could find about NPS. I sat and sobbed at what I found. There were other people who had my thumb nails. There were children who were suffering from the skeletal deformities. They could not straighten their arms more than 90 degrees, some were in wheelchairs, and some kept breaking bones and weren't allowed to run or play. I found pictures of a few with deformed feet just like our Grace had. I read stories about children who were blind from glaucoma. I was devastated that I passed a gene to my child that could do all of this.

It was a short conversation; we both knew the quality of life for this child would be horrible. My husband had asked me about my feelings about termination before we even became pregnant the first time. He told me that he absolutely would not feel good about bringing a sick child into this world. I told him I did not know if I would be able to terminate a pregnancy for a problem that was compatible with life. He asked me to think long and hard about my position. I thought he was a monster for his beliefs, but decided to let it go since I assumed I would never be in that situation. I would never have to make such a decision so it would be a nonissue. I was wrong, and I surprised myself at how quickly I decided that letting her go would be kinder than letting her suffer.

We decided to terminate. We called to let our OB know what we had decided, and we were given the phone number and address for the abortion clinic in town that does "these types of abortions." I thought my OB would take care of me, and I did not realize I would have to go to a clinic. It was the same place I had gone for my D&C from pregnancy one. Since we were so far along we were separated from the other women who were there, I can only assume, to end unwanted pregnancies. We were told it was too hard for them to look at me. "What? I did not realize any of this experience was about them." I was in such a daze that I really did not care about where they wanted me to wait. I just wanted it to be over with.

Our very tiny daughter Grace was born at 22 weeks gestation on August 3, 2005 at an abortion clinic by dilation and extraction. I was sedated for each procedure along the way. This clinic really did specialize in my type of situation. I was not happy to be at an abortion clinic, but I was happy to not have pain during the process.

She weighed less than a pound, and we donated her remains to the International Skeletal Dysplasia Registry at Cedars-Sinai Medical Center. In order to donate her remains, the termination took an extra day to dilate my cervix sufficiently for her to pass. It was the worst three days of my life. I begged my husband to come with me to see her and to say goodbye. He couldn't do it, so I went alone. I held her, I kissed her, and I told her I loved her. I felt so numb being in there alone with my little daughter. I remember wondering what I was supposed to do after I had told her all I wanted to say. I felt awkward sitting there with her alone. The nurse came in a short time later and took her from me.

The doctor from Cedars-Sinai who gave us the first diagnosis of NPS called me regularly before the termination. She was the one who encouraged us to donate our daughter's remains to her registry. After the termination was complete and she received the remains, she neither sent us the report outlining the findings, nor did she send Grace's DNA for analysis like she had promised. I am still angry with the way she treated the situation. It was as if she was just courting me to get the remains. I had to fight and fight to get the DNA tested, and I have yet to receive the final report.

After the termination we went home and started the healing process. My husband's mother was born in Nicaragua, and he and I had been building a beach house there, so I dove into getting that house completed in time for the Christmas party that my husband and I spontaneously planned after the loss of Grace. I worked day and night trying my best to forget about what had just happened. I went to two therapists to try to work through what had happened, but there was no way to speed up the grieving process. I just needed to work to take my mind off things and to cry my heart out when I couldn't forget anymore.

Prior to the termination we did not ask for our families' opinions; we did not feel it was their decision to make. We made the phone calls, and sent the e-mails informing every one of what had happened and what our decision would be. We wanted to be upfront with everyone about what had happened. That was a big mistake. Looking back on things, I could have saved myself so much sadness had I just told them the baby died and we induced labor. At the time, I did not realize that so many of our friends and family would judge us for what we had decided. I am glad that I now know who our "real" friends are, but I really regret testing our relationships at a time when I really needed any and all support I could get.

The distance between my husband and I and those who had judged us began to grow. Some never even called to share their condolences. Some called and told me outright that what I had decided was wrong. I cried and my husband ran away to work as much as he could. I needed every friend I had, and I felt so lonely and angry that some of my closest friends had judged me for doing what I thought was best for me and my family. I cried every day for two months. I remember my husband feeling very frustrated that I was still so sad eight weeks after we lost Grace. He wanted to fix me and he couldn't.

I had a really hard time accepting that I had a genetic disorder and somehow I was not normal like everyone else. All of the funny things that I had like crooked elbows, weird thumb nails, and tiny kneecaps all of a sudden became things I was embarrassed about. I did not want my husband to see me naked. I did not want him to touch me at all. I kept waiting for him to leave, but he never did. It took me about six months to realize that he loved me just the way I was before we found out about the NPS.

Johns Hopkins Hospital

While I was working hard to forget what just happened to me by diving into completing the house in Nicaragua, I started the process to locate the NPS gene on my DNA so that testing could be developed for chorionic villus sampling (CVS) or preimplantation genetic diagnosis (PGD) for a future pregnancy. There are over 130 different known mutations that cause NPS. We were told it could take anywhere from four weeks to one year to locate the mutation on my DNA.

We met with Iain McIntosh, the head researcher looking at NPS, at The Johns Hopkins Hospital. We actually met with him before Grace was born, and he gave us a lot of useful information about NPS. He helped us make an informed decision about what our daughter would be facing. I mailed my blood sample over to him, and in early December my mutation had been located and confirmed. My family shares the same mutation with five other families. We were lucky it only took a few weeks to find it.

Shortly after learning about the mutation, I was scheduled to participate in a study at Johns Hopkins. I flew out to Baltimore and went through three days of testing. I had over 100 x-rays taken, a bone density scan performed, a glaucoma check, a dental check-up, an evaluation of every joint movement in my body, and an interview with a genetic counselor. My kidneys are normal and I don't show any signs of glaucoma. I am lucky. I found out that I am mildly affected, and that any OB I asked should have offered me genetic counseling. I was mad to hear what should have happened. It stung to hear that all my suffering could have been avoided.

My dad had promised to go with me to Johns Hopkins to be evaluated too since he lived only 45 minutes away. At the last minute, he backed out. So I went alone. He did not even drive over to have dinner with me. I still have not spoken to my dad since he backed out of going. Two years later, I am still having a hard time forgiving him for not being there for me.

About a month after Grace was born, my husband had some business to do in Hong Kong and I had never been to Asia, so we planned our much-delayed honeymoon vacation around his business trip. We found out at the same time that only one other family affected by NPS had tried to rule it out in their children using in vitro fertilization (IVF) with PGD. They had some severe manifestations in that family. They used the Sydney IVF clinic to do their IVF/PGD. Since we were going to be on that side of the world, we decided to pay the clinic a visit. That clinic was far more advanced than any clinic we had seen in Los Angeles. They were very confident and had the statistics to back it up. We slapped our money down to have the genetic tests worked up to do an IVF/PGD cycle should we decide to do so in the future.

Pregnancy Three

Now we had new odds…50/50 odds!

My husband and I decided we didn't want to have a baby with NPS. The severity of NPS cannot be predicted, so we did not want to wait again until a 20-week ultrasound to be told that, yet again, the baby was severely affected. We were told it could be risky to my health to do another 22-week termination. We did not need to be told that to decide against it, it was horrible, and I never would intentionally decide to do it again. Now that we knew about the mutation, we had to decide what route to take to get pregnant. We could try to get pregnant the natural way and test the baby for the NPS gene by CVS at 11 weeks gestation or we could try IVF with PGD to test the embryos for any problems before they were transferred.

We found ourselves right back where we started in December of 2004. It was one year later, two losses later, but our desire to have a baby was the same if not stronger. My cycle began on January 6th, and the thermometers and charts for trying to conceive were pulled out again. I was not too dedicated to charting my cycle exactly right, but nonetheless I still managed to get pregnant for the third time in a row on the first try. Again, I remember feeling so proud of our fertility.

At that point my husband and I were in total shock that three times we tried to conceive and three times in a row we succeeded in the first month. We thought "This is impossible, this time has to work out. The third time is a charm, right?"

There was no bleeding during that pregnancy, just some light spotting at the beginning. I felt really sick, but that faded quickly, and by 10 weeks I was feeling like my old non-pregnant self again. It was a new feeling for me, as I had never had that easy of a time with morning sickness and intense hunger. Things were looking up again, but we were scared.

Finally, March 21st came, the day of the CVS test. The day we knew our life would change again. Funny how for us a home pregnancy test no longer qualified as something that would change our lives, but a CVS test would. So there we were, back at Dr. P's office looking at our baby on the ultrasound monitor again. There we were, nervous and scared.

The CVS went off without any problems. I had some slight spotting and some mild cramping, but for the most part, all was okay. We decided to go to our OB's office to confirm the pregnancy was still looking good four days after the CVS. At that ultrasound, we saw the clearest picture of the straightest legs and correctly positioned feet you could ever dream of. My husband had jumped and landed on cloud nine. He was pulling me along with him, but I was resistant. I was scared; not just a little scared, but scared for real. I was scared that I might not be able to pull myself together to try again if this baby had NPS too. I don't think I had totally accepted the NPS diagnosis for myself.

Days ticked by, then one week had passed since the test, then more days ticked by, and we were dying to find out. I was beginning to feel signs of movement. I wanted to know my fate, my baby's fate. Finally, when I was 12 weeks and six days pregnant, the news came back that this baby had the NPS gene, the same gene that had caused our sweet Grace so many problems. The same gene that gave me the immense guilt I felt for deciding Grace's fate, for not giving my husband a perfect healthy child, and now for failing a second time. We found out it was a boy. It took me a good day before I could really cry and accept that we had failed again and that it was my genes, my imperfection, and my fault all of this was happening. This time my husband did not run to work, but stayed by my side. He took care of me this time. I am glad he did, I needed him to. My mother had completely fallen to pieces at this point and was incapable of doing anything for me. She cried every time I talked to her. I needed my husband to step up and he did.

We knew we had 50/50 odds going into the pregnancy, but I suppose we never imagined that whoever was in charge upstairs would be so cruel. I thought the natural way would prevail over IVF, that I could avoid that scary stomach poking journey all together. But I was wrong.

That year on Good Friday we were not in Santa Barbara. We were at our dream house mourning the loss of yet another child. We terminated the pregnancy on April 13th and made plans for IVF.

IVF / PGD

After the third loss, we started thinking hard about what to do next. Would IVF be worth it? The Sydney IVF clinic had given us 50/50 odds despite my track record of conceiving on the first try. Our odds were so low because of the PGD. Hadn't my body been through enough? I had been pregnant three times in 13 months and lost three pregnancies in 16 months. Would it be the best thing for me physically or emotionally to get all hopped up on hormones, fly to Australia, get those eggs surgically removed, then fertilized, then tested for NPS, and then after all that, if we were lucky, get one transferred, and if we were really lucky, get a baby at the end of it all?

<u>Our Fourth Attempt</u>

We decided to go for it and started all the IVF medications at home. We were monitored at a local clinic until about eight days into the stimulation part of the cycle. That was when we boarded a plane to fly halfway across the world to Australia to get pregnant.

Stupid Home Pregnancy Tests

Our IVF cycle began on Mother's Day of all days. The birth control pills came first, then the hormone suppression shots, and then the follicle stimulating shots. My husband and I fought like crazy over who would give the shots. I was terrified of needles, and he was not too happy about having to administer them. We about killed each other with divorce threats, but we made it through.

We arrived in Sydney on Father's Day of all days. We had the eggs retrieved and tested, and on the day before my birthday we transferred one perfect embryo. Of the seven embryos that made it to day five, one had an abnormal number of chromosomes, and four of the six which had the normal number of chromosomes were affected with the NPS gene. That left us with two good embryos. Sydney IVF would only transfer one at a time, so we froze the other embryo. Our testing day for pregnancy was on my husband's birthday, of all days. I couldn't believe the significance of all the days involved in this cycle. Unfortunately, they were not a sign of good things to come.

On July 6th, I went to my OB's office in Los Angeles where they tested my blood. I loved to take those home pregnancy tests, so for three or four days prior to the blood test I was peeing my heart out, waiting for the double line. No double line. "Hey, what is wrong with these tests? I always get a double line after an attempt. It must be the tests, right? Please let it be the tests!" "Is there a God?" I had my doubts most of the time, but everyone said there was one. "Where is he?" I went to the store to buy different home pregnancy tests, to find the one that would detect the lowest amount of the pregnancy hormone possible. I found the test, and I got a double line, a faint one, but a double line. I was hopeful on the day of the blood draw, but not confident. I had never failed in getting pregnant yet, and I was terrified that this time, the most expensive time so far, I would fail.

The dreaded call came on July 7th, my husband's birthday, and my heart sank, again. "Hello, is there anybody up there? God…can you hear me? Hello?"

How many failures is one person expected to endure before going completely insane?

Our 5th Attempt and Pregnancy Four

After the failed IVF cycle, my husband and I decided to take a break, a long break. We both felt like this was taking over our lives. We both felt like we were losing ourselves in the desire to have children. We were. We had been trying nonstop for two years. Even though we were on a break from starting a family, both of us still seemed preoccupied with our future plans. I am not sure we ever *truly* took a break.

Five months later, there we were again, another December cycle. Except this time, it was 2006, two years after the first December cycle when we conceived. This would be the third December we attempted to get pregnant, and it would be the third December that we would become pregnant naturally. Again, just like all the other times we tried the natural method, we succeeded in the first month trying. Even so, I was still shocked to see the positive home pregnancy test. So was my husband, for that matter. I remember not feeling particularly lucky since I knew that the baby could be affected just like the previous two babies and four of my seven embryos from the failed IVF cycle.

The pregnancy went along without much morning sickness or intense emotions about whether the baby would test positive for NPS or not. I couldn't accept that again we would have bad luck. We were supposed to have 50/50 odds on this genetic problem, right? The CVS test was scheduled for February 19th. February 19th two years prior was the day we had the D&C performed after the miscarriage of the first pregnancy. It was strange how dates seemed to keep resurfacing. You would think living through the pain once would be enough. The constant reminders were enough to drive me insane.

This go around with the CVS, I had to have it done transabdominally. That meant the huge needle would need to pass through my stomach instead of my cervix. I hate needles and especially those that must go in my stomach. I did not look at the needle for fear that I would back out of the test. Things went well and I had little to no problems afterwards. I stayed in bed for an entire week, anticipating good news. I was thinking "This had to be the one, right?" This was our fifth go around at having a baby. This was our fourth time being pregnant. Bad things don't happen 100 percent of the time, do they?

For all of you who have a strong belief in your religious faith, I am convinced you have never experienced this sort of thing in your life. Wouldn't this experience shake even the strongest faith? My belief in religion was never really strong, but I always felt sure there was a God. I was in shock when, once again, we received bad news about our pregnancy journey. I was unsure if there was a God at that point.

I truly thought that we were nearing the end of the journey, whichever way it ended up. If we had a child without NPS or another severe problem, that would be terrific. If we never conceived a child without NPS or another problem, that would be fine too. Things always work out for the best, right? But even I doubted that things would work out.

The decision to terminate that pregnancy was the hardest, even harder than the first. I struggled with the question of whether the risk of not being able to carry a healthy child to term due to all the terminations was enough of a motivation to not terminate a pregnancy I knew could bear a child with some type of problem. What was the purpose for all this sadness in our life as a married couple? How could any one couple be tested in this way?

We both considered bringing a sick child into the world to satisfy our own fears about not having a family. We were a wreck. Finally, we decided that the decision to terminate the previous two pregnancies could not be in vain. We had to continue in our commitment to have a healthy child. We had to keep going, and we had to do what was right for this child. It was not right to bring a child into the world to suffer for our selfish desires. I vowed to have my tubes tied to prevent me from going crazy and thinking that trying things with 50/50 odds was a good a decision ever again. We terminated the pregnancy after days of discussion.

Our Future Plans

After my fourth pregnancy, my husband and I agreed that maybe it was time to look into other avenues to have a healthy baby. We decided that our best chance was to look into egg donation. This was a very difficult decision for me because I was only 33 years old at the time. I was young, and I had good quality eggs.

I found myself mourning the fact that we would never be able to make a baby together in the privacy of our bedroom. I was also very sad that I would be sacrificing seeing myself in my children if I ever managed to have any. In the beginning, when I agreed to this new plan, I did not anticipate the grief and depression I would deal with as a result. I knew it was the best plan, so I worked though my grief.

We found an egg donor who looked like she could be my sister. Maybe our family members wouldn't be able to tell? Maybe no one would know? I don't plan on keeping it a secret from my children, but I would like to be the one who tells them. I would like the opportunity to answer all their questions and explain my decisions to them before anyone else has a chance to fill their innocent minds with judgments.

We finally conceived the second time we tried using frozen embryos from the donor. I am currently six months pregnant with what appears to be a healthy baby. We still have our one embryo from Australia in storage. We flew it over to the U.S. shortly after the last frozen embryo transfer. If we decide to try for another child in the future, we plan on pairing the Australian embryo with another embryo from the same egg donor we used to achieve this pregnancy. Maybe we will get lucky and conceive a child with our DNA (from the Australian embryo), but our chances are slim.

Regrets and Realizations

This journey of trying to have a healthy child has taught me many things about myself, and it has changed how I see the world around me. Before any of this happened, I was very sensitive to what others had to say, how they reacted to me, and if they liked me or not. I was a people pleaser, I admit it.

Now, I am stronger about what I believe and a lot less sensitive to what other people think about me or my beliefs. I have learned who I can rely on in the tough times. I have been surprised that it has been my friends and not my family. I have realized that everyone has their own journeys and they should not be judged for how they react to or handle situations.

I learned that my marriage is strong and my husband has the ability to take care of me when it really counts. Most importantly, I have learned to be kind to myself and to appreciate every day as a new experience. We should never take our time here for granted or spend it worrying about what has happened in our lives.

I regret that I was not more assertive with my first OB about getting genetic counseling. I regret being upfront with certain people about what happened with Grace. I regret wasting six months of my married life feeling sorry for myself for having NPS. I regret not using donor eggs sooner.

I do not regret trying my hardest and doing everything in my power to bring a healthy baby into this world. I do not regret donating my daughter's remains to research. I do not regret doing all I can to help future generations with NPS learn as much as possible about how the disorder affects them and their unborn children. I do not regret choosing the very best for my unborn children. I do not regret feeling confident in my decision to prevent suffering in their lives.

42

Tammy's Story "Too Special for Earth"

In January of 2006, my husband Jeff and I started trying for what would be our third and final child. We were the proud parents of a 12-year-old boy named Max from Jeff's first marriage and a wonderful two-year-old boy named Garrett who we had together. We had planned it out perfectly so that our youngest two children would be just less than three years apart. We didn't anticipate any problems getting pregnant and my pregnancy with Garrett had been so uneventful that I was ready to dive in without hesitation. I had started taking prenatal vitamins and went off birth control months in advance to prepare for our big journey. The table was set and we were ready. My sister was trying to get pregnant at the same time and I was excited because our first children were born only three weeks apart and I wanted that again. She got pregnant very quickly, but I did not. She miscarried early and went on to get pregnant again very quickly. I found out shortly after she did that I was pregnant as well. Our due dates were only four days apart. We were so excited. Then, she miscarried again. I had so badly wanted our children born together. I was sad that wasn't going to happen.

My pregnancy continued with no major problems while my sister dug in her heels to try again. I noticed that I felt very different during this pregnancy than I had felt with my son. This time I was so very tired. No amount of sleep was enough. My morning sickness was really 24-hour sickness. All day long I felt like I was about to throw up, but I never did. I never had that relief. Then there were the nightmares. They were horrible, vivid nightmares of the deaths of my family members. I would awake in the middle of the night tangled in my sheets, drenched in sweat, with my heart racing a hundred miles an hour. I had vivid dreams while pregnant with Garrett, but they were always happy-go-lucky dreams. Something wasn't right. I felt it deep down. I forced myself to pass it off as nervousness because a friend of mine had just had a miscarriage at 16 weeks for no apparent reason. I never mentioned it to anybody except my husband and only then did I mention it in passing, "Man, I sure feel different this pregnancy." He thought it was because this time I was chasing after a two-year-old and not sleeping whenever I wanted to.

At 13 weeks I had a gush of pinkish fluid and rushed to the emergency room. They were able to quickly find the baby's heartbeat. Relief washed over me and I couldn't wait to get an ultrasound so that I could see my gorgeous little bean. After the ultrasound the doctor told us that my placenta was laying a little low which caused the bleeding, but other than that everything looked great with a completely normal-looking 13-week fetus. I went home on cloud nine thinking that that was the worst to come. Three days later, on my four-year wedding anniversary, I had more bleeding. Jeff was in bed with the flu and our dinner reservations had already been cancelled. I lay down as much as possible while still caring for my two-year-old. In the morning, my doctor wanted me in right away for an ultrasound so that he could see for himself what was happening. Jeff was still very sick so I took Garrett to my sisters' and went to the appointment alone.

When I got there, I was nervous, but felt that everything was going to be fine. I mean, after all, it is just my placenta lying too close to my cervix, right? I entered the ultrasound room and handed the technician my video tape so that I could have all of my ultrasounds on video. I wanted to see my baby again. I was happy to get another peek in there, no matter the reason. Before all this happened I wasn't scheduled to have an ultrasound until 20 weeks. The first thing I asked was if the baby's heartbeat was okay. "Yep, it's great. 167" she said. Baby moving? "Flipping all around." How low is my placenta? "It's not." What? "No, it is high and in the back. Great location." Then where is the blood coming from? "Don't know yet." The technician was slow and diligent, taking her time looking at everything. The whole time I was getting more and more nervous. Something wasn't right. She started asking questions about family members and if anyone in our families had birth defects or anything wrong with their spine. Nope, no one. Why, what is wrong? "I'm just having trouble finding where the spine enters the base of the skull" she said.

There it was. My world crashed and I began crying. The technician knew that I was a nurse and we were on a very friendly level. More so than with most patient/technician relationships. She said to me that while they aren't supposed to do this that she would tell me what she was seeing. The baby had no skull and no discernable brain. It is called anencephaly. How do you cope with news of that magnitude when you are half-clothed, your feet in stirrups, and wholly alone? The tears began in a tidal wave. She stood up, gave me some Kleenex, and said she was going to get the doctor. They ushered me quickly into an exam room and shut the door. As my doctor was not there that day the doctor on call appeared after a few minutes and introduced herself. She had spoken to my doctor on the telephone and he suggested that I have the diagnosis confirmed with a level II ultrasound at the local perinatologist's office. She then continued to explain to me the prognosis and options I had available should the diagnosis be correct. There is NO chance of survival. NONE. NADA. ZILCH. And for my options? Carry to term and the baby would die within minutes of birth or terminate the pregnancy. What? This was my baby, what do you mean terminate? Kill my baby? How is either one of those options okay? I sat there in stunned silence with tears coursing down my face. Jeff was at home, sick, and in bed. I was by myself and hearing the worst news that had ever befallen me.

They let me collect myself and then I left the building through the back door so that I would not have to face the waiting room full of happy women expecting healthy babies. Thank God for small favors. I made my way to my car and picked up my cell phone. I called Jeff and as soon as he answered I began sobbing uncontrollably. He was barely even able to understand what I was saying. Somehow through the crying he was able to discern that there was something wrong with the baby. He wanted to come and get me, but I was 45 minutes away with my own car that we would have to come back and get later and I still had to go pick up Garrett. We spoke for only a few minutes as I was crying too hard for him to make much sense of what I was saying. I called my sisters who sat in stunned silence as I tried to tell them what was wrong. Nothing like this had ever happened to anyone in our family. We were not prepared for this.

I drove to my sisters' house to pick up Garrett and stayed there until I thought that I could drive the rest of the way home. Once I finally made it home Jeff and I sat on the couch in disbelief. Things like this didn't really happen, did they? This was all a mistake. My OB's office had made me an appointment with the perinatologist for a confirmation the next day. I wanted to believe so badly that the level II ultrasound would show a healthy little baby and all this would be for naught. Deep down I knew though. I had felt it the whole time. Of course this was real. Of course they were right. We continued to call family members and let them know what was happening and to get the prayers started. Boy, did we need them.

The next morning Jeff and I dropped Garrett off at my sisters' again and then headed to the perinatologist's office. With sweating palms and fast-beating hearts we barely spoke as we waited for our turn. We were led to our room and the ultrasound began. The technician asked me why we were there and I told her that we were there to confirm a diagnosis of anencephaly. She turned and looked at me and said "I am so sorry, but, yes, your baby is anencephalic." I asked if I could have some pictures of him as the only ones that I had were of a six-week fetal pole. She complied with a huge stack of pictures of my beautiful baby. I then asked if she could tell the sex. She was 90 percent sure that it was a little boy. My little baby boy, my Sprout. My sadness was deeper than I can explain. She left the room to get the doctor and Jeff held me and rocked me back and forth. He told me how much he loved me and that we would make it through this. When the doctor came in he held my hand and explained what the diagnosis meant. Our little boy had no brain and no skull. He had no breathing center and would never take a breath on his own. Death would come within minutes of birth. The majority of anencephalic babies don't make it to term at all. We could opt for termination, but did have a limited time to make that decision due to state law. We asked about organ donation, but due to Sprouts defects he was not a candidate for donation.

After our appointment with the perinatologist we went to see our OB for a consultation. In his 25 years of practice we were only his second set of parents to have an anencephalic baby. He gave us the information about termination and gently encouraged us in that direction. He made it very clear that it was nothing I did or didn't do to make this happen. How could I not feel like a failure though? I was Sprout's mama and I didn't grow him right and I could not make him better.

Within two hours of leaving the office we had an appointment at a women's clinic across the state line (the state in which I reside does not allow second trimester terminations) to end the pregnancy in three days. Jeff and I quickly came to the conclusion that we could not continue with the pregnancy. I don't think that I could have endured the next five months knowing what was to come. Also, we had two boys at home who would be forced to go through the loss of a sibling. This way we could make it a little less tragic for them. We felt that this was the best route for everyone involved. I had already called into work for the weekend and now I just had to wait. It was going to be the longest three days of my life.

I made it through the weekend somehow and on the day of the termination, Jeff drove me to the clinic to check in one hour before our appointment. As I walked in I was astounded at the number of women in the waiting room. I searched their faces for someone who showed the despair that I felt inside. As soon as I signed in the receptionist ushered us to a private room and told us that we could wait in there so that we didn't have to sit in the waiting room with the rest of the women. That alone confirmed to me that our situation was very different. Were there really that many women who were ending an unwanted pregnancy? The idea made me feel even sadder, if that was possible.

Due to the gestational age of my pregnancy (14.5 weeks) a dilation and evacuation (D&E) was considered the quickest, easiest, and lowest risk of the procedures available. The doctor who performed the procedure, while highly recognized for his skills, was one of the most awful people I have ever been in company with. His bedside manner was nothing short of cruel and the things that he said to me were too awful to repeat. The procedure was over quickly and despite the medications that I had received, I remember it all. The feeling, the sound, the smell. We left the clinic in silence, holding hands, with me wondering how many other married couples would be forced to share such an awful experience.

I healed physically very quickly with no complications. Mentally and emotionally? Well, now, that's another story.

I was an emotional wreck. I didn't function well. I slept a lot and I quit doing anything fun. Normally I am a very outgoing, generous person and I was surprised by some of the emotions that I began experiencing. When I saw another pregnant woman the most awful pangs of hatred and jealousy would course through me. When I saw another woman with her newborn it would take considerable effort on my part to not run up to them and make sure they knew how lucky they were that their babies were healthy and alive. I didn't understand these feelings as I had never experienced anything even remotely close to this. At night I would cry myself to sleep. Not just a sad cry either. It was the kind of cry that exhausts you physically. It was often the only way that I could fall asleep and it went on for months.

All that I was feeling was compounded by the fact that the faith I have spent all of my 30 years in did not support my decision. It was so hard to be rejected by my faith the one time that I needed it the most. I never really talked about how I felt until I met my friends on the *BabyCenter* message boards. No one in my life would have been able to understand fully. The group of women that I met there essentially saved my life. It was amazing to communicate with someone who had been in your shoes. Someone who had made the same painstaking choice. Someone who understood the guilt that goes along with the decision that was made. It was heaven to have found that group. A place where I wasn't that different. A place where people didn't tiptoe around me and whisper behind my back "Did you hear what was wrong with her baby?" I was online for hours every day talking with those women. I was consumed by it. To this day they are the only people who remember when I have an anniversary coming up. The anniversary of the bad news, the anniversary of Sprout's passing, the anniversary of his due date.

There is always a note of "We're thinking of you and we love you." on these days addressed to me. They helped me be whole again.

Jeff definitely didn't understand what I was feeling. He was sad and hurt and although we had made the decision together, it was very different for him. I was the one who had carried Sprout and had felt all the physical changes that came with being pregnant. I was the one who could feel the baby move if I lay perfectly still and in just the right position. I was the one who signed the consent form for the procedure. And I am now the one with a surgical history of an elective abortion. How could he be expected to understand what I was going through? He supported me the best that he could while trying to deal with his own feelings and emotions of the situation.

My OB was amazingly supportive and helped me to believe that I could go on to have another healthy child. He was very attentive and kind in the appointments that followed.

I realize that I was very early in my pregnancy and that I had not ever held or fed or rocked my baby, but I daydreamed of those things every second of my pregnancy. To me it was as if those things had really happened. I cannot put into words how the loss of that has affected me forever.

I have gone on to have another child, a daughter, Reece. I endured a frighteningly scary pregnancy with her, to the point that she was really not expected to make it. She is one year old now and perfect in every way. Every day that I look at her I thank God that he let me have her and then I wonder if Sprout would look like her and Garrett. I wonder what color his hair would have been and if his eyes would be bright green like mine or deep brown like his daddy's. Would he be a snuggler like Reece or a play-til-you-drop baby like Garrett? I don't go a day without thinking of him.

Sprout's two year angelversary is in just a few weeks and I have finally found peace in what happened. Only recently have I stopped sectioning my life into "before Sprout" and "after Sprout." Instead of being my tragedy, he is finally just my angel that I look forward to meeting in Heaven. My husband helped me make it to this point when he told me that these things had to happen to make the world go round and that we were chosen because God knew that we could handle it and would make the right decision.

Laying my sweet baby to rest was undeniably the hardest decision that I have ever had to make. And I am finally completely at peace with it. I don't wonder anymore if I made the right decision, I know that I did. He is happy, healthy, and whole where he is. He must be an unbelievably special boy for God to want him before he was even born. I can't wait to meet him someday.

43

Tania's Story "Surviving Jacob's Broken Heart"

It's pretty bizarre, how far I've come over the past four years. A whole lifetime it seems. A whole new world, a new outlook and a new understanding of things I never would have dreamed of even trying to comprehend.

On July 24th, 2003 I found out I was pregnant. I remember it clearly since it was my future brother-in-law's birthday. My period had been late for two days, but I wasn't really thinking that I might be pregnant. I worked from home and that day, like the previous couple of days, I had dozed off to sleep during my lunch hour. I couldn't seem to stay awake at all. I had an appointment at my chiropractor's office for an adjustment that day. When I mentioned to him how I kept falling asleep during the daytime, he made a joke that maybe I was pregnant. He knew my husband and I were thinking of trying for a child. I told him that I didn't think I was pregnant since I really felt like my period was coming at any moment, and I had only been off the pill for six weeks. Something told me to drop by the pharmacy, just in case, and pick up a home pregnancy test. So I did. My husband was to go in to work at 1:00 PM that day, so he was in the shower when I got home. I decided to take the test right then. I read the instructions and peed on the stick. I kept watching the wick getting wetter and the urine creeping its way up to the control line. Then I watched as the result line showed up as plain as day, without the five minute wait! I kept telling myself, "Holy cow, holy cow, holy cow!" My husband came out of the shower and I showed him the test. He didn't quite know what to make of it, so he asked "What is it?" I said, "It's a home pregnancy test! It's positive…I'm pregnant!" Not quite knowing what to say or how to react he said "Congratulations!" My next words were, "What have we done?" All of a sudden, I got a very panicky feeling.

I had wanted all my life to be a mom. At that point, I had been able to think of nothing else. I had been taking my prenatal vitamins religiously, and I had been practicing taking my basal body temperature for at least three months prior to stopping the pill in order to optimize our chances of conceiving. We had been married a couple of years, had been together 14 years, had our new house, two cars, etc. Having a baby was the next thing on our list. So why was I so nervous?

The first thing I did following the positive pregnancy test was get on my computer and search for a pregnancy calendar to figure out when the baby would be due. I was supposed to give birth to our baby around March 30th, 2004—that was my estimated due date. I figured that by Christmas I would be pretty big and pretty proud! After figuring out my due date, I started to make some telephone calls. I was getting so excited. I called my doctor's office and got in for an appointment within a week. I then got referred to the OB clinic since all pregnant women in my area of Canada are referred to the clinic to have our pregnancies followed. My first appointment was at 10 weeks. It was such a long wait!

I was accompanied by my husband for my first routine prenatal appointment. We were told that they were going to try to listen for the baby's heart with a Doppler, but not to get too worried if they couldn't hear it since we were still pretty early. After what seemed like an eternity, all of sudden we heard a rhythm which was mesmerizing. Our jaws dropped. It was our baby's heart, beating like crazy.

The pregnancy was wonderful. I didn't suffer one bout of morning sickness and my energy was pretty good. I felt really wonderful and couldn't wait to start showing. I had my AFP testing done at 14 weeks, and the results came back fine.

The next step was our first ultrasound at 18 weeks. We would finally get to see our baby. My husband was out of town for work during my 18th week so we rescheduled it to week 19. We went in and everything looked great. The only problem was that they couldn't get a good look at the baby's heart. We were told that happened all the time, and so they scheduled us for another ultrasound two weeks later.

Two weeks later, my husband and I met up at the hospital. It was November 19th. I had diligently drunk all the water required before the ultrasound and I waited for my turn. We were very pleased to see our little one again. We were playfully trying to figure out if we were seeing a boy or a girl as the ultrasound technician took measurements and made small talk with us. I secretly wanted a girl so much. At the hospital, the technicians were not allowed to confirm or comment on the sex of the baby. They also weren't allowed to mention anything to the patient should they see something potentially problematic with the baby. Once the ultrasound was over, my husband and I parted with a kiss, and headed back to our respective workplaces.

Later that same afternoon, I got a call from the OB clinic. Apparently, they had been waiting for us. The ultrasound technician had failed to tell us that we were supposed to go upstairs to the clinic to discuss the ultrasound. So I drove back to the clinic alone to meet with the OB on duty, only to get a taste of the news that was to come over the next week. The doctor explained to me that they still weren't able to take all the measurements they wanted of the baby's heart. They couldn't see the baby's atriums correctly and it seemed the pulmonary artery was a bit larger than the aorta, which could possibly mean a septal defect. But not to worry at all…it might still mean nothing. I was told that they didn't quite have the technology to see those things very well. I was asked if I would consider a referral to IWK Children's Hospital or to Saint John Hospital, whoever would have a spot for me first. I said, "Of course!"

Next I had to explain the situation to my husband without him jumping to the wrong conclusion too quickly. I was trying to keep positive. After all, they fix babies' heart problems every day! We got a call the next day to drive up to IWK Hospital for an appointment.

On Friday, November 21st, we learned that our lives would never be the same. "There's something very wrong with your baby's heart," the perinatologist said. It took him about three minutes of going over my belly with the ultrasound probe to tell us exactly what we didn't want to hear. My brain just went to another place as I heard "Double outlet right ventricle, transposition of the great arteries, subpulmonary ventricular septal defect," etc. I kept hearing my heartbeat inside my head as if I was totally in another dimension. This couldn't be happening!

They arranged for us to meet with a pediatric cardiologist that afternoon. We went out for lunch, but couldn't stomach anything. We were certain about one thing—whatever we needed to do, we'd do it. We had faith that they could fix whatever was wrong. The pediatric cardiologist was great at explaining the nature of what was wrong and what it meant in terms of surgeries, life expectancy, quality of life, etc. He also arranged for us to meet with another specialist the following Monday. Since it was Friday afternoon, most people had already gone home.

We drove back from the hospital and every time I felt my baby move, I'd choke up. I had the feeling that my life would never again be the same.

On Monday, we met with the pediatric radiologist. As she performed yet another ultrasound, she had an additional list of identified problems with our baby. After that, we all met in a room and the doctors kept mentioning

"If you bring this baby to term…" and they'd explain the procedures and steps they would take to try and save our little one's life. It was all mind-numbing.

My husband and I looked at each other several times on the drive home. We didn't want to say it out loud, but we both knew what the other was thinking.

We drove back up to IWK Hospital on November 26th, and shared our decision with the group of doctors. I couldn't believe it when we had to utter the words "We've decided to interrupt the pregnancy." I don't think I had slept more than an hour per night since the diagnosis. I had been reading and researching everything I could find on such heart malformations. I even spent hours on end consulting medical journals and research papers since I had access to all that information through my work. Everything I found wasn't good. Maybe my baby would survive by some miracle, but what type of quality of life would he or she have?

We spent that night at a hotel. The hospital could fit us in the next day, on Wednesday, for the termination. I was 22 weeks and three days along. Where we lived we had until 24 weeks to legally terminate a pregnancy for medical reasons. Our health care coverage covered the costs and we were told that we didn't have to worry about a thing. The next morning, I met with part of the team that would look after us through the "procedure." They would inject a liquid called potassium chloride into the baby's heart to stop it from beating. Apparently, it would be less traumatic for everyone at birth. I will never forget that. I think that was the most painful moment for me because I would never again hear my baby's heartbeat. The sweet sound of my baby's heartbeat from a heart that was so sick and tangled that only my own heart would be able to keep him alive unless extensive and invasive medical interventions were attempted.

We had an amniocentesis performed first. We wanted to ensure that our baby's heart problems weren't due to some unknown chromosomal defect. Then they did the KCl shot, as they called it. I couldn't watch. We were all in tears and I was trying to keep my sobs inside because the procedure required me to be extremely still. I couldn't believe what we had just done. Just like that, my baby was gone, no longer alive, no longer twirling carelessly in my womb, no longer with a heartbeat.

We were then escorted to a wing of the hospital which cared for "complicated pregnancies." They didn't want us stationed on the same floor as labor and delivery since it would have been a cruel reminder that we weren't leaving with our baby. As if it wasn't cruel enough to actually have to give birth to him or her.

The procedure started that evening with the insertion of Misoprostol every four hours behind my cervix. My body temperature started to become slightly elevated. I was uncomfortable and my lower back was so painful. I kept thinking it was the bed, only to find out much later that it was the start of "back labor." Thursday night came and went. Friday did too. I was in agony and my temperature was pretty high by that point. By midnight on Friday, my temperature had spiked to 41 degrees Celsius (105.8 degrees Fahrenheit). I was shaking so much my bed was rattling. The nurses were starting to get nervous and kept putting wet compresses on my head. All I kept thinking was that I deserved every minute of it. In my mind, it was a small price to pay for having done what I did. A pattern of contractions had also emerged at that point and I eagerly accepted an IV shot of morphine to dull the pain. I kept dozing in and out of consciousness.

Saturday morning came and I felt the urge to push. I pushed twice and my baby was born. It was 9:59 AM, on November 29th, 2003. They whisked the baby away to clean him off. We were told we had a baby boy. That was another cruel realization for me. I was fixated on a girl so much; it never occurred to me that I'd lost a little boy. My son! They dressed him, and asked if I'd want to hold him. I didn't think I wanted to but an impulse came over me and I said that, of course, I wanted to see him. He had the cutest little hat and was dressed in a tiny doll-sized nightgown and wrapped in a blanket. He looked perfect. I just kept staring at him in wonderment. He looked like his dad. He had a crooked little finger like my grandfather. He was just precious. It was a surreal moment. This was the little one that had been growing inside me and whose heart had been so sick. My husband and I had been playing with names for little boys and "Jacob" had come up as one of our favorites. We looked at our son and knew he was Jacob. That was his name. We wouldn't be saving it for another, it was all his. We asked for him to be blessed and then told our nurse she could take him. They took pictures of him and made the arrangements to have him cremated. We were grateful. My temperature had somehow gotten back down and we were ready to leave by lunchtime.

As we prepared to leave for the two and a half-hour drive back home, we were escorted to the elevator by our wonderful nurse and the lady who coordinated our procedure. As I stepped inside the elevator, I felt a sense of panic and tearfully threw myself into their arms. Nobody said anything. There was nothing to say. We left. We drove. I cried.

My darling husband was as supportive as he could be. He was hurting so much as well. I think he was most worried about me having to deal with the throes of post-partum depression on top of everything else. My milk came in even though I didn't have a baby to nurse; my body was telling me over and over that I had just had a baby, but my arms were empty. What a difficult journey.

I received a telephone call from the hospital a few days after we got home. They needed the name and address of a funeral home close to where I lived in order to make arrangements to ship Jacob's ashes. He had been cremated at a funeral home nearby the hospital which had an ongoing service relationship with the hospital. The funeral home did this free of charge for people in situations such as ours. There was even a local pottery maker who made the beautiful urns used to store babies' ashes. I proceeded to contact the closest funeral home to where I lived and expected the call to be fairly simple. I was supposed to provide their coordinates to the hospital and get Jacob's ashes shipped there so I could pick up his remains when they arrived. However, all I was able to say to the owner when she answered the phone was my name. To my surprise, I started sobbing on the phone and I had a hard time trying to explain to her why I needed her address. This is when I met an Earth Angel.

She asked if I could manage to get to her office because I needed to sign some documents for the release of Jacob's remains. If I couldn't, she would send someone to pick me up. I drove to her office and she greeted me with a hug and told me how sorry she was for the loss of my son Jacob. She was the first person, outside of the staff at the hospital, who had acknowledged Jacob by his name. Not only did she patiently listen to me through my sobbing fits, but she said they would take care of everything and I wouldn't have to worry about trying to make these calls myself. She took it upon herself to call the other funeral home, she sent a driver to pick up Jacob's ashes instead of having his remains shipped over, and she had her Funeral Director deliver Jacob's remains to me personally at my home. I couldn't believe how sensitive and compassionate this perfect stranger was. When I tried to arrange for the payment of her services, she refused any money. She said I had been paying enough already and that I didn't owe her a thing. I was in awe of how wonderful this woman had been. In the midst of losing all control of my emotions and completely pouring my heart out to her, she had left me with a little ray of hope that I would be okay through all this. In the space of a 30-minute meeting, this Earth Angel, with whom I had received such solace and comfort, had understood what I feared the most and told me how I already had all the strength I needed to get through this. I proceeded to rely on her wisdom and a wonderful online support network to get through the difficult weeks that followed.

Two and a half months after Jacob was born I wrote the following in my journal:

"I can't believe 2.5 months have gone by. Today I can feel so much better. I still don't know and still search to make sense of why we had to lose you so dramatically and traumatically. You were such a gift, Jacob. I never knew such love in my life. You represented everything I hoped and wanted in my life. I'm so sorry for putting such pressure on you. It was never about me. Now I look at your pictures and I feel nothing but love and gratefulness. I miss you so much. As I was carrying you, I had found a renewed sense of purpose, of value.

I have now found some sense of peace with everything. I have found joy and happiness again and I've realized that it doesn't mean I have forgotten you or "gotten over" your loss, but I've come to realize that you, my dear son, are now okay. You are not suffering and even if your heart isn't beating anymore and you're not inside me growing as you still should be, I've realized that your soul is very healthy and that I feel your presence every day. I find it somehow comforting to carry you so strongly in my heart. I'm sorry for having to make the horrible choice I did. I couldn't bear the thought of having you here with me, selfishly, when you would have struggled so much to live. I love you too much, I love you that much."

March 30th came. It was my due date. I wrote this poem to my son, one of my last journal entries:

As Today Comes to a Close,
You My Darling Angel I Still Hold in My Heart so Close.
You Should Have Been Just About Here for Me and Your Father to Love.
Instead, We Need to Find Comfort in the Fact that You Are Happy With Loved Ones Up Above.
As Today Comes to a Close,
I Can Only Say Thank You My Angel for Loving Us Enough To Choose Us as Your Parents and Making Us Realize We Could Love So Much.
You've Left an Imprint on My Heart Which I Carry with Motherly Pride.
The Kind That Only another Mother Realizes You Can Never Hide.
As Today Comes to a Close,

I find Peace in Knowing You Are Free of Any Suffering or Pain.
And The Hope of Reuniting with You One Day Will Always Remain.
For Today, I Still Have Work to Do To Honor Your Memory.
In The Meantime My Precious Son, Remember How Loved You Are by Your Mommy.

Life goes on. Time slowly works its magic and puts things in perspective. When I look back, I am so thankful and grateful for all the gifts I've received. I feel privileged in a way it's hard to describe. In losing Jacob, I've found an inner strength and peace I had never experienced. I've been let in on a secret, a new way of looking at life, a new understanding of the true meaning of love, faith and selflessness. So after all, maybe Jacob's purpose in life played itself out exactly as it was supposed to.

44

TJ's Story "An Unexpected Diagnosis of Down Syndrome"

I thought I was safe. I was 32 years of age at conception and would be 33 at delivery. I had not yet crossed that magical threshold of 35 years that labels you as "advanced maternal age." So when I found out I was pregnant in early January, I simply started planning for a September baby, one that would be due only six days after my son's third birthday. I worked in the medical field and really believed that the statistics were still on my side. I never imagined that I would be the one faced with a diagnosis of a chromosomal disorder.

It was only our second month trying to conceive, and since we were in the middle of an interstate move, I never expected to actually get pregnant. My husband and I weren't even living together at the time we conceived; we were only together on weekends because of his new job, so we had no real hopes for success in December. I had to call him at 6:30 AM on the day the movers came to tell him that my period was late and that there were, in fact, two lines on all three pregnancy tests I had taken. All we could do was laugh. This baby was wanted and planned for, but still a bit of a surprise. Despite our unexpected news, I had a household to get packed up and one toddler and four cats to move to another state, so I hung up with my husband and went about my business.

Within days the family was reunited and we were living in our new home in a new state. Those first few weeks were a whirlwind of unpacking and settling into our new neighborhood. Truthfully, I didn't think much about being pregnant, with the exception of avoiding foods on the forbidden-for-pregnant-women list and trying to stay awake despite the overwhelming exhaustion. It wasn't like my first pregnancy, when I thought about being pregnant every single minute. I assumed my detachment was simply a by-product of the chaos of moving and the fact that I'd been through it all once before; I never considered that it would be a harbinger of things to come. I found a new OB and had my first prenatal appointment at eight weeks gestation, where they confirmed my dates and offered to schedule me for a new test called the nuchal translucency (NT) screen. I was a big believer in medical testing, seeing as I worked in the medical field, so I accepted every test they offered me.

Unlike a lot of parents-to-be, my husband and I had discussed during our pregnancy with our son what we would do if any tests detected a problem. We felt strongly that if any of the testing found a chromosomal problem or a problem incompatible with life, we would end the pregnancy. We never thought we would be in a position to make that kind of decision, but we had the discussion just in case. When we became pregnant once again, we had a quick recap chat of our feelings, to see if anything had changed, and we agreed that we still felt the same.

Our NT screen was scheduled for the beginning of March with a local perinatology group. I was just shy of 12 weeks. I was able to see the baby moving, I could see all four chambers of its little heart beating away, and all of the major organs appeared to be normal-sized and healthy. The actual nuchal translucency, a measurement of the thickness at the back of a fetus's neck, was within the normal range and, though it wasn't factored in to my risk assessment, the perinatologist was able to visualize a nasal bone, which is frequently absent in fetuses with Down syndrome at that stage. I got my blood drawn for the blood work component of the test and walked out of the office, ultrasound pictures in hand, a very happy woman without a worry in the world about the pregnancy.

Eight days later, I got the phone call that shook my very foundation. Even after a perfect looking ultrasound, the blood work showed that my baby had a one in five risk of having Down syndrome. I called my husband at work and gave him the bad news. I called my parents to prepare them that there might not be a new grandchild come Christmas after all. Then I just sat there, stunned. I called the genetic counselor back because I needed to know what my actual blood work results were, not just the risk. When I found out just how skewed the hCG and PAPP-A levels were, I immediately knew that I would, in fact, be the "one." We made an appointment with the perinatologist to discuss what was next. Unfortunately, I was too late for a chorionic villus sampling and too early for an amniocentesis, so I had to wait over two weeks to get a confirmatory diagnosis.

I probably cried more in those few weeks than I had in the previous 33 years of my life. I tried everything I could to stay positive. I developed what I refer to as my "umbrella analogy." If I were to see a 20 percent chance of rain on the weather forecast, I would hardly even think to throw an umbrella in the car before I went out; I would assume it would not rain that day. Similarly, I had only a 20 percent chance of something being wrong with my baby's chromosomes and an overwhelming 80 percent chance that everything was just fine, so I just prayed for that sunny day. I clung to that analogy, even though deep down I knew I was probably just deluding myself. You play games like that with yourself when you are facing an unthinkable diagnosis.

My husband and I rehashed the conversation about continuing or ending the pregnancy, although this time, it wasn't just a conversation. It was a life-altering decision we were now contemplating. We probably had the exact same conversation, covering the exact same points, at least one hundred times during that two-week wait. We talked with our parents, who fully supported us and agreed that they would have likely made the same decision if they were in our shoes. My poor husband had to face his co-workers every day and act as if nothing was happening, as he never told any of them about our situation. I, at least, was home with our son and could cry all I needed to. It was very hard caring for my son during those weeks and I'm not sure how I did it, but obviously I managed. Those weeks were just a blur of tears.

Our biggest consideration in all of those conversations was our son. He was two-and-a-half years old at the time and clearly loved his carefree life. We became very afraid of what impact a disabled sibling would have not only on his childhood, but also on his adult life. We didn't want to see his childhood diminished by his sibling's medical problems, physical therapy appointments, and developmental delays. We didn't want to burden him with not only our care when we are older, but also the care of his sibling. The risks to our son's life just seemed so great and who were we to take that risk with his life? I understand from mothers of children with Down syndrome that many times, the other children are not detrimentally affected, but I have heard stories to the contrary as well.

We also considered the potential for medical problems with our disabled child. Many children with Down syndrome have heart defects or bowel defects that require surgery either immediately or within months after birth. Vision and hearing problems are common, as are problems with the thyroid. Individuals with Down syndrome are at greater risk of developing leukemia and frequently develop early-onset Alzheimer's. There were indications that my placenta was not functioning as it should have been and a pre-term birth was a very real possibility. Both pre-term birth and Down syndrome each have their associated medical problems; how could we ask a child to begin his or her life facing the challenges of both? What would the quality of life even be for our child?

I will freely admit a bit of selfishness in my decision as well; raising a disabled child was not something I wanted for my life either. Were I to be put into the situation due to some misfortune such as a birth accident, I would dig deep and find a way to do it. But given the choice I chose a happier life for myself, too. I felt like there were days when I could barely keep it together while parenting a well-behaved, healthy toddler. How could I possibly be a good mother to a child whose needs would be that much greater? What would that do to me as a mother to my existing child? Would I come to resent my disabled child? Would I come to resent both of my children? Would I simply shut down because I was in over my head? They were very real, very frightening possibilities to me.

Finally, at the end of March, at 15 weeks gestation, I was able to have the amniocentesis. They did an ultrasound first, and the ultrasound technician took a lot of measurements and pictures. We made small talk and I asked her about all of the internal structures, making sure everything looked okay. The baby just looked so normal; so much like my son did on ultrasound. How could there be anything wrong with a baby that is growing right on target and is put together perfectly? The perinatologist came in and prepped my slightly swollen belly. I was expecting something more technical and precise, but he literally came in, looked at the ultrasound, found his pocket of amniotic fluid and popped the needle in. He drew off the tubes of fluid they needed and when he was done, put a Mickey Mouse bandage over the spot where the needle went in.

Since we were already at 15 weeks, we opted to pay out-of-pocket for a fluorescent *in situ* hybridization (FISH) test, a rapid test that would count chromosomes 13, 18, and 21 and the sex chromosomes. It wouldn't be the final report, but it was highly accurate and would tell us within two to three days whether or not our baby had that extra chromosome 21. We got the call late on the second day from the same genetic counselor that indeed, our unborn child did have Down syndrome. We made an appointment to meet with the perinatologist again the very next day. Most providers recommend that you wait for a full confirmatory karyotype before making any decision regarding continuing or terminating a pregnancy, but we felt between the blood work from the NT screen and the FISH results from the amniocentesis, we had two independent tests performed by two separate laboratories that both strongly suggested the same conclusion: Down syndrome.

My husband and I made our final decision at that point. The best way I can describe it, and it sounds so terribly insensitive and cold, is that I just wanted to cut my losses and move on to another pregnancy. This pregnancy was no longer "useful" to me; it wasn't going to provide me with another child, and so I just wanted it over. I feel so bad referring to another human being, especially one that was inside of me and shared my genetic material, in such an uncaring manner, but I think my detachment was somewhat of a survival reflex. To this day, over a year later, I still haven't found out the gender of my unborn child; the words "son" and "daughter" are simply filled with too much meaning for me to apply them to my lost child. Someday, I hope to have the strength to find out.

Because we had spent so much time in those few weeks discussing the issues, by the time we had to actually make that decision, I think we were comfortable with it. Choosing to end the pregnancy wasn't an easy decision, but we both felt it was for the best and neither of us had lingering doubts. We loved our children, both born and unborn, and we couldn't ask either to suffer.

Our appointment with the perinatologist went well. We never for a moment felt we were being judged for our decision. We already had decided to terminate the pregnancy via dilation and evacuation (D&E) rather than labor and delivery and the perinatologist provided us with the name and telephone number of a provider in a clinic to which they frequently referred cases. He also called my current OB practice to see if there was anyone who performed the procedure in that office. Mercifully, one of the providers in my current OB practice did perform D&E's and so we were able to have the procedure in a hospital rather than a clinic, which made us much more comfortable.

I met with my OB on Friday morning, when he explained all of the risks of the procedure, what to expect from it, and what preparations I should make before it. We also discussed the impact on my future fertility, as we did want to have more children and didn't want to jeopardize our ability to do so. I left the office an hour later, still comfortable with my decision, and with a prescription for a pill to soften my cervix that I was to get filled and bring with me to my appointment the following Monday.

My husband and I spent the weekend saying our goodbyes to our unborn child and trying to live as normal of a life as we could for the sake of our son, who had seen far too many tears in recent weeks. I stopped wearing maternity clothes and squeezed myself back into regular clothes. We called all of the people in our everyday life that knew what we were going through and gave them the final decision. We found everyone to be very supportive, and the neighbors we feared would have the most negative reaction due to their deep-seated religious beliefs actually turned out to be the most compassionate. The worst part of the weekend was that I had just started to feel flutters of baby movement and I knew that it would all be coming to a crashing end within days.

Come Monday, we went to the OB's office for the beginning of the procedure: the insertion of the laminaria sticks to dilate my cervix. I cried and cried and cried because that was the point of no return; once the laminaria are in, you are committed to complete the procedure. I went home, had a small dinner, and took some painkillers and a sleeping pill. Sadly, the rule of not taking certain medications during pregnancy no longer applied to me. I was free to dull the pain, both emotional and physical, however I wanted to. I was to return to the hospital the following day around lunchtime for the actual procedure.

I never made it to the appointment. During the middle of the night I woke up with terrible cramps, which I quickly realized were evenly spaced. Despite my OB's assurances that it wouldn't happen, I was in labor. As I got up to use the restroom, my water broke all over the bed and carpet. I became a hysterical mess; this was my biggest fear regarding the procedure, the one thing that made it not a clinical procedure but the end of a very real pregnancy. I had been through labor before and it was supposed to be a happy time with a happy ending. My husband called the OB who instructed us to go straight to the ER. They were waiting for us and took us right up to the obstetrical floor, where I was given some strong sedatives. Thankfully, I remember nothing more from that point until when I woke up in recovery.

I was discharged home and spent the next week babying myself while my mother took care of my son for me. To prevent my milk from coming in, I bound my breasts in a sports bra and an Ace bandage for five days, taking it off only to shower or readjust it. I was lucky and my milk never did come in. I slowly re-entered the world of the living and tried to get back into a normal routine. My friends were all supportive, inquiring as to how I was doing, getting me out of the house, even if it was just to have our kids play in the driveway. It was hard, I still had moments of intense grief, but I just stayed focused on the future and started thinking about my next pregnancy. Our final amniocentesis results came in two days after we said goodbye to our unborn child, and confirmed the diagnosis of Down syndrome.

Physically, my recovery appeared to be uneventful until the bleeding started up again a few weeks later. I would get cramping and then bleeding for a few hours every day to every other day. Each time I thought my period had finally resumed, but then the bleeding would abruptly stop. After a few weeks of this, I returned to my OB, who performed an ultrasound and discovered that I had retained tissue still in my uterus; something he assured me was not common, but not entirely uncommon either. I required another procedure to remove the offending tissue and shortly thereafter, my normal menses resumed. After one more cycle, I was cleared to try to conceive again.

Emotionally, I had moments of extreme guilt over our decision in those first few weeks. I felt I was incredibly selfish and that life wouldn't really have been as bad as I perceived it to be. I didn't regret my decision, I didn't wish I had chosen otherwise, I just had to deal with the tiny lingering "what-ifs" that plagued my thoughts. And then I took my son to lunch at a fast food restaurant where there was a grown woman with Down syndrome working, cleaning the tables. She talked to herself incessantly and quite loudly. While I was happy to see that she was a woman healthy enough and with enough mental capacity to hold a job, I was sad to realize that this kind of job might be as good as it would ever get for her. I looked at my son, thoroughly enjoying his cheeseburger and realized that if he chose to flip those burgers for a living, it would be entirely his choice. This woman didn't have a choice. And from that moment I have been completely, unequivocally at peace with our decision.

During my decision-making time, I also discovered an Internet message board with a community of women who were all facing the same decision I was or had already made their decision. Immediately after my D&E, this community became my lifeline. There were women who had walked many miles in my shoes, could comfort me like no one else could, and made me feel like what I was going through was a normal part of the recovery process. It was an amazing community to become a part of and saved me thousands of dollars in therapy bills. I am forever grateful to the kindness of those strangers who helped me through probably the most devastating experience any woman can go through. I am still a part of that community, though now my role is to support other women who are making heartbreaking choices.

I am now over a year out from my heartbreaking choice. I am not a horrible person for having made the choice I made; I am simply a person who made the best decision I could when faced with a horrible situation. Making this choice changes you forever, but your life adjusts to a new normal. Your lost child is permanently woven into the tapestry of who you are and is part of your history. You learn to appreciate things differently and when you hear that a friend or family member is pregnant, your first thought is "Please, let her baby be healthy."

45

Wendy's Story "Broken Dreams"

We were a happy family with two young boys—Baxter was six and Louie had just turned five. Before the boys were born I had owned my own business. When Baxter turned five I realized that I could not go on being the kind of mum I wanted to be if I continued working the way that I had been. My husband and I wanted another baby, but three children and having to work 40 hours plus a week was not conducive to being a successful parent with happy, well-adjusted children. My husband, James, also owned his own business, so life for us had been chaos.

We made some major life changes; I sold my business, we paid off our mortgage, took the boys on a great holiday to Europe and tried to make baby number three.

I always knew I wanted to have three children, whether it was because I was one of three or not, I don't know. But to me, three seemed perfect.

After getting pregnant the first time we tried with the boys I felt a bit frustrated that the third baby was taking so long to conceive. But after 10 months of trying we were delighted that number three was on its way.

I went in for the 13-week nuchal scan, which measured the fluid at the back of the baby's neck, and everything was perfect. I felt very blasé and assumed that once we were out of the first trimester we would be home free. However, being quite superstitious, we did not tell anyone except close family until we were about 18 weeks gestation. At 18 weeks we also told the boys—they were so excited. Baxter said, "I know it is a boy." There was no doubt in his mind.

The following are excerpts from my diary:

347

Tuesday 4th October

It was the school holidays; I went to my usual *aqua aerobics* class, left the boys at crèche and totally forgot about the scan. The boys had a lovely morning and we were all in high spirits. When I got home there was a message on my phone advising me that I had indeed forgotten and that they had an opening at 2:15 PM, if I would like it.

At the allotted time we arrived at Radiology, the boys were so excited, Baxter especially as he was convinced we were having a boy. Baxter wouldn't sit down and kept asking to see the baby's *bottom* so we would all know he was right. The doctor eventually said "Okay Baxter you can see it is a boy." Instantly I had a vision of Baxter, Louie and little Archie running along–with Archie trying to catch up. In my vision Archie was wearing a t-shirt and nappy and had short, fat legs, like Baxter used to have.

The boys soon got restless and went out to the waiting room to read some books. I thought the scan was taking a wee while too long and the doctor kept doing a head measurement. All of a sudden I felt this cold fear come over me. I looked over at the computer and saw the time read 3:10. I asked if everything was okay. That was the minute my life changed forever, when the doctor said "Don't panic, it could be my machine, but for some reason his ventricle is measuring 13 mm and it should measure 10 mm, and it looks like he has spina bifida." I thought that can't possibly be me she is talking to. I realized things were really bad when the receptionist said not to worry about paying. I left there in a total blur, but managed to drive home.

6:00 PM – James came home—told him, me very upset.

6:20 PM – Mum and Dad popped in—they said they would support us whatever we decided to do.

I had a sleepless night—Archie was kicking a lot. I felt like he was saying "I'm okay." I had huge hopes that Wednesday would make everything okay. All night I kept thinking I would wake up and it had all been a terrible nightmare. I lay there watching my bedside clock all night waiting for the morning.

Wednesday 5th October

We waited for Radiology to open to get a second opinion. Our appointment was scheduled for 10:45. I picked up James from his work. Waiting in the waiting room was just agony—I felt I would collapse.

I was called in and as soon as the scan started the doctor said, "I'll do the scan and we'll talk about it after." I knew we were in deep trouble.

After the scan he said, "This is not good," and said that our baby definitely had spina bifida, Arnold Chiari brain malformation, as well as ventriculomegaly. He then said, "There is nothing mild about this."

I said to him, "Is there any point in doing an amnio?" He said no. We left there, barely able to walk. We had to walk through a waiting room full of pregnant ladies who were happy, smiling.

James drove home. They had obviously contacted my obstetrician when we left. I had two phone calls from doctors at the practice as well as a midwife. They were so kind and so sad for us, but confirmed that the prognosis was very grim. We told them we could not continue with the pregnancy and would have to terminate.

Easy decision given the prognosis—hardest thing ever to do.

I was told a counselor from the hospital would contact us for counseling before we terminated.

When we came home, I was still in disbelief, all of our hopes and dreams broken. We had been so excited at the thought of Archie's arrival. Louie insisted on all the baby clothes going into his room. Louie said that when Archie comes home he would be the "bottle man" and Baxter said that he would make the baby laugh and be the "funny man." I made a counseling appointment for 11:00 AM Thursday.

I told the boys that Archie had died. Both very upset, Baxter cried continuously for three hours, he was inconsolable. I tried to ring my sister who lived in London, couldn't, too upset to speak.

James went to collect some sleeping pills the doctor had arranged.

Thursday 6ᵗʰ October

We went to the hospital—I cried all the way up to the second floor. We discussed everything. We were told that he would probably die in utero, or soon after birth. We were also told there was every chance Archie would be born alive, and they asked if we wanted to hold him until he died. Of course we did, he was our baby. We discussed labor. We said we would take Archie home with us. The hospital would give us special clothes for him, which a lady makes just for such occasions.

Friday 7ᵗʰ October

Another terrible night—I've had no sleep now for three nights. I felt totally sickened by what was going to happen. Archie was very quiet, without much movement.

When we arrived at the hospital, James had to literally drag me from the carpark up to the second floor. We met the counselor at the lifts as arranged. I was still hysterical; the doctor said she wasn't going to do the termination because I was "too traumatized." I said, "Who wouldn't be?" I remember it made me sober up. The doctor returned and agreed to do it.

I had the first medication at 10:20 AM —a time I will never forget.

After an hour the stomach tightening pains began. My OB called in on his day off to see how I was doing. The staff throughout the day was lovely to me. I had a special midwife just for me. They were all so kind.

The day passed in a blur. My mother popped in, as did the boys. Lots of medications, lots of pain.

3:10 AM, 8th October 2005

Archie entered the world—he was 21 weeks old and born sleeping. The midwife wrapped him in a towel and passed him to me. I cuddled him tight. He looked just like Louie—he had Louie's same nose. His head was swollen on one side from his brain. I turned him over and could see his spina bifida. The midwife dressed him in the most beautifully made outfit with matching blanket. She took ink prints of his feet. His hands were all curled up so I said not to uncurl them. Had a shower, but just wanted to cuddle my baby.

James told me my sister Kate had been given compassionate leave from her job in London and would be coming home to New Zealand the next day. I couldn't believe she would do that for me.

I tried to sleep—I had not slept for days. I kept sobbing, cuddling my precious Archie, so tiny, and so innocent and so cold. I kept forgetting he was dead—kept trying to be quiet so as not to wake him up.

9:00 AM – Left the hospital.

Arrived home. Mum and Dad were there, lots of tears; everyone had a cuddle of Archie. Baxter and Louie had a quick look, but were a bit frightened of him, as he was getting quite discolored.

1:30 PM – Dropped him off at the funeral home—so, so hard.

Monday 10th October

Today we buried our baby. It was a lovely service: immediate family only, I did not want any friends there to witness my grief. I was still in a state of shock. Putting my baby in his coffin and closing the lid was just the most terrible thing I hope I ever have to do.

In the days and weeks following my termination, I wished I could just curl up in a ball and stay there. I spent many hours in bed after I had taken my children to school. It was so hard to function, just to get through the day.

At the end of October my best friend who lives in the Cayman Islands had her baby. I knew it was going to be a boy beforehand and I just dreaded it arriving. When he did arrive I was sent some lovely baby photos and a note from my friend saying how happy they were, which just destroyed me. Of course I was happy for my friend, but could not believe she would send me photos. Now I realize that some people just don't think; she never, ever would have intentionally hurt me. There was also my friend who said to me, "Thank goodness it was not a girl. That would have been so much worse." These are the sorts of things that cut me to the core.

I was very lucky that seven weeks after my termination I became pregnant again. I was told to wait three months, but I was obsessed, I could not wait. Of course it was an exceptionally stressful time—thinking it could happen again. I was taking five milligrams of folic acid, which I started one month after my termination.

I had about 10 scans throughout my pregnancy, all showed a perfectly healthy baby, and we did not want to find out what it was. I secretly wanted a boy, possibly to replace Archie. The whole nine months really went by in a blur—lots of appointments, and then the baby was in a lovely breech position!

On the 24th August 2006, Fergus (Gussie) entered the world. He is and continues to be our little ray of sunshine. Not that he has made everything perfect in my life again—he was never a replacement for Archie, but boy, did he help.

In January 2006 I decided to do some personal research on folic acid as I realized that spina bifida and other neural tube defects can be an avoidable condition. I was horrified to discover that the folic acid I had been taking only had 300 mcg of folic acid in it when the recommended health department guidelines say it should be 800 mcg. I took this to the media, as I was totally outraged and heartbroken by what I discovered. We were involved in a national current affairs program; to this day I have not watched it. There has been a good outcome though, as apparently the awareness for women taking folic acid has increased dramatically, as well as an increase in lower fetal spine examinations much earlier in pregnancy. So I feel that if we have stopped one family from going through what we went through by baring our hearts and souls on television, it was worth it.

Writing this over two and half years later brings it all back, all the feelings of helplessness and despair. If you are reading this and are about to go through, or have recently been through what myself and other ladies have gone through, I can honestly say that it does get better. You will never forget your precious baby, but time does heal.

So I conclude—this, Archie my precious, is for you. We will never forget you, we will always love you. You will always be our baby. You will always be Baxter and Louie's brother. Archie, you will always be in our hearts.

Archie, born sleeping 8th October 2005.

46

Zaylie's Story **"Having Hope"**
© *2008*

December 31st, 2005 marked the beginning of what we thought was our dream finally coming true. My husband and I had been trying for 16 months and we were getting increasingly frustrated that we weren't becoming pregnant. I started to research fertility specialists, as it just did not seem like it would happen naturally. We were traveling the month before and so were not thinking about trying. Much to our joyful surprise, the pregnancy test I took that day was positive. We were so happy! It had been a long road and yet there we were, expecting our first.

We scheduled our first doctor's appointment for early February, where we breathed a sigh of relief when the doctor said the baby looked perfect. For some reason I still worried a little, but we got more good news at our nuchal translucency (NT) test in early March.

We scheduled our 20-week ultrasound for late April and were eager to find out if we were having a girl or a boy. We had no preference, but were very curious. We both thought it was a girl, but were not entirely certain.

We watched the screen with great interest, amazed at the little being growing inside. The ultrasound technician left the room and we marveled at the fact that we were having a daughter.

After a while, the doctor came in and said our little girl had hydrocephalus. He had no bedside manner and explained nothing. He told us to search on the Internet and said he had spoken to our midwife practice and we could go back to them; they were waiting. We drove the five minutes to their office, not really understanding what was happening, but thinking that things might be bad.

The midwives did not have much information but helped us schedule an appointment with the best perinatologist. As it was Friday afternoon, we had to wait until Monday to get more information and a second opinion. My mom is a doctor and so we called her and she called the doctor we had just seen. She called back and told us we had to end the pregnancy. There were no ifs for her. She was convinced. I could not believe she was telling me that. I was not ready to consider it and still did not really understand what hydrocephalus was.

We spent the weekend on the Internet trying to understand the diagnosis. We were in tears trying to comprehend the decision we might have to make. A friend who works as a radiologist saw us on Sunday to perform another ultrasound. She thought the baby was in great distress. It was unbelievable. Our little girl was all we thought about—how much we loved her and how much we wanted her.

On Monday we saw the perinatologist. He did the ultrasound and spent a great deal of time looking at our baby. He thought he saw additional problems with the heart and suggested both a fetal echocardiogram and an MRI. We were able to schedule those appointments for Wednesday.

The waiting was long and filled with worry and the tiniest sliver of hope. Unfortunately, Wednesday brought even more bad news—the condition was grave. The doctors had all given us little hope that our baby could lead a normal healthy life. She would suffer seizures, might not know hot from cold, would have severe developmental delays, countless surgeries, and her chances of survival were not great. In addition, as her head was already measuring two weeks ahead of the rest of her there was a chance that my health would be at risk and that delivery, even via c-section, would be difficult.

With such a grim prognosis, and everyone telling us the same thing, we felt we could not let our little girl suffer. We had consulted all the best doctors and done all the research. We did not take it lightly. I strongly believe that all life is sacred, yet my living will says not to leave me on a respirator if there is no hope. I knew that I could not let my baby suffer in a way I was unwilling to suffer myself. I cried out in so much pain. I prayed for a miracle. I tried to make sense of it. I kept reading on the Internet, looking for stories of hope. I could not find much to give me any solace.

So we scheduled the induction for the following week. My kind friend did a repeat ultrasound the day before the procedure to make sure that our miracle had not happened. She was shocked to see how much worse things looked in the matter of a week. In some sense that gave me peace. It made the decision easier, because instead of her condition staying the same or improving, it had gotten much worse. The trend was clear—and there was no maybe. Everyone we saw told us the same exact thing. None of the specialists we saw thought otherwise. I could not believe that the first decision my husband and I had to make as parents was to let our little girl go.

I was petrified of what was to come. I had never gone through labor and delivery. I read about other people's experiences and was terrified. Not only did I have to say goodbye to my beautiful girl, but I also had to go through the physical delivery. I had to get an IV and an epidural. I feared that my placenta would not come out and I would have to go in for a D&C. I worried about any complications that might occur. I was scared of the physical pain as well as the emotional pain.

The delivery was difficult, not so much physically, but ever so much mentally. My little girl kicked me so many times during the hours leading up to her birth. We spoke to her and cried. We wished that things would happen quickly but also wanted to treasure every moment we had with her. It was nearly 12 hours from start to finish, and now, two years later, I can remember lying in the bed, unable to get up because of the epidural, not sure how to pass the time. I cried a lot. I told her I loved her a lot. I wondered why this was happening to me.

After she was born, I held her in my arms and cradled her. My husband sang to her. We tried to make the two hours we had with her very special. We took a family picture. I kissed her cheeks and held her hand. She was so little and seemed so fragile. Slowly her body started to get cold and my husband thought it was time that we said goodbye. We got hand and footprints of her and I wrapped her in a blanket that I then took home with me. I still will pull out this blanket every now and then and cry into it. It is the only thing I have that touched her. We left the next morning before breakfast. I needed to go home, to get away. I knew once I was home that the healing could begin.

Of course there were still things to be done. We had our daughter cremated and had to find an urn for her. We had to send out an announcement letting all the people we had told about our pregnancy know that our little girl had passed away, so that we would not have awkward and painful moments. I also wanted to finish her scrapbook so that I would have something filled with all the letters and poems I had written to her, starting on the day I found out she was growing inside me.

There were so many tears in the weeks and months that followed. Our sadness was compounded by the fact that friends and family did not understand, and that I felt a need to keep what really happened a secret. Even without knowing the details, some of our loved ones were able to say that they were sorry or to ask how we were weeks and months later. Others, however, ignored the birth announcement, and never called to ask about us, never sent an e-mail to express their sorrow for our loss, never even sent a pre-written Hallmark card expressing sympathy.

I was going through the most difficult thing in my life, and rather than providing me compassion, those people added to my sadness. Not only did I lose my precious first daughter, but I also lost friends and family members who I doubt I will ever forgive. Even my parents thought I should forget and move on—they did not see my little girl as something real. They could not understand that we had so many hopes for our little girl and so much love for her already.

However, there were others who I expected nothing from who offered me so much support. Most surprising, I found support from strangers on the Internet message boards at *BabyCenter* and *A Heartbreaking Choice*. I made virtual friends who understood what I was going through and offered me so much support; support that I often could not find in real life. I spent hours and hours on those boards, offering others support and seeking solace in the words of women further along in the grieving process. While I started posting on those boards with the screen name "Whyme" I soon changed it to "havinghope," as we thought what happened to us was a fluke. We believed we could get pregnant again with a healthy child. We had hope underneath all the sadness.

After my body had healed, my husband and I decided to try again. The idea of trying again helped ease the pain of all that we had lost. We expected another long journey, and were joyfully surprised when we conceived in our second month of trying. That was before the due date of my first daughter. It gave me great comfort that the new being that I was carrying would not have been possible were it not for losing our first. While I would rather not have lost her at all, I knew I would love my second child with all my heart, so it provided me a silver lining. I was meant to bring home this child; there was a reason for my loss.

I was worried for this pregnancy though, since lightning had struck us before. We switched from our midwife practice to a high risk OB. We prayed and hoped that all would be well. Still we worried. Early on things looked good and, before we knew it, it was time for our 12-week nuchal translucency test. The nuchal test had come back perfect with our first, so we were not expecting problems. We were so wrong.

Our second little girl had a gaping black spot in her abdomen and there were possible heart defects. We did a chorionic villus sampling (CVS) to see if there was a chromosomal problem and scheduled weekly visits to the perinatologist's office. The chromosomes turned out to be fine but the black spot was growing, and our little girl was not urinating. Every night we sang songs. Instead of "Twist and Shout," we sang, "Pee it all out." We doctored other songs just to say she was perfectly healthy.

We had weekly appointments that provided us a mix of hope and worry. We tried to stay optimistic. If surgery would correct the problem, if she could live with a tube to drain her bladder—it would not be ideal, but we could adjust. Surgery could fix most heart defects, so we kept going to our appointments and waited. At 18 weeks, we received a fatal diagnosis: her kidneys were not functioning. There was no amniotic fluid left so her lungs would not develop and she had hydrocephalus. She had no chance. There was no hope. Her condition was even worse than her sister's was. All that praying, all that hoping and we were faced with making another choice, of saying goodbye to our precious second daughter.

We scheduled the induction with an ultrasound immediately beforehand. Once again, we prayed for a miracle. We prayed that her condition would improve, that the new doctors at the hospital would see something that would give them hope. Instead, the new doctors wanted their associates to look, as her condition was so unique and so beyond words.

The procedure began. Since I had been through an induction before, I was a bit demanding and the procedures seemed different from my last experience. We spoke to the doctors about various issues and reached tentative agreements. We would begin with an epidural. The anesthesiologist came in and my husband asked if he had performed many epidurals. He said he watched a video once and we laughed. Then, as he prepared my back for the injection, I lost it. I cried and cried and everyone waited. I could not believe I had to say goodbye to my second much loved daughter, too soon. The epidural was the first step in saying goodbye. I quieted down and the doctor put in the epidural. We then waited. Once again, I felt her kick. We asked her what name she preferred and took her kicks as answers.

I then told her it was time for her to say goodbye, that she should leave her body and go be with her sister. I told her that she would always be healthy, happy, and joyful and that she would live in my heart forever. I just kept talking and told her how much I loved her. My husband lost it in middle of my conversation with her, and I just kept talking. I did not want her to suffer through the labor and delivery. I did not want her to suffer for even a second.

When she was born, the nurses tried to take her away to clean her up and I demanded to hold her immediately. I wanted my baby girl in my arms. I needed her there, so they gave her to me and I held her. She looked so very peaceful, my happy-go-lucky little girl. One of the nurses came in, asked to hold her, and said she was perfect. It was the kindest gesture and meant the world to my husband and me. We kept her with us until we left the hospital some six hours later. We took pictures and dressed her in a little 'onesie' that was very big on her.

Most of our friends and family did not know we were pregnant again. Their reactions to our first loss disappointed me so much that I could not share our second with them. While the message boards that I spoke so highly of before were my lifeline after my first loss, I could not turn to them now. I was different; I was the worst nightmare of my friends there—so many would say things to that effect. If someone had a miscarriage, they would be grateful that it was not another termination. If someone did not get pregnant, they would see a silver lining that at least they did not have to make another heartbreaking choice. The day before I said goodbye to my second daughter, someone started a thread saying "no baby" with a tears emoticon next to it …. What she meant was that her induction of her healthy baby was postponed by a day … that is not what no baby means—what I went through was "no baby."

So I became silent. I retracted into myself. I wrote poetry to reflect my pain.

Grief © 2006
From deep within
The pain it starts
The waves of grief
They pound my heart

I cannot live
I do not die
I sit and ask
Why me? Why? WHY?

Searing sorrow
Crushing despair
Takes hold of me
No joy to spare

Two daughters lost
Nothing is left
Great hopelessness
I am bereft

My two angels
Both now are free
Yet shackles bind
This life to me

Without my girls
I am alone
I have become
A sad old crone

I want my girls
I want my bliss
Instead I cry
My girls I miss

Will there be joy?
And can I cope?
Is my future
Filled with hope?

A healthy child
For whom I pine
Will I not have
This dream divine?

And if I do
I still will crave
My girls I lost
And could not save

How am I here?
How is this me?
I do not want
This misery

The waves of grief
With time will wane
But that won't keep
Me free from pain

_____ and _____
Daughters of mine
I love you girls
To me you shine

Your memories
Live in my heart
Always forever
My dear sweethearts

For the first time in my life, I did not want to be me. It was a shock to my system. While I felt that I had learned things after my first loss—I learned who I could count on; I learned that I had strength; I learned compassion and kindness; I learned what loss could be—now there was nothing left to learn. It made no sense why I would have to go through such pain again. So in the course of a year, I had been pregnant 40 weeks and had two angels rather than one healthy baby.

My husband and I decided we needed a change. We packed the car and drove cross-country. We stayed with friends while we looked for work and tried to sell our house. I grieved constantly and just withdrew into myself. It was such a dark time and I kept asking my husband when things would get better. He would give me a date weeks out, and I would patiently wait, hoping that I would be less miserable then. He revised the date many times. I also found a small e-mail support group—three others who had suffered through losses at the same time as my first loss and who had seen me through my second loss, while they still kept trying to conceive. We all were struggling and we started e-mailing each other off-line. My support network included a couple of other women as well. They all helped me through a very difficult time.

Six months later I somehow landed my dream job and that definitely gave me hope. And with the new job, the sale of our house, and the real beginning of a new life across the country, we felt that maybe our luck was changing. So we decided to throw caution to the wind and try to conceive again. I kept up with my off-line support network and they offered me hope and advice and believed it would work.

My first month trying, I tried to dream big. I was so optimistic. I was shocked when I did not get pregnant. My second month, I self-medicated with Clomid and tried to take a more relaxed attitude. I refused to get worked up and tried to keep my hopes in check. I was blessed that month and found out I was pregnant. Of course, living in a new place, I did not have an OB or know who the best perinatologist was. I did not know how things worked if disaster were to strike again—maybe the practices would be different. To make matters worse, three days after my positive test, I started spotting.

So I did online research and tried to find recommendations for a caring OB and for the most skilled perinatologist in my area. I found both. My

OB was willing to see me as often as I wanted and to do ultrasounds at each appointment. I went in every two weeks or so, constantly worried. A friend sent me a baby bootie, infused with good luck. I carried it with me to each appointment. I prayed every day. I hoped. I must admit, I felt different than with the first two pregnancies. People often say they knew something was wrong with the pregnancies they had to terminate. As they were my first two, I had no basis of comparison. However, this pregnancy seemed different—and better. Even with the early spotting, I still believed my baby would be okay. Of course, that feeling would waver close to an appointment—but generally, I had hope.

We made it through each appointment with good news. It was unbelievable. At 16 weeks, we learned we were having a boy. I was shocked as I had lost two girls and so I was somewhat expecting a girl. Overall, I was just thrilled that things looked healthy. When we crossed the 22-week threshold—the gestational age of my oldest daughter, I breathed a sigh of relief. I was finally able to start believing we would be bringing home a healthy baby. I finally was ready to share our news with others.

Now, I am 35 weeks pregnant and feel completely and utterly blessed. I still do not understand why I had to go through everything that I did. I still find it difficult to explain why a second loss was necessary. Nevertheless, I am ever so grateful that I was able to conceive again and that this time my baby is healthy. I am counting the days until I meet him. I am savoring every kick. I tell my husband at least once a week how lucky we are. There is joy in my life again.

After four years of trying, three pregnancies, and two broken hearts, I am finally bringing home one perfectly healthy bouncing baby. I truly wish my road to this end had been easier, had been filled with less pain. I know our experiences, good or bad, shape who we are. I would not be the person I am today had it not been for everything that brought me here. A year ago, I did not want to be me, but that is no longer the case.

I still have the pain. That will be with me forever. Angel days are particularly hard as they bring the sadness to the forefront. I still can cry out of the blue because I just miss my daughters so much. I still think that the little boy I am carrying should be the youngest child, not the oldest. I still flip through the scrapbooks I lovingly made for my girls, which include all the letters and poems I wrote to them. I have the sonogram photos and their birth photos. I have the vivid memories of all that I went through. Thinking about them makes it feel like yesterday. The details are etched into my mind.

Someone recently asked me if being pregnant eases the pain; there is no doubt that it does. It does not make it go away. Nothing will do that, and I wouldn't want it to, but now there is hope. In a few weeks I will be cradling my baby and watching him grow. I also hope that he will have living siblings. I vow to let him know about his sisters, his two wonderful guardian angels who will always be with him, and will always be a part of this family. I miss you and love you little girls; you are always with me.

AFTERWORD

The following was written by a member of an online support board. Her words were inspiring to many of us, and with her permission, we elected to include them here, for you, too.

"Hope for the Newly Bereaved"
By Sara

I am so sorry for your losses. You *will* get through and life *will* be good again. Please know that you can handle anything now. Not much could be worse than what we have all been through. I still think of my baby every day, but it doesn't break my heart anymore. It just is, there, in the background. I have moved along, dealt with my loss and accepted it.

My new outlook on life is a little less naive, but stronger. I no longer expect that things will be okay, I accept that what will be will be, and I have the strength to take it on. I feel confident to face what may lie ahead. I'm ready to take the punches. Once upon a time I never dreamed that a punch would come anywhere near me. Now, I've got my gloves on, and I am fighting fit. Bring it on.

The women I met online got me through the hardest part of my life. I want to pay it forward. This is my way to honor my child. Help others with my experience. And remember my lessons—lessons not to judge, not to criticize. Lessons not to take a moral stance based on the idea that my morals would never be tested.

So, I want you to know, each of you, that you will emerge from this hell like newly tempered steel. You've been blasted and bashed so much that you are now much stronger, much more useful, and much more valuable than the soft metal that went into the furnace.

And when the pain eases and the clouds part; when the sun tentatively streams back into your life and you can once again smile without guilt. When you can once again wake without horror at finding your baby gone, and you can walk past the baby aisle in the supermarket without breaking down. When the inept comments of others seem simply that, rather than as viciously sharpened spears aimed at your heart. When you can sit in the doctor's office without having a panic attack. When the world stops spinning and crashing down around you, and the dust settles, and there is peace. Then, go forward and honor your child. Live a life.

This hurts like hell. This destroys you. But you will get through. And when you do, you will be better than you were before. This is your angel's gift to you.

APPENDIX A

PRENATAL TESTING, ABORTION LAW AND THEIR IMPLICATIONS

A Brief History of Prenatal Testing

During the mid 1960's ultrasounds were used increasingly in the field of obstetrics and gynecology. In 1968, the first paper was published regarding the visualization of fetal anatomy via ultrasound (Garrett, Robinson, and Kosoff 1968). In 1970, the first paper was published regarding a fetal malformation visible via ultrasound (Garrett, Grunwald, and Robinson 1970). Professor Stuart Campbell of the University of Glasgow published the first papers regarding a prenatal diagnosis of anencephaly (Campbell, Johnstone, Holt, and May 1972) and spina bifida (Campbell, Pryse-Davies, Coltart, Seller, and Singer 1975) via ultrasound in 1972 and 1975, respectively. The diagnosis in each of those cases led to the elective termination of the pregnancies. The early 1980's witnessed the expanded use of ultrasound from hospitals to private clinics and doctor's offices for obstetrical purposes, including the prenatal diagnosis of birth defects.

The first use of a procedure whereby amniotic fluid was extracted and examined in the diagnosis of genetic disease was reported in 1956 (Fuchs and Riis 1956). That report concluded that it was possible to determine fetal sex from cells found in amniotic fluid. A 1966 paper demonstrated that cultured amniotic fluid cells were suitable for karyotyping in order to determine genetic disease of a fetus (Steele and Breg 1966). Several controlled studies were conducted in the late 1960's and in the early 1970's to evaluate the safety of amniocentesis. Subsequent to these studies, amniocentesis became an accepted standard of care for women in the second trimester of pregnancy. Amniocentesis is used to detect chromosomal abnormalities as well as neural tube defects, generally from 13–18 weeks gestation, with 99.4 percent accuracy.

Chorionic villus sampling (CVS), in which small samples of the placenta can be biopsied for genetic analysis, has been performed since 1968 using various cannulas, forceps, catheters, and needles (Mohr 1968). The procedure has been perfected over the years, and now carries almost the same low miscarriage risk as amniocentesis (1.93 percent for CVS versus .83 percent for amniocentesis) (Caughey, Hopkins, and Norton 2006)) and a similar accuracy rate of 98 percent (Hahnemann and Vejerslev 1997). CVS allows for the earlier diagnosis (from 10–13 weeks gestation) of chromosomal abnormalities.

The late 1980's saw the development of non-invasive biochemical screening tests (Triple screen, AFP) which were offered to all pregnant women between 15–21 weeks gestation in order to test for abnormal levels of specific proteins and hormones in the mother's blood. An abnormal result could indicate the possibility of neural tube defects, chromosomal defects, and other birth defects in the fetus. The improved quadruple screen test, available since 2001, has shown a higher accuracy rate for detecting fetuses with trisomy 21 (Down syndrome).

In the early 1990's, another non-invasive screening test (the nuchal translucency screen) started being used in the first trimester of pregnancy. The nuchal translucency screen combines a maternal blood test and a special ultrasound which measures the amount of fluid accumulation behind the neck of the baby. The nuchal translucency screen can identify those at increased risk of having a baby with Down syndrome, Patau syndrome (trisomy 13), Edwards syndrome (trisomy 18), or congenital heart defects. It has been reported that it can detect about 82 to 87 percent of pregnancies affected by Down syndrome and up to 95 percent of those affected by Edwards syndrome (March of Dimes 2007).

The Implications of Prenatal Testing

The improved resolution of ultrasound equipment, the increasingly safer use of amniocentesis and CVS testing for genetic determination, and the introduction of the non-invasive nuchal translucency screening test has led to an earlier and more accurate detection of many fetal anomalies. This earlier and more accurate level of diagnosis has led to an increasing number of parents facing the dilemma of what to do with those test results. Do they proceed with the pregnancy or do they terminate? A 2006 study found that among 833 patients who had fetuses with seven common aneuploidies (trisomies 21, 18, and 13; 45, X; 47, XXX, 47, XXY, and 47, XYY), the overall rate of

366

termination was 81 percent (Shaffer, Caughey, and Norton 2006). Although some studies have found the termination rate of fetuses diagnosed prenatally with Down syndrome to be as high as 90 percent, a more recent study has found the rate to be closer to 73 percent (Mansfield 1999 and Perry 2007, respectively).

In January of 2007, The American College of Obstetricians and Gynecologists (ACOG) recommended that all pregnant women, regardless of their age, should be offered both screening and diagnostic testing for Down syndrome and other chromosomal abnormalities (ACOG 2007). Previously, women were automatically offered genetic counseling and diagnostic testing for Down syndrome and other chromosomal abnormalities (by amniocentesis or CVS) only if they were 35 years and older. The 2007 ACOG guidelines recommended that all pregnant women first consider less invasive screening options (such as the nuchal translucency) for assessing their risk for chromosomal abnormalities, to be followed with the option of diagnostic testing if the screening test indicates an increased risk for a chromosomal abnormality. There has been criticism that the January 2007 ACOG recommendations were an attempt to widen the net to catch more Down syndrome cases prenatally and that ACOG was thereby encouraging the termination of fetuses found to have Down syndrome. Despite this criticism, it should be clear that the new recommendations were an attempt to allow universal access to prenatal testing for all expectant parents so they can make their own informed decisions based on individualized risk assessment. No prenatal testing is ever mandatory.

Maternal Health Complications

There are circumstances wherein a woman chooses to interrupt a pregnancy due to complications with her own health.

Idiopathic dilated cardiomyopathy is a rare condition in which the muscle fibers of the heart become thinner, causing one or more chambers of the heart to become enlarged or dilated. This weakens the heart and affects blood flow. During pregnancy, this condition can lead to heart failure, stroke, a pulmonary embolism, or even death.

HELLP syndrome is a variant of pre-eclampsia in which a woman exhibits hemolysis (breaking down of red blood cells), elevated liver enzymes, and a low platelet count. HELLP syndrome affects kidney and liver function, can cause severe high blood pressure, protein in the urine, seizures, and can be fatal to both the mother and the baby.

Hyperemesis gravidarum is a rare disorder of severe and persistent nausea and vomiting during pregnancy. The frequent nausea and vomiting can lead to dehydration and vitamin and mineral deficits, resulting in the progressive weight loss of more than five percent of a woman's pre-pregnancy weight. Weight *gain* is essential in order to sustain a pregnancy, and hypermesis gravidarum can make that almost impossible.

The presence of cancers which need to be treated with surgery, chemotherapy, and/or radiation can also impact a woman's decision to continue a pregnancy or not. While some surgeries to remove cancerous cells do not impose an inherent risk to a fetus, some cancers (such as rectal and gynecological cancers) cannot be treated with surgery during pregnancy. Chemotherapy to treat cancer during the first trimester is toxic to a fetus and can cause birth defects or miscarriage. Radiation involves high-energy x-rays and can be harmful to a fetus, especially in the first trimester. If a woman decides to continue a pregnancy despite a cancer diagnosis, delaying treatment can result in an unfavorable prognosis for her and her baby.

In situations such as those discussed above, ending the pregnancy— either by previable termination or pre-term delivery—is often the only way to remedy the situation and preserve the mother's health.

A Brief History of Abortion Law

Before the mid 1800's, abortion in the United States was legal. With no codified laws against abortion, Americans followed the common law of England which allowed abortions up until the point of "quickening"— the point at which a woman could feel fetal movement. Abortions were commonly performed by midwives, doctors, apothecaries, and homeopaths and were even openly advertised in newspapers. Attitudes toward abortion began to change in the mid 1800's. The strongest force behind the push to make abortion illegal came from the exclusively male physicians who would establish the American Medical Association in 1847. Feeling threatened by the midwives, apothecaries and homeopaths, the physicians wanted an exclusive right to perform abortions, so they launched a campaign to criminalize abortion under the view that it was both immoral and dangerous and should only be performed by physicians with medical degrees, and only in order to save the life of the mother. The Comstock laws of 1873 made it a crime to send any obscene, lewd or lascivious materials for the prevention of conception, or for causing unlawful abortion through the mail. After the Civil War, state legislation began to replace the common law. Eventually the quickening distinction lost favor and by 1910, all states but one had passed laws outlawing abortion except in the rarest of circumstances. By the end of the 1950's, a large majority of the states had banned abortion, however and whenever performed, unless done to save or preserve the life of the mother.

A pattern toward less stringent laws followed the 1959 publication of the American Law Institute's Model Penal Code, which recommended that states allow licensed physicians to perform abortions if two physicians certify in writing that a pregnancy threatens the woman's physical or mental health, results from rape or incest, or if the fetus is gravely deformed. Colorado was the first state to liberalize its abortion law in 1967, modeled after the Model Penal Code, followed shortly thereafter by thirteen other states over the next five years.

In *Griswold v. Connecticut,* 381 U.S. 479 (1965) the U.S. Supreme Court struck down a Connecticut law (passed in 1879) which banned the distribution or use of "any drug, medicinal article or instrument for the purpose of preventing conception" by married couples (Conn. Gen. Stat. § 53-52). Justice Douglas, in his majority opinion, stated that a marital relationship is a relationship "lying within the zone of privacy created by several fundamental constitutional guarantees," and that though the Constitution does not explicitly protect a general right to privacy, the various guarantees within the Bill of Rights create penumbras, or zones, that establish a right to privacy (381 U.S. at 484). The same right to privacy would be extended to unmarried couples in *Eisenstadt v. Baird,* 405 U.S. 438 (1972). These constitutionally protected rights to privacy and access to contraceptives would prove to be crucial to the future of women's reproductive rights.

In *United States* v. *Vuitch,* 402 U.S. 62 (1971), the U.S. Supreme Court, in deciding on what grounds a physician had the right to perform an abortion, approved a broader definition of the word "health" to include psychological health as well as physical wellbeing.

Two years later in *Doe v. Bolton,* 410 U.S. 179 (1973), the Court held that "medical judgment may be exercised in the light of all factors—physical, emotional, psychological, familial, and the woman's age—relevant to the wellbeing of the patient." (410 U.S. at 192). It also struck down a provision of a Georgia abortion statute that required two independent physicians to confirm the attending doctor's determination that the continuation of a pregnancy would endanger the woman's life or injure her health (Guttmacher 1997). "The attending physician's 'best clinical judgment that an abortion is necessary'…should be sufficient," the Court said (410 U.S. at 199).

The landmark case of *Roe v. Wade,* 410 U.S. 113 (1973) would give women access to safe and legal abortions, under most circumstances, nationwide. It would also deem unconstitutional all previous state bans on abortion during the first trimester of pregnancy. The Court held that Americans' constitutionally protected right to privacy included the right of a woman, in consultation with her doctor, to decide whether to have children without state interference or intrusion. The Court held that during the first trimester, the abortion decision must be left to the medical judgment of the pregnant woman's attending physician. For the stage subsequent to approximately the end of the first trimester, the State, "in promoting its interest in the health of the mother, may, if it chooses, regulate the abortion procedure in ways that are reasonably related to maternal health." (410 U.S. at 164). For the stage subsequent to viability, "the State in promoting its interest in the potentiality of human life may, if it chooses, regulate, and even proscribe, abortion except where it is necessary, in appropriate medical judgment, for the preservation of the life or health of the mother." (410 U.S. at 165). The Court noted that while it was acceptable in 1973 to refer to the point of viability as at about seven months or 28 weeks gestation, the point of viability could change as medical advances make it possible for viability to occur earlier.

The Court held three years later in *Planned Parenthood of Missouri v. Danforth*, 428 U.S. 52 (1976) that "it is not the proper function of the legislature or the courts to place viability, which essentially is a medical concept, at a specific point in the gestation period. The time when viability is achieved may vary with each pregnancy, and the determination of whether a particular fetus is viable is, and must be, a matter for the judgment of the responsible attending physician." (428 U.S. at 64). The Court reaffirmed those principles in *Colautti* v. *Franklin,* 439 U.S. 379 (1979) when it held that "Viability is reached when, in the judgment of the attending physician on the particular facts of the case before him, there is a reasonable likelihood of the fetus' sustained survival outside the womb, with or without artificial support. Because this point may differ with each pregnancy, neither the legislature nor the courts may proclaim one of the elements entering into the ascertainment of viability—be it weeks of gestation or fetal weight or any other single factor— as the determinant of when the State has a compelling interest in the life or health of the fetus." (439 U.S. at 388).

In *Thornburgh v. American College of Obstetricians and Gynecologists,* 476 U.S. 747 (1986) the Supreme Court ruled that a woman may not be required to risk her health to save a fetus even after the point of viability, and it granted the attending physician the right to determine when a pregnancy threatens a woman's life or health. The court also ruled that when performing a post-viability abortion, a physician must be permitted to use the method most likely to preserve the woman's health, even if it might endanger fetal survival.

In *Planned Parenthood of Southeastern Pennsylvania v. Casey,* 505 U.S. 833 (1992), the court reaffirmed the essential tenets of *Roe* and added, "Although subsequent maternal health care advances allow for later abortions safe to the pregnant woman, and post-Roe neonatal care developments have advanced viability to a point somewhat earlier, these facts go only to the scheme of time limits on the realization of competing interests. Thus, any later divergences from the factual premises of Roe have no bearing on the validity of its central holding, that viability marks the earliest point at which the State's interest in fetal life is constitutionally adequate to justify a legislative ban on nontherapeutic abortions. The soundness or unsoundness of that constitutional judgment in no sense turns on when viability occurs. Whenever it may occur, its attainment will continue to serve as the critical fact." (505 U.S. at 835).

The *Partial-Birth Abortion Ban Act of 2003* (PBA ban), was passed by the United States Congress and signed into law by President Bush on November 3, 2003. The main focus of the PBA ban was to prohibit one form of late-term abortion known in the medical community as an intact dilation and extraction (intact D&E or D&X). Congress decided that, despite testimony from expert witnesses, the intact D&E procedure is never medically necessary and therefore should be banned, except to save the woman's life. Critics of the PBA ban concluded that it was unconstitutionally vague, it posed an undue burden on a woman's ability to choose a second trimester abortion, and it lacked an exception to protect the health of the mother. After the PBA ban was signed into law, it was deemed unconstitutional by three separate federal district courts, and by the Second, Eighth and Ninth Circuit Courts of Appeal. The United States Supreme Court heard the appeals from the Eighth and Ninth Circuit Courts of Appeal in the cases of *Gonzales v. Carhart*, 550 U.S. ___ (2007) and *Gonzales v. Planned Parenthood Federation of America, Inc.*, 550 U.S. ___ (2007), respectively. In April 2007, the Supreme Court issued one opinion to cover both cases and upheld the PBA ban despite the fact that there was no exception to save the *health* of the woman, only an exception to save her *life*.

The Implications of Abortion Law on Terminations for Medical Reasons

If a woman receives poor prenatal test results or experiences serious health problems of her own, she essentially has only two options—to carry the pregnancy to term or to interrupt the pregnancy. Parents must take several factors into consideration when making such a critical decision. They must consider their own religious or moral beliefs about electively ending a pregnancy and the impact such a decision could have on their spiritual and emotional health. They must consider their financial situation, specifically their ability or inability to care for a child who might need extensive surgeries, hospitalizations, therapies, medications, etc. The parents must think about the logistical and emotional impact of carrying such a pregnancy to term on other members of the family, especially siblings, both in the short- and long-term. Caring for a baby or a child who has moderate to severe health issues can take time, resources, and attention away from other members of the family. A child with serious health issues can also impact a parent's employment status if the parent has to be frequently absent from work. Parents must investigate how strong (or absent) of a support network is available to them should they carry to term. They must determine if the help available—be it from friends, family members, or medical professionals—would be adequate in caring for their child's needs . Parents must also consider who would care for the child after their own deaths. Finally, they must consider any suffering the child would likely face if carried to term and whether subjecting the child to any level of suffering is appropriate in their eyes.

If a family chooses to carry a pregnancy with a poor prenatal diagnosis to term, it can be a relief to take the responsibility of making a life-or-death decision out of their hands and off of their consciences. Some parents find carrying such a pregnancy to term, even in cases of diagnoses incompatible with life, to be a memorable and invaluable experience. In some circumstances, putting the child up for adoption after birth can be an option. Parents who wish to carry their pregnancies to term should be given every opportunity to do so, and should be supported however possible.

Other families ultimately decide that interrupting the pregnancy is the wisest course of action for their situation. After the decision to interrupt a pregnancy is made, they must consult with their doctor to determine what procedures are available to them. The procedures available vary, depending on the gestation of the pregnancy, the willingness of the doctor to assist, and the place of residence of the parents. In the United States, each state has its own requirements in terms of gestational limits, physician involvement, hospital requirements, private insurance coverage, state-mandated counseling, and waiting periods.

Each state in the United States has a different threshold for when an abortion can legally be performed. Some states have a threshold of 24 weeks, some have a threshold of the beginning of the third trimester, and still others at the point of "viability." (Guttmacher 2008). Viability, which is the point at which a fetus is capable of "meaningful life" outside of a woman's body, is hard to define in specific gestational terms. The United States Supreme Court has held that because viability is a point that varies with each pregnancy, states may not declare that it occurs at a particular gestational age (*Planned Parenthood of Missouri v. Danforth*, 428 U.S. 52 (1976)). Viability is a *medical* term, not a legal term, and it can only be determined by a physician on a case-by-case basis. Despite this, 36 states have passed laws which prohibit abortion after a certain fixed point in gestation, and eight states have laws prohibiting abortion after 20 or 24 weeks. (Guttmacher 2008).

Twenty-three states have a threshold of "viability" which is the most proper threshold given the Supreme Court decisions in *Danforth* and *Colautti*. It is common practice in obstetrics to have an ultrasound done for dating purposes at approximately eight weeks gestation, and an anatomy scan at 20 weeks gestation. Because of this, many women are not alerted as to their baby's serious condition until well into the second trimester. Given the varied nature of the gestational cut-offs, some women who choose to end a pregnancy find themselves having to travel 100 or more miles to receive proper care. And regardless of the state's legal cut-off, finding an abortion provider can be near impossible in some areas of the United States. According to Stanley Henshaw of the Guttmacher Institute, in 1988, 61 percent of women from Wyoming who were seeking abortions had to travel out of state to get them. By the year 2000, the figure had climbed to 95 percent. In Mississippi, where the number of places that offer abortion services has dropped from six to one, 60 percent of women traveled to neighboring states to terminate their pregnancies in 2000, up from 33 percent in 1988. In Kentucky, the percentage jumped from 22 percent in 1988 to 41 percent in 2000. In South Carolina, the rate jumped from 19 percent to 35 percent. (Henshaw 1992). In 2008, three states—North Dakota, South Dakota, and Mississippi—have only one abortion clinic each.

According to the Guttmacher Institute, in 2005, 87 percent of counties in the United States did not have an abortion provider, and only 24 percent of all abortion providers offered abortion services at or after 21 weeks gestation (Jones, Zolna, Henshaw and Finer 2008). In contrast, approximately 50 percent of counties in the United States do have providers for general gynecological/obstetrical care (Henshaw and Finer 2003). Overall, the number of abortion providers in the United States has fallen 37 percent since 1982 (Henshaw and Finer 2003).

Low-income or uninsured women face the additional challenge of being able to afford an abortion. A surgical abortion performed during the second trimester can cost upwards of $3,000 (Henshaw and Finer 2003). A labor and delivery termination can cost close to $10,000. The Hyde Amendment, first enacted by the United States Congress in 1976, forbids the use of federal funds such as Medicaid for abortion services except in cases where the mother's life is in danger, or in cases of rape or incest. Meanwhile, Medicaid does cover routine prenatal care and other services related to childbirth. This disparity in coverage is a form of discrimination and is a huge injustice to women. Other groups denied access to federal funds for abortion services include members of the United States military and their dependents, federal employees and their dependents, Native Americans, Peace Corps volunteers and federal prisoners.

Private insurance companies vary in their coverage of the costs of terminating a pregnancy. Insurance coverage varies depending on the provider and the limitations of the particular policy as determined by the employer. In 2000, only 13 percent of abortions were paid by Medicaid and another 13 percent were billed directly to private insurance (Henshaw and Finer 2003). In Idaho, Kentucky, Missouri and North Dakota private insurance companies are forbidden from providing coverage for abortion services unless the mother's life is in danger (Guttmacher 2008). It is wise to check with an insurance company before scheduling a termination to determine what coverage is available.

If the gestational requirement is met and a provider is found, parents who wish to terminate must then determine from their provider whether they have a choice between an induction labor and delivery (L&D) termination, a dilation and curettage (D&C) termination, or a dilation and evacuation (D&E) termination. A D&C is the surgical option until 12 weeks gestation. A D&E is the surgical option after 12 weeks gestation. Some physicians offer both a surgical option and an induction option to their patients, and some offer only one of the two options. Some physicians are able to perform the procedure themselves, while others have to refer their patients to another doctor. This can be due to moral beliefs about terminating a pregnancy, a lack of training in performing D&E's, or because of the doctor's hospital privileges. For example, a doctor who only has privileges at a Catholic hospital will not be able to assist his patient in obtaining a termination in that hospital. He would have to refer her to a doctor who can assist her in a non-Catholic hospital.

Many physicians offer L&D terminations only after a certain point in gestation (approximately 15 weeks). Many parents choose L&D so that they are able to see and hold their baby after delivery. There are situations where an L&D termination is necessary in order to be able to donate the baby's remains to a medical college for research (such as in the case of skeletal dysplasias, where only intact remains can be sent to an international skeletal dysplasia registry). An L&D termination usually requires a hospital stay of one to three nights, which can cost several thousand dollars. There are a small handful of clinics in the U.S. which can accommodate a woman terminating for medical reasons, using induction methods, even into the third trimester.

Some physicians recommend D&E terminations to their patients. This can be because of the potential dangers to the mother's health caused by an induction of labor. A D&E is also suggested for patients who do not wish to be hospitalized and who wish to avoid the experience of giving birth in such devastating circumstances. A D&E procedure can be done in a hospital or in a clinic and can be significantly less expensive than an L&D termination.

Depending on the gestation of the pregnancy, a D&E termination can be either a two day or a three day procedure.

Not all women are given the option of having a D&E done in a hospital. Some are given no other option than to go to an abortion clinic. There are physicians who actually recommend their patients go to clinics for their D&E since the clinic doctors are much more experienced in performing D&E's. There are other physicians who, for moral reasons, will not perform D&E's. Those patients are also often referred to abortion clinics. And some patients choose to have their D&E performed in a clinic because it is frequently less expensive than a D&E performed in a hospital.

Whether a person chooses to have a surgical termination or an induction termination, they are often allowed to decide on the disposition of their baby's remains. Some families choose to have a funeral and/or memorial service complete with burial in a cemetery for their baby. Some families choose cremation with or without burial, and still other families choose to allow the hospital or clinic to dispose of their baby's remains in a respectful manner.

The final decision a parent must make is how to carry on and heal oneself, both physically and emotionally, after the termination is over. Physically, the recovery from a termination for medical reasons is very similar to the recovery from a late-term miscarriage or a pre-term delivery. A woman should have a check-up with her physician two to four weeks after the termination. Emotionally, the recovery process can seem like a roller coaster of emotions and can take anywhere from a few months to a few years. A parent should not hesitate to speak to a professional if they are feeling "stuck" in their grief, if they feel no longer in control of their life, if they're engaging in addictive or destructive behaviors, or if their grief is significantly interfering with daily functioning (such as eating, sleeping, etc.). There are several resources available online which allow parents to anonymously connect with others who have walked a similar path. Having this type of connection and support can often help with the feelings of isolation, guilt and sadness that are so common following a termination for medical reasons (see Appendix B).

It is important for both partners to understand that they may not handle their feelings of grief in the same way. No two people will grieve in exactly the same manner, but the differences between men and women are vast. Due to societal expectations, men often feel like they are supposed to be stoic, in control, brave, and productive. Many men feel overlooked in comparison to their partner, and are often pressured to return to work and to "normal" life very soon after their loss. Men should be encouraged to express their feelings about the loss and to seek and accept support in order to work through their grief.

If there are other children in the family, their feelings of loss will depend on their age. Most children under three years old will only be aware of the changes in Mommy or Daddy's behavior and mood. Parents with children under three years old should try to be consistently nurturing and patient in order to help their toddler to cope. Children from about three years old to seven years old view death as either a magical place the baby is visiting and will return from, or as a form of sleep. They are often unable to grasp the abstract concept of a spirit as something separate from the body. Parents should try to honestly and patiently explain to the child, in simple terms, what death means and be reassuring if their child exhibits anxiety about their own mortality or the death of other close family members or friends. Children from about seven years old to 10 years old are often consumed by curiosity about what happens to the body and the spirit after death. Parents should welcome these questions and stress the importance of not hiding one's feelings in an attempt to seem "grown up." Children over 10 years old have a more sophisticated understanding of death, but often still have lots of questions about the spiritual aspect of death. They may wonder what life after death is like for their lost sibling and what their own life would have been like had the baby not died.

There are many tough decisions to be made when faced with a poor prenatal diagnosis or a serious threat to the mother's health. Each of those decisions can lead to repercussions felt by the entire family and to criticism from outsiders. But regardless of the choices a parent makes, if they are made with love, after serious consideration, and in the best interest of their child, the parent should never be judged or condemned by others. As Justice Blackmun so eloquently stated in *Thornburgh*, "Few decisions are more personal and intimate, more properly private, or more basic to individual dignity and autonomy, than a woman's decision—with the guidance of her physician and within the limits specified in Roe—whether to end her pregnancy. A woman's right to make that choice freely is fundamental. Any other result, in our view, would protect inadequately a central part of the sphere of liberty that our law guarantees equally to all." (476 U.S. at 772).

APPENDIX B*

SUPPORT RESOURCES

FOR THOSE WHO ARE CONSIDERING A TERMINATION DUE TO MEDICAL REASONS

Internet Resources

Genetic Counseling:	http://www.nsgc.org
Antenatal Results and Choices:	http://www.arc-uk.org
Prenatal Diagnosis Information:	http://www.poorprenataldiagnosis.com
	http://www.rarediseases.org
	http://www.marchofdimes.com/pnhec/188.asp
	http://www.birthdefects.org/index.htm
Abortion Law Homepage:	http://www.hometown.aol.com/abtrbng
Abortion Clinics On-line:	http://www.gynpages.com
Planned Parenthood:	http://www.plannedparenthood.org
Bereavement Photography:	http://www.nowilaymedowntosleep.org

Information by diagnosis:

Amniotic band syndrome	http://www.amnioticbandsyndrome.com
Acrania/Anencephaly	http://www.anencephaly.net
Arnold-Chiari malformation	http://www.pressenter.com/~wacma

Arthrogryposis	http://www.emedicine.com/ped/TOPIC142.HTM
Cat eye syndrome	http://www.nt.net/a815/cateye.htm
Choroid Plexus cyst	http://www.choroidplexuscyst.org
Cri du Chat syndrome	http://www.fivepminus.org
Congenital diaphragmatic hernia	http://www.cdhsupport.org
Congenital heart defects	http://www.congenitalheartdefects.com
Cystic fibrosis	http://www.cff.org
Cystic hygroma	http://www.novanews.org
Cytolomegalovirus infection	http://www.cdc.gov/cmv
Dandy Walker syndrome	http://www.dandy-walker.org
Down syndrome (trisomy 21)	http://www.ndsccenter.org/index.php
Ebstein's anomaly	http://www.americanheart.org/presenter.jhtml? identifier=11075
Edwards syndrome (trisomy 18)	http://www.trisomy18.org
Encephalocele	http://www.ninds.nih.gov/disorders/encephaloceles/encephaloceles.htm
Fetal obstructive uropathy	http://www.fetalcarecenter.org/fetal-surgery/obstructive-uropathy
Gastroschisis	http://www.nlm.nih.gov/medlineplus/ency/article/000992.htm
Holoprosencephaly	http://www.ninds.nih.gov/disorders/holoprosencephaly/holoprosencephaly.htm
Hydrocephalus	http://www.hydroassoc.org
Hyperemesis gravidarum	http://www.hyperemesis.org
Hypoplastic left heart syndrome	http://www.hopeforhlhs.com
Klinefelter syndrome	http://klinefeltersyndrome.org
Meckel-Gruber syndrome	http://www.emedicine.com/ped/TOPIC1390.HTM
Multifetal pregnancy reduction	http://www.climb-support.org

Oligohydramnios	http://www.healthline.com/ galecontent /oligohydramnios-sequence-1
Omphalocele	http://www.nlm.nih.gov/medlineplus/ ency/article/000994.htm
Osteogenesis Imperfecta	http://www.oif.org
Patau syndrome (trisomy 13)	http://www.livingwithtrisomy13.org
Pentalogy of Cantrell	http://www.bchealthguide.org/kbase/ nord/nord939.htm
PBD-Zellweger syndrome spectrum	http://www.emedicine.com/neuro/ TOPIC309.HTM
Polycystic kidney disease	http://www.pkdcure.org
Potters syndrome	http://www.emedicine.com/ped/ TOPIC1878.HTM
Renal agenesis	http://www.healthline.com/ galecontent/renal-agenesis
Sirenomelia	http://www.healthline.com/ galecontent/sirenomelia-1
Skeletal dysplasia	http://www.csmc.edu/9934.html
Smith-Lemli-Opitz syndrome	http://www.smithlemliopitz.org
Spina bifida	http://www.spinabifidaassociation.org
Thanatophoric dysplasia	http://www.emedicine.com/ped/ topic2233.htm
Triploidy	http://www.healthline.com/ galecontent/triploidy
Turner syndrome	http://www.turnersyndrome.org
VACTERL association	http://www.cincinnatichildrens.org/ health/heart-encyclopedia/disease/ syndrome/vacterl.htm
Ventriculomegaly	http://www.childrenshospital.org/az/ Site562/mainpageS562P0.html
Wolf-Hirschhorn syndrome	http://www.geneclinics.org/profiles/ whs

Overview of state-by-state abortion laws:
http://www.guttmacher.org/statecenter/spibs/spib_OAL.pdf

Clinics that offer information regarding a termination for medical reasons:
http://www.drtiller.com/mainpg.html (Women's Health Care Services, P.A., Wichita, Kansas)
http://www.drhern.com (Boulder Abortion Clinic, P.C., Boulder, Colorado)
http://www.choicemedicalgroup.com/our_services_special.htm (Choice Medical Group, California)
http://www.hopeclinic.com/MedicalReasons.htm (Hope Clinic, Illinois)
http://www.womenscenter.com (Orlando Women's Center, Florida)
http://www.gynpages.com/ACOL/category/late.html (State-by-state listing of abortion providers past 20 weeks gestation)

Book Resources

"Empty Cradle, Broken Heart: Surviving the Death of Your Baby" by Deborah L. Davis
"Trying Again, a Guide to Pregnancy after Miscarriage, Stillbirth or Infant Loss" by Ann Douglas
"Living When a Loved One Has Died" by Earl A. Grollman
"I'll Hold You in Heaven" by Jack Hayford
"Precious Lives, Painful Choices: A Prenatal Decision Making Guide" by Sherokee Ilse
"Unspeakable Losses, Understanding the Experience of Pregnancy Loss, Miscarriage and Abortion" by Kim Kluger-Bell
"A Silent Sorrow: Pregnancy Loss – Guidance and Support for You and Your Family" by Ingrid Kohn, Perry-Lynn Moffitt, and Isabelle A. Wilkins
"Pregnancy After a Loss, A Guide to Pregnancy After a Miscarriage, Stillbirth or Infant Death" by Carol Cirulli Lanham
"A Mother's Dilemma" by Wendy L. Lyon
"A Time to Decide, A Time to Heal" by Molly A. Minnick, Kathleen Delp, and Mary Ciotti
"How to Survive the Loss of a Child" by Catherine Sanders
"We Were Gonna Have a Baby But We Had an Angel Instead" by Pat Schweibert (a book for surviving siblings)
"Empty Arms: Hope and Support for Those Who Have Suffered a Miscarriage, Stillbirth, or Tubal Pregnancy" by Pam Vredevelt

Face-to-Face/"In Person" Resources

The Compassionate Friends 1-877-969-0010
Chapter locator: http://www.compassionatefriends.org/Chapter_Locations/states.shtml

Mothers in Sympathy and Support Foundation (M.I.S.S.) 1-888-455-MISS
Support group locator: http://www.misschildren.org/group/index.html

SHARE Pregnancy & Infant Loss Support, Inc. 1-800-821-6819
Group Listing: http://www.nationalshareoffice.com/resources_share_groups.shtml

SUPPORT RESOURCES
FOR THOSE WHO HAVE TERMINATED
DUE TO MEDICAL REASONS

Internet Resources

A Heartbreaking Choice - Grief support after terminating a much-wanted pregnancy for medical reasons
http://www.aheartbreakingchoice.com

BabyCenter Termination for Medical Reasons message board - Grief support after terminating a much-wanted pregnancy for medical reasons
http://community.babycenter.com/groups/a6325/termination_for_medical_reasons

P.A.S.S. - Post abortion healing and help
http://afterabortion.com and http://www.passboards.org/index.php

I'm Not Sorry - Positive experiences with abortion
http://www.imnotsorry.net

The Compassionate Friends - Grief support after the death of a child
http://www.compassionatefriends.org

M.I.S.S. Foundation - Providing crisis support after the death of a child from any cause
http://www.misschildren.org

Share Pregnancy & Infant Loss Support, Inc. - To serve those touched by the death of a baby
http://www.nationalshareoffice.com/index.shtml

Afghans for Angels - Non-profit group which provides free hand-made baby afghans and caps
http://www.afghansforangels.net

A Place to Remember - Support materials and resources for those touched by a crisis pregnancy or the death of a baby
http://www.aplacetoremember.com

The Comfort Company - Sympathy gifts, books, cremation jewelry, keepsakes, etc.
http://www.thecomfortcompany.net

Centering Corporation - Education and resources for the bereaved
https://www.centeringcorp.com/catalog/index.php

Grief Watch - Resources for bereaved families and professional caregivers
http://www.griefwatch.com/Default.asp

Book Resources

"Empty Cradle, Broken Heart: Surviving the Death of Your Baby" by Deborah L. Davis
"Trying Again, a Guide to Pregnancy after Miscarriage, Stillbirth or Infant Loss" by Ann Douglas
"Living When a Loved One Has Died" by Earl A. Grollman
"I'll Hold You in Heaven" by Jack Hayford
"Precious Lives, Painful Choices: A Prenatal Decision Making Guide" by Sherokee Ilse
"Unspeakable Losses, Understanding the Experience of Pregnancy Loss, Miscarriage and Abortion" by Kim Kluger-Bell
"A Silent Sorrow: Pregnancy Loss – Guidance and Support for You and Your Family" by Ingrid Kohn, Perry-Lynn Moffitt, and Isabelle A. Wilkins
"Pregnancy After a Loss, A Guide to Pregnancy After a Miscarriage, Stillbirth or Infant Death" by Carol Cirulli Lanham
"A Mother's Dilemma" by Wendy L. Lyon
"A Time to Decide, A Time to Heal" by Molly A. Minnick, Kathleen Delp, and Mary Ciotti
"How to Survive the Loss of a Child" by Catherine Sanders
"We Were Gonna Have a Baby But We Had an Angel Instead" by Pat Schweibert (a book for surviving siblings)
"Empty Arms: Hope and Support for Those Who Have Suffered a Miscarriage, Stillbirth, or Tubal Pregnancy" by Pam Vredevelt

Face-to-Face/"In Person" Resources

The Compassionate Friends 1-877-969-0010
Chapter Locator: http://www.compassionatefriends.org/Chapter_Locations/
states.shtml

Mothers in Sympathy and Support Foundation (M.I.S.S.) 1-888-455-MISS
Support Group Locator: http://www.misschildren.org/group/index.html

SHARE Pregnancy & Infant Loss Support, Inc. 1-800-821-6819
Group Listing: http://www.nationalshareoffice.com/resources_share_groups.
shtml

*** These support resource lists can also be found on the Our Heartbreaking
Choices web site at http://www.ourheartbreakingchoices.com**

APPENDIX C

Special Poems

LITTLE FOOTPRINTS©
By Dorothy Ferguson

How very softly
You tiptoed into my world
Almost silently,
Only a moment you stayed.
But what an imprint
Your footsteps have left
Upon my heart.

© 1990 Reprinted with permission from Centering Corporation, Omaha, NE, www.centering.org

WHAT MAKES A MOTHER?
By Jennifer Wasik

I thought of you, I closed my eyes, and prayed to God today.
I asked "What makes a mother?" and I know I heard him say
A mother has a baby, this we know is true.
But God, can you be a mother when your baby's not with you?
"Yes you can," he replied with confidence in his voice.
"I give many women babies, when they leave is not their choice.
Some I send for a lifetime; and others for a day.
And some I send to feel your womb, but there's no need to stay."
I just don't understand this God, I want my baby here.

He took a breath and cleared his throat; and then I saw a tear.
"I wish I could show you, what your child is doing today.
If you could see your child smile with other kids and say
'We go to earth to learn our lessons of love and life and fear.
 My mommy loved me oh so much, I got to come straight here.
I feel so lucky to have a mom, who had so much love for me.
I learned my lesson very quick, my mommy set me free.
I miss my mommy oh so much, but I visit her each day.
When she goes to sleep, on her pillow's where I lay.
I stroke her hair and kiss her cheek; and whisper in her ear
Mommy don't be sad today, I'm your baby and I'm here.'
So you see my dear sweet one, your children are okay.
Your babies are here in my home; And this is where they'll stay.
They'll wait for you with me, until your lesson is through
And on the day that you come home; they'll be at the gates for you.
So, now you see what makes a mother, it's the feeling in your heart.
It's the love you had so much of; right from the very start.
Though some may not realize you are a mother,
Until their time is done.
They'll be up here with me one day,
And know you're the best one!

In memory of Zachery Wasik 1/29/98-1/29/98
Reprinted with permission from Jennifer Wasik, Phoenix, AZ

UP IN HEAVEN
By Kathryn

I never got to see your face
Because I chose to send you to a happier place.
I hope one day we will meet again
But who will hold & rock you until then?
When I think of you
I try to imagine you
But, will I ever recognize you?
Will you look in on me
So that you will know me?
What if you never know me?
How will we know if and when we meet again?
Up in heaven

Does time pass by?
Will you remain my little baby?
If so, will I even recognize your cry?
My arms never held you
Now I wonder if they ever will.
Up in heaven
Does time stand still?
I never got to say "hello" or "goodbye."
I just can't help but wonder, if and when I get to heaven
Will you just pass me by?

Excerpts from WHEN GOD CALLS
By Cindy O'Connor

Perhaps God tires of calling the aged to his fold,
So he picks a rosebud, before it can grow old.
God knows how much we need them, and so he takes but few
To make the land of Heaven more beautiful to view.
…
So when a little child departs, we who are left behind
Must realize God loves children, angels are hard to find.

MEMORIES
Author unknown

If we could have a lifetime wish,
A dream that would come true.
We'd pray to God with all our hearts
For yesterday and you.
A thousand words can't bring you back,
We know because we've tried.
Neither will a thousand tears,
We know because we've cried.
You left behind our broken hearts
And happy memories too.
But we never wanted memories,
We only wanted you.

A PAIR OF SHOES
Author unknown

I am wearing a pair of shoes.
They are ugly shoes.
Uncomfortable Shoes.
I hate my shoes.
Each day I wear them, and each day I wish I had another pair.
Some days my shoes hurt so bad that I do not think I can take another step.
Yet, I continue to wear them.
I get funny looks wearing these shoes.
They are looks of sympathy.
I can tell in others' eyes that they are glad they are my shoes and not theirs.
They never talk about my shoes.
To learn how awful my shoes are might make them uncomfortable.
To truly understand these shoes you must walk in them.
But, once you put them on, you can never take them off.
I now realize that I am not the only one who wears these shoes.
There are many pairs in the world.
Some women are like me and ache daily as they try and walk in them.
Some have learned how to walk in them so they don't hurt quite as much.
Some have worn the shoes so long that days will go by
Before they think of how much they hurt.
No woman deserves to wear these shoes.
Yet, because of the shoes I am a stronger woman.
These shoes have given me the strength to face anything.
They have made me who I am.
I will forever walk in the shoes of a woman who has lost a child.

UNTITLED
Author unknown

The Mention of my child's name
May bring tears to my eyes,
But never fails to bring
Music to my ears.
If you are really my friend,
Let me hear the beautiful

Music of his name.
It soothes my broken heart
And sings to my soul.

UNTITLED
Author unknown

The angel, in the book of life
Wrote down my baby's birth
And whispered as she closed the book
"Too beautiful for earth."

BIBLIOGRAPHY

Preface

Center for Reproductive Rights, "Unconstitutional Assault on the Right to Choose: Federal Abortion Ban is an Affront to Women and to the U.S. Supreme Court." 2003 http://www.reproductiverights.org/pdf/pub_bp_uncon_assault.pdf

Dailard, Cynthia, "Courts Strike 'Partial-Birth' Abortion Ban; Decisions Presage Future Debates." The Guttmacher Report on Public Policy, 2004, volume 7, number 4 http://www.guttmacher.org/pubs/tgr/07/4/gr070401.html

The Guttmacher Institute, "State Facts About Abortion: New York." 2006 http://www.guttmacher.org/pubs/sfaa/new_york.html

Henshaw SK, "Unintended Pregnancy in the United States." Family Planning Perspectives, 1998, 30(1):24–29 & 46.

Jones RK, MR Zolna, SK Henshaw, LB Finer, "Abortion in the United States: Incidence and Access to Services, 2005." Perspectives on Sexual and Reproductive Health, 2008, 40(1):6–16.

National Public Radio (NPR), "Doctors Weigh Next Move on Legality of Abortion." 2007 http://www.npr.org/templates/story/story.php?storyId=9692283

Strauss, LT et al., "Abortion Surveillance—United States, 2004." <u>Morbidity and Mortality Weekly</u>, November 23, 2007; 56(SS09):1–33.

Appendix A

American College of Gynecologists Practice Bulletin No. 77: "Screening for Fetal Chromosomal Abnormalities." <u>Obstetrics and Gynecology</u>, 2007 Jan; 109(1):217–27.

Campbell, S, FD Johnstone, EM Holt, P May, "Anencephaly: Early Ultrasonic Diagnosis and Active Management." <u>The Lancet</u>, 1972 Dec 9; 2 (7789):1226–7.

Campbell, S, J Pryse-Davies, TM Coltart, MJ Seller, JD Singer, "Ultrasound in the Diagnosis of Spina Bifida." <u>The Lancet</u>, 1975 May 10; 1(7915):1065–8.

Caughey, AB, LM Hopkins, ME Norton, "Chorionic Villus Sampling Compared With Amniocentesis and the Difference in the Rate of Pregnancy Loss." <u>Obstetrics and Gynecology</u>, 2006 Sep;108 (3 Pt 1):612–6.

Colautti v. Franklin, 439 U.S. 379, 388–89 (1979).

Davis, Deborah L., <u>Empty Cradle, Broken Heart</u>. Golden, CO: Fulcrum Publishing, 1996.

Doe v. Bolton, 410 U.S. 179 (1973).

Eisenstadt v. Baird, 405 U.S. 438 (1972).

Fuchs, F, and P Riis, "Antenatal sex determination." <u>Nature</u>, 1956 Feb 18; 177(4503):300.

Garrett, WJ, DE Robinson, G Kosoff, "Fetal Anatomy Displayed by Ultrasound." <u>Investigative Radiology</u>, 1968 Nov-Dec; 3(6):442–9.

Garrett, WJ, G Grunwald, DE Robinson, "Prenatal Diagnosis of Fetal Polycystic Kidney by Ultrasound." <u>The Australian and New Zealand Journal of Obstetrics & Gynecology</u>, 1970 Feb; 10(1):7–9.

Gonzales v. Carhart, 550 U.S. __ , 127 S. Ct. 1610; 167 L. Ed. 2d 480; 75 U.S.L.W. 4210 (2007).

Gonzales v. Planned Parenthood Federation of America, Inc., 550 U.S. __ , 127 S. Ct. 1610; 167 L. Ed. 2d 480; 75 U.S.L.W. 4210 (2007).

Griswold v. Connecticut, 381 U.S. 479 (1965).

The Guttmacher Institute, "Get 'In the Know': Questions About Pregnancy, Contraception, and Abortion." 2007 http://www.guttmacher.org/in-the-know/providers.html

The Guttmacher Institute, "Issues in Brief. Late-Term Abortions: Legal Considerations." 1997 http://www.guttmacher.org/pubs/ib13.html

The Guttmacher Institute, "State Policies in Brief. An Overview of Abortion Laws." 2008
http://www.guttmacher.org/statecenter/spibs/spib_OAL.pdf

The Guttmacher Institute, "State Policies in Brief. Restricting Insurance Coverage of Abortion." 2008 http://www.guttmacher.org/statecenter/spibs/spib_RICA.pdf

The Guttmacher Institute, "State Policies in Brief. State Policies on Later-Term Abortions." 2008 http://www.guttmacher.org/statecenter/spibs/spib_PLTA.pdf

Hahnemann, JM, and LO Vejerslev, "Accuracy of Cytogenetic Findings on Chorionic Villus Sampling." Prenatal Diagnosis, 1997 Sep; 17(9):801–20.

Henshaw, S, "Abortion Trends in 1987 and 1988: Age and Race." Family Planning Perspectives, Vol. 24, No. 2 (Mar.–Apr., 1992), pp. 85–96.

Henshaw SK and Finer LB, "The Accessibility of Abortion Services in the United States, 2001." Perspectives on Sexual and Reproductive Health, 2003, 35(1):16–24.

Jones RK, MR Zolna, SK Henshaw, LB Finer, "Abortion in the United States: Incidence and Access to Services, 2005." Perspectives on Sexual and Reproductive Health, 2008, 40(1):6–16.

Mansfield C, Hopfer S, Marteau TM, "Termination Rates After Prenatal Diagnosis of Down Syndrome, Spina Bifida, Anencephaly, and Turner and Klinefelter Syndromes: a Systematic Literature Review." Prenatal Diagnosis, 1999; 19:808-812.

The March of Dimes, "Maternal Blood Screening for Birth Defects." 2007 http://www.marchofdimes.com/professionals/14332_1166.asp

"Midtrimester Amniocentesis for Prenatal Diagnosis. Safety and accuracy." JAMA, 1976 Sep 27; 236(13):1471–6.

Mohr, J, "Foetal Genetic Diagnosis: Development of Techniques for Early Sampling of Foetal Cells." Acta Pathologica et Microbiologica Scandinavia, 1968; 73(1):73–7.

National Abortion Federation, "History of Abortion." 2008 http://www. prochoice.org/about_abortion/history_abortion.html#1

Partial-Birth Abortion Ban Act of 2003, 18 U.S.C. §1531 (2000 ed., Supp. IV), (2003).

Perry S, Woodall AL, Pressman EK, "Association of Ultrasound Findings with Decision to Continue Down Syndrome Pregnancies." Community Genetics, 2007; 10(4):227-30.

Planned Parenthood of Missouri v. Danforth, 428 U.S. 52 (1976).

Planned Parenthood of Southeastern Pennsylvania v. Casey, 505 U.S. 833 (1992).

Roe v. Wade, 410 U.S. 113, 163 (1973).

Shaffer, BL, AB Caughey, ME Norton, "Variation in the Decision to Terminate Pregnancy in the Setting of Fetal Aneuploidy." Prenatal Diagnosis, 2006 Aug; 26(8):667–71.

Steele, MW, and WR Breg, Jr., "Chromosome Analysis of Human Amniotic Fluid Cells." The Lancet, 1966 Feb 19; 1(7434): 383–5.

Thornburgh v. American College of Obstetricians and Gynecologists, 476 U.S. 747 (1986).

United States v. Vuitch, 402 U.S. 62 (1971).